Manual of
Oral Histology and
Oral Pathology

Second Edition

COLOR ATLAS and TEXT

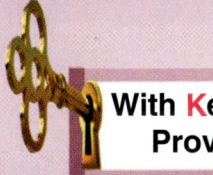

**With Key Points of Identification
Provided with Each Figure**

Manual of
Oral Histology and
Oral Pathology

Second Edition

COLOR ATLAS and TEXT

Maji Jose MDS, PhD

Professor and Head
Department of Oral Pathology
Yenepoya Dental College and Hospital
Yenepoya University
Daralkatte, Mangalore 575018, Karnataka, India

Email majiajoyin@yahoo.co.in

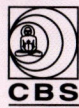

CBS Publishers & Distributors Pvt Ltd

New Delhi • Bengaluru • Chennai • Kochi • Kolkata • Mumbai
Hyderabad • Jharkhand • Nagpur • Patna • Pune • Uttarakhand

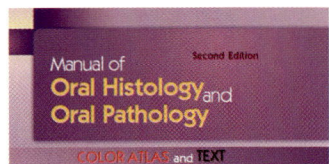

ISBN: 978-81-239-2798-5

Copyright © Author and Publisher

Second Edition: 2016
Reprint: 2017, 2019, 2021
First Edition: 2006
Reprint: 2006, 2007, 2008, 2009, 2010, 2011, 2012, 2013, 2014, 2015

Published by Satish Kumar Jain and produced by Varun Jain for

CBS Publishers & Distributors Pvt Ltd
4819/XI Prahlad Street, 24 Ansari Road, Daryaganj, New Delhi 110 002, India
Ph: 011-23289259, 23266861, 23266867 Fax: 011-23243014   Website: www.cbspd.com
e-mail: delhi@cbspd.com; cbspubs@airtelmail.in.
Corporate Office: 204 FIE, Industrial Area, Patparganj, Delhi 110 092, India
Ph: 011-4934 4934   Fax: 011-4934 4935   e-mail: publishing@cbspd.com; publicity@cbspd.com

Branches

- **Bengaluru:** Seema House 2975, 17th Cross, K.R. Road,
  Banasankari 2nd Stage, Bengaluru 560 070, Karnataka, India
  Ph: +91-80-26771678/79   Fax: +91-80-26771680   e-mail: bangalore@cbspd.com
- **Chennai:** 7, Subbaraya Street, Shenoy Nagar, Chennai 600 030, Tamil Nadu, India
  Ph: +91-44-26680620, 26681266   Fax: +91-44-42032115   e-mail: chennai@cbspd.com
- **Kochi:** 42/1325, 1326, Power House Road, Opp KSEB, Power House, Ernakulam 682 018, Kochi, Kerala, India
  Ph: +91-484-4059061-65/67   Fax: +91-484-4059065   e-mail: kochi@cbspd.com
- **Kolkata:** 6/B, Ground Floor, Rameswar Shaw Road, Kolkata 700 014, West Bengal, India
  Ph: +91-33-22891126, 22891127, 22891128   e-mail: kolkata@cbspd.com
- **Mumbai:** PWD Shed, Gala No. 25/26, Ramchandra Bhatt Marg, Next to JJ Hospital, Gate No. 2,
  Opposite Union Bank of India, Noorbaug, Mumbai 400 009, Maharashtra, India
  Ph: 022-66661880/89   e-mail: mumbai@cbspd.com

Representatives

• **Hyderabad**	0-9885175004	• **Jharkhand**	0-9811541605	• **Nagpur**	0-9421945513
• **Patna**	0-9334159340	• **Pune**	0-9623451994	• **Uttarakhand**	0-9716462459

Printed at: Magic International Pvt. Ltd., Greater Noida, UP, India

to

my husband
Ajoy S Joseph
and
my children
Joe and Jiya

Foreword

Dental science has registered commendable growth in over the last few decades with specialization in almost all its branches. Modern-day dental students have to shoulder a greater responsibility by passionately involving themselves in mastering these specializations so as to justify their role as guardians of community oral health. Knowledge of oral histology and oral pathology provides the students an overall insight to the understanding of oral diseases so that they become efficient clinicians who can impart effective and safe patient care.

Dentistry and its specialized fields like oral pathology and oral histology have become more information-oriented and students are overloaded with too much information that they find it difficult to keep pace with. Facing examination seems to be a Herculean task as it is hard and confusing for them to understand what exactly to study and to write in the examinations. It is essential to secure good marks in practical examinations too, apart from theory papers, to score an overall high percentage. Being a diagnostic science, the study of histopathology with the help of microscopic slides is of paramount importance in learning oral pathology and facing the examination successfully.

Dr Maji Jose has come out with a detailed practical manual of oral histology and oral pathology, specially suited for BDS students. What this book uniquely provides is an opportunity to learn and understand these subjects with the help of histological diagrams and photomicrographs, which will be of immense help for the students to face the examination more confidently. The comprehensive text added, makes it more student-friendly.

I have no doubt that this book will be of definite help to the students of dentistry, making an otherwise difficult subject easy to learn. This book represents a great deal of effort and the author deserves appreciation for this monumental work.

I wish this book all success.

BH Sripathi Rao MDS
Principal
Yenepoya Dental College and Hospital
Yenepoya University, Mangalore

Preface to the Second Edition

Manual of *Oral Histology and Oral Pathology* is a textbook designed to cover the essential aspects of oral histology and oral pathology, especially for the undergraduate dental students. The photomicrographs and hand-drawn diagrams, along with brief description linked to them, help a student to understand the subject, learn well and face the examination confidently.

In two sections, this book covers various topics in oral histology in 11 chapters and oral pathology in 10 chapters. More than 125 hand drawn diagrams on various topics are included in this textbook, of which 60s are supported by photomicrographs to make learning easier. The text added is explained in simple, lucid language to help an undergraduate student to develop a comprehensive knowledge which makes a sound base for learning pathologic basis of diseases.

I am gratified that original edition has received a good response. A positive feedback on the first edition of the book and various encouraging comments received from students and teachers, who have used the book, has encouraged me to come out with second edition. The second edition is a revised and updated version with more diagrams to further ease the learning process. A section on special stains included in this edition will be useful for students to develop an understanding about the special stains that may be used in histopathology laboratory.

I offer this book to the dental students, hoping that this will satisfy the readers and ensure an enjoyable and rewarding learning.

Maji Jose

Preface to the First Edition

There had been a long-standing demand from BDS students for *Manual of Oral Histology and Oral Pathology* which would help them in microscopic slide identification and drawing histology and histopathology diagrams in the record book. These practical exercises are very important in understanding and learning oral histology and oral pathology and also for facing the examination successfully.

By providing histology and histopathology diagrams in card forms in the practical classes along with the microscopic slides, in our college, we observed that the students understanding of the subject, and quality of the diagrams have improved drastically. The leap to publication was provoked by an innocent comment from a friend, who suggested that the publication of this would help many students and teachers all over the country.

This book is structured to cover the essential aspects of oral histology and oral pathology, especially for undergraduate students. The handdrawn pictures are designed to facilitate better understanding of the subject so that the reader is able to link them with the theory.

This book contains 21 chapters in two sections. The first section is devoted to explain oral histology. Fist two chapters provide a foundation for study of oral histology and oral pathology. The subsequent 9 chapters deal with detailed histological structure of oral tissues. In section 2 oral pathology topics are discussed.

I have tried my level best to include almost all topics prescribed in the syllabus of various universities as well as Dental Council of India and to express it in simple language. Of particular importance is my handdrawn colored illustrations used in all the chapters to support the learning. A total of 101 colored diagrams are included of which 60s are supported by photomicrographs. The diagrams, photomicrographs, key identification points along with the text added will definitely make the learning of the subjects easy.

With pleasure I offer this book to the dental students of India. I hope this book will reduce the burden of students in learning oral histology and oral pathology and they will find it useful for a rewarding study of these subjects.

I will feel amply rewarded if the book satisfy the readers, and will be grateful to them if they provide me the feedback to improve the text further.

Maji Jose

Acknowledgments

Every author owes a great deal to others, and I am not an exception. First and foremost I bow in gratitude to the almighty for His blessing.

- I owe a deep sense of gratitude to Dr BH Sripathi Rao, Principal, Yenepoya Dental College, Mangalore, for writing the Foreword to this book and for his wholehearted encouragement.

- I can never forget the help, encouragement and scholarly advices I received from my teacher and friend Dr Heera R.

- My deep appreciation is due towards my colleagues. In particular, I would like to acknowledge the total support provided by Dr Girish KL, Dr Vani and Dr Ajeesha Ahmed.

- CBS Publishers & Distributors, New Delhi, deserves a special acknowledgment for the care and promptness with which they have brought out this book.

Maji Jose

Contents

Oral Histology

Preparation of Oral Tissues for Microscopic Examination

- Study of dental hard tissues
  - Ground sections
  - Decalcified sections
- Study of oral soft tissues
  - Routine tissue processing

A sound knowledge of the structures of oral tissue is very much essential for understanding of this region. The knowledge about these structures gives the clinician an insight into the understanding of the disease mechanism that may develop in these tissues and predict the reaction of tissues to various factors, etc.

Microscopic examination is the method adopted to study the histological structures of the oral tissues. To study the histological structure, the tissue should be appropriately prepared for microscopic examination.

STUDY OF DENTAL HARD TISSUES

The structure of dental hard tissues can be studied using ground sections or decalcified sections. The exception is enamel, where decalcified sections are not of much use because 96% of enamel is mineralized, which is lost while decalcification.

Decalcification

Decalcification is the process by which calcium in the mineralized tissue is removed so that the tissue becomes soft enough to make sections. Decalcification is achieved by using acids, chelating agents or by electrolysis. The commonly used method is acid decalcification.

Frequently used acid for decalcification is 5% Nitric acid. 15% Formic acid may also be used. Nitric acid may cause yellowing of the tissue, that may interfere with further staining procedure. To avoid this 0.1% urea is added to nitric acid.

Procedure

Hard tissue to be decalcified should be fixed in 10% formalin or formal saline. To reduce the time for decalcification tissue may be cut into smaller pieces. Then place the tissue in a container with 5% nitric acid. The acid should be changed daily for few days. The specimen is then tested for completion of decalcification.

Methods to check the completion of decalcification

1. **Checking the consistency of the tissue:** Completely decalcified tissue will be soft without any hardness being felt (Experienced hand can tell by the feel of the tissue.).

2. **Piercing the tissue with a needle:** If it enters the tissue without resistance, the tissue is completely decalcified. This is not recommended because it may cause damage to the tissue.

3. **Judicious bending or trimming of the tissue:** This can be done to ensure completion of decalcification.

4. **Taking radiograph of the specimen:** In the radiograph, if radiopaque specks are found, tissue is not completely decalcified.

5. **Chemical test:** The basis of this test is to identify calcium in the decalcifying solution in which the specimen was kept. Sodium hydroxide or strong ammonia is added to 5 ml of decalcifying fluid, to neutralize the solution. Then 5 ml of saturated ammonium oxalate solution is added. After this, check for turbidity. Absence of turbidity after 5 minutes indicate the fluid is free from calcium and thereby decalcification is complete. Turbidity is observed due to precipitation of calcium. If precipitation is observed after addition of sodium hydroxide, it indicates large amount of calcium is present in fluid. Precipitation seen only after addition of ammonium oxalate suggests decalcification is nearly complete.

Checking the end point of decalcification is important because incomplete decalcification makes further cutting of specimens difficult. Prolonged decalcification is also not desirable because it may affect the staining procedure. Once the decalcification is complete the tissue should be washed in running water to remove all acids. Then the steps of processing can be continued like soft tissue processing which includes dehydration, embedding, sectioning and staining.

Ground Sections

Ground sections are of particular importance in the study of structure of dental hard tissues especially enamel. In this method the tooth is made into thin sections by grinding, using abrasive stones.

Procedure

The tooth to be examined should be cut into 2–3 sections using dental hand piece and diamond impregnated or carborundum disc.

These sections should be ground using an Arkansas stone or by simply rubbing on a glass plate using abrasive slurry. Grinding should be continued till it is approximately 25–50 microns thick. Fine abrasives should be used for the final polishing. Most suitable abrasive is domestic scouring powders followed by soapy water. Once the desirable thickness is attained the section should be washed and dehydrated and mounted on a glass slide using synthetic resin or Canada balsam as mounting medium and is allowed to dry.

Grinding of the tooth can also be done using a laboratory lathe. Initial grinding is done by holding the tooth in fingers and pressing it against the rotating coarse abrasive wheel of a lathe. When the tooth is thin, it is difficult to hold with fingers. Therefore a wooden block wrapped with adhesive plaster with sticky side directed outward can be used. Stick the tooth on to the plaster and press the wooden block to the rotating wheel of the lathe so that the tooth is ground thin. Then change the coarse wheel to fine wheel and continue grinding till the section is sufficiently thin. To remove the adhesive plaster the sections can be soaked in water. The section removed from the plaster is then mounted on a glass slide using a mounting medium.

Precision equipment like hard tissue microtomes are now available for the preparation of ground sections.

STUDY OF ORAL SOFT TISSUES

The most commonly used method of preparing soft tissue for the light microscopic study is by embedding the tissue in paraffin, and cutting and mounting the section on slides and staining.

Preparation of Sections of Paraffin Embedded Specimens (Soft Tissue Processing)

1. **Obtaining the specimen:** Specimens for microscopic study are obtained through either biopsy or autopsy.

   Biopsy is the removal of tissue from a living organism for the purpose of microscopic examination and diagnosis. If tissue is taken for the same purpose from dead organisms it is called autopsy.

2. **Fixation:** After the removal, specimen should be kept in fixative solution at the earliest. The amount of fixative should be approximately 25 times the size of the specimen. Depending on the size and density of the specimen the fixation time can vary from few hours to days. Usually 24-hour is sufficient for small specimens.

Commonly used fixative is 10% buffered formalin. Other fixatives used are methyl alcohol, ethyl alcohol, etc.

The aims of fixation are
- To preserve the cells and tissue constituents in life like condition as closely as possible without loss or derangement.
- To prevent the process of autolysis and bacterial action or putrefaction of tissues.
- To coagulate the proteins, thus reducing the change in shape or volume during further processing of tissue and to make the tissue more readily permeable to the subsequent application of reagents.

After fixation the specimen is washed in running water.

3. **Dehydration of specimen:** Dehydration is the process by which the water content from the tissue specimen is removed to allow the penetration of paraffin. Dehydrating agents commonly used are alcohol and acetone. Gradual dehydration is done using increasing grades of alcohol (40, 60, 80 and 95% and absolute alcohol). To ensure complete removal of water, the specimen is placed in 2–3 changes of absolute alcohol. After dehydration the water in the specimen is completely replaced by alcohol.

4. **Clearing:** Alcohol is not miscible with paraffin. So impregnation of the tissue by paraffin is not possible unless alcohol is replaced by a fluid that is miscible with both alcohol and paraffin. The fluid used for this purpose is xylene. Xylene is an organic solvent, miscible with alcohol and paraffin.

This process is called clearing because tissue becomes transparent or clear after the treatment with xylene. This occurs because the refractive index of xylene is similar to that of proteins in the specimen. Other clearing agents used are toluene, chloroform, benzene, etc.

5. **Impregnation of specimen with paraffin:** After clearing the specimen should be transferred to a dish with molten wax and this should be kept in an oven where temperature is adjusted to around 60°C. The xylene in the specimen is gradually replaced by paraffin. To ensure complete impregnation 2–3 changes of molten paraffin is required.

6. **Embedding:** The specimen is embedded in paraffin after impregnation. For this a paper box or Leuckhart's 'L' pieces fixed to form a cube can be used. Fill the cube with molten wax and the specimen can be embedded in to this with the help of a warm forceps. Allow the wax to cool and solidify. When the 'L' forms are removed the tissue is found embedded in a cube of solidified wax block.

7. **Cutting the specimen:** The tissue specimen embedded in the paraffin wax is clamped to a rotary microtome to take sections of desirable thickness of 4–10 microns.

8. **Mounting the cut sections on microscopic glass slides:** Sections taken using a microtome is floated on warm water and mounted on to a microscopic slide coated with adhesive. The slide is then placed on a slide warmer adjusted to a temperature of 40°C which helps to adhere the sections to the slide.

9. **Staining the section:** The sections are now ready for staining. Routinely used stain is hematoxylin and eosin. After staining mounting is done using a mounting medium. Commonly used mounting medium is Distrene dibutyl phthalate xylene (DPX). After mounting it is allowed to dry, before microscopic examination.

2

Cells, Tissues and Stains

- Epithelial tissue
  - Stratified squamous epithelium
  - Pseudostratified ciliated columnar epithelium
- Connective tissue
  - Fibroblasts and fibrocytes
  - Fat cells
  - Bone cells
  - Cartilage cells
  - Endothelial cells
  - Muscle
  - Defence cells
  - Giant cells
- Cells of odontogenic apparatus
- Routine stain
- Special stains

Cells are the basic structural units of the body. A group of cells performing the same function forms a tissue. Two important basic tissues of the body are epithelium and connective tissue.

EPITHELIAL TISSUE

Epithelium is an ectoderm derived tissue that forms a protective covering of connective tissue. Although there are different types of epithelia in the human body, the main types important for students of dentistry are stratified squamous epithelium that forms the lining of oral cavity and pseudostratified ciliated columnar epithelium lining the maxillary sinus and respiratory tract.

Stratified Squamous Epithelium (Fig. 2.1)

In stratified squamous epithelium the cells are arranged in different layers or strata. The basal cells are cuboidal in shape with central nucleus, arranged in single layer on the basement membrane. The superficial cells are squamous or polyhedral in outline with centrally placed nucleus. All these cells are attached to each other by desmosomal junctions.

Pseudostratified Ciliated Columnar Epithelium (Fig. 2.2)

The cells of the ciliated columnar epithelium are columnar in shape, of varying sizes arranged in a single layer on a basement membrane. The nuclei of the cells are placed at different levels giving the erroneous appearance of stratification. The cells on the superficial aspect have cilia which help in the movement of the mucous secretions. Among the columnar cells unicellular secretory organs called goblet cells are also noticed. Goblet cells are goblet shaped with a basally placed nucleus and apical cytoplasm filled with secretory products.

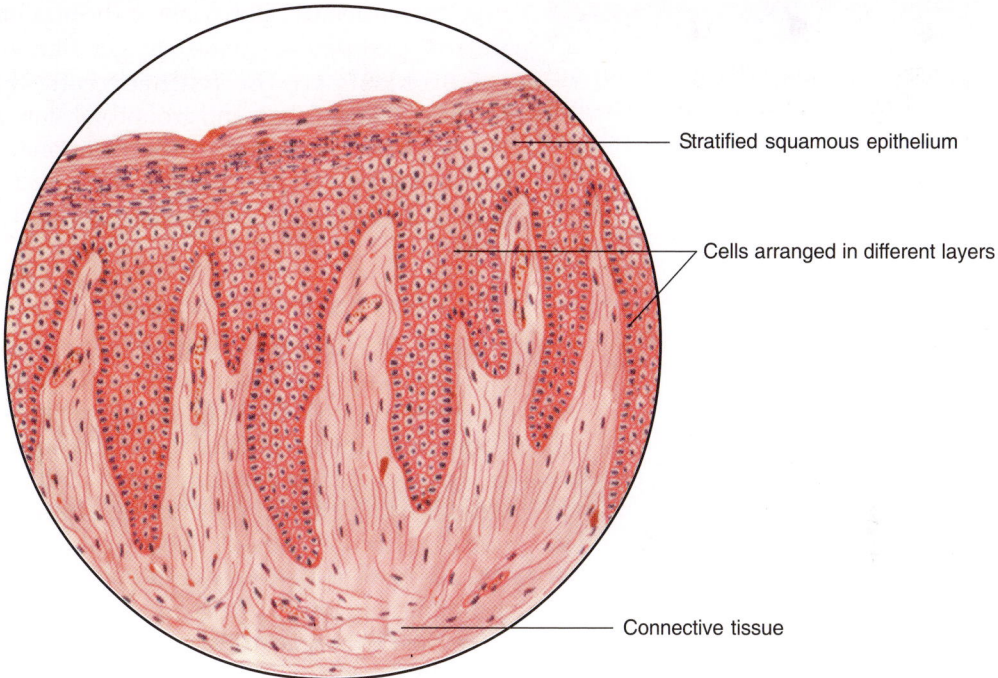

Stratified squamous epithelium

Cells arranged in different layers

Connective tissue

Fig. 2.1: Stratified squamous epithelium

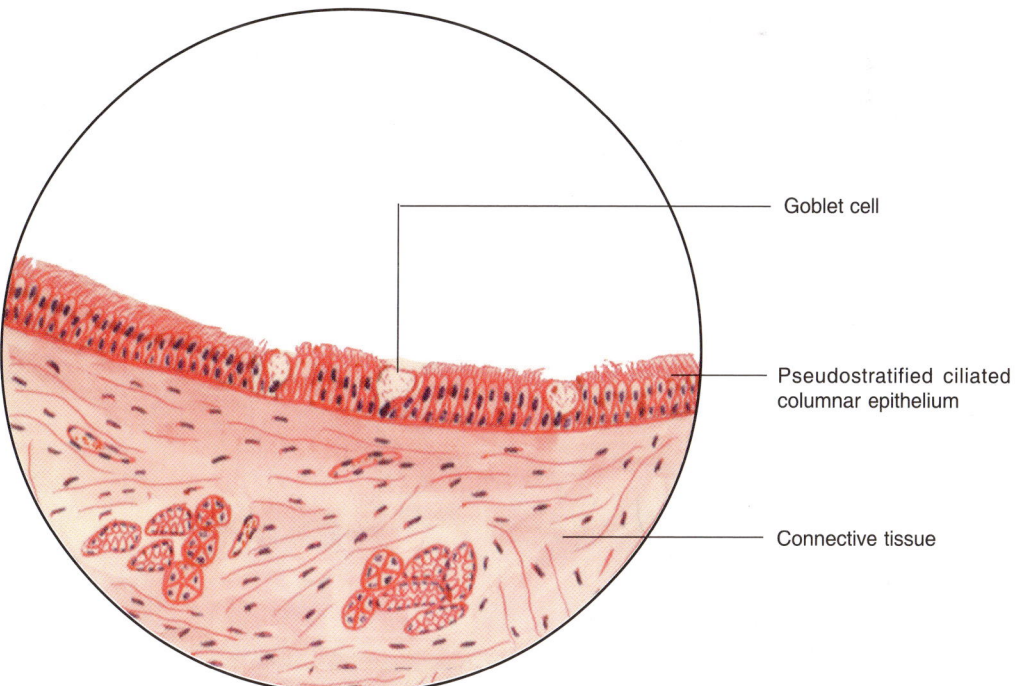

Goblet cell

Pseudostratified ciliated columnar epithelium

Connective tissue

Fig. 2.2: Pseudostratified ciliated columnar epithelium

CONNECTIVE TISSUE

Connective tissue is of mesodermal origin and comprises of fibers, ground substance and cells. The primary groups of fibers are collagen fibers. Collagen fibers are arranged to form bundles and stain pink in H and E stained sections. Collagen fibers and cells are embedded in ground substance, rich in proteoglycans and glycoproteins. Fibers and ground substance together constitute the extracellular component. Cellular components are:

Fibroblasts and Fibrocytes (Fig. 2.3)

These are the primary cells of the connective tissue. **Fibroblasts** are ovoid or star shaped cells with multiple cytoplasmic processes. The cell has large, round and vesicular or open face nucleus and abundant cytoplasm exhibiting slight basophilia indicating that they are highly active in protein synthesis. **Fibrocytes** are spindle shaped with flat deeply staining,

close face nucleus. Fibroblast and fibrocytes are arranged parallel to the collagen fibers.

Fibroblasts are the synthetic cells that produce collagen fibers and ground substances. They also help to degrade these components, thereby helping in remodelling of connective tissue. Fibrocytes are resting cells in connective tissue.

Fat Cells or Adipocytes (Fig. 2.4)

These are the cells those synthesize and store fat. These cells are spherical or ovoid with a flattened nucleus displaced to the periphery. These cells filled with fat are usually seen as groups where they are compressed with each other giving rise to polyhedral shape. In routine H and E stained histological sections fat cells appear as empty cells because fat is dissolved during processing. Fat cells can be stained by a special stain called Sudan III. Fat cells are distributed in the submucosal tissue.

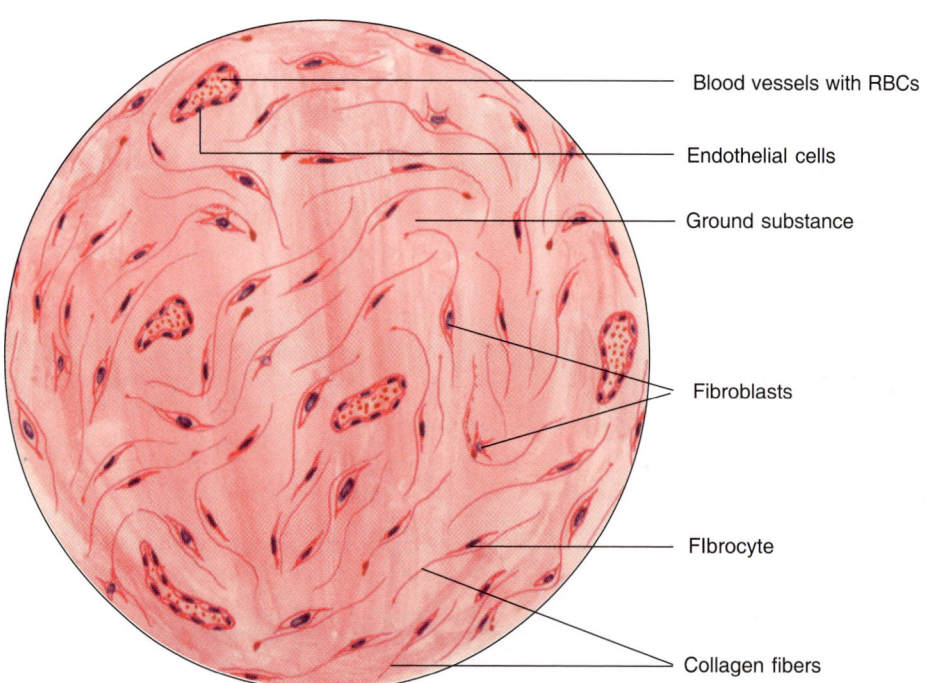

Blood vessels with RBCs

Endothelial cells

Ground substance

Fibroblasts

Fibrocyte

Collagen fibers

Fig. 2.3: Fibroblasts, fibrocytes and endothelial cells

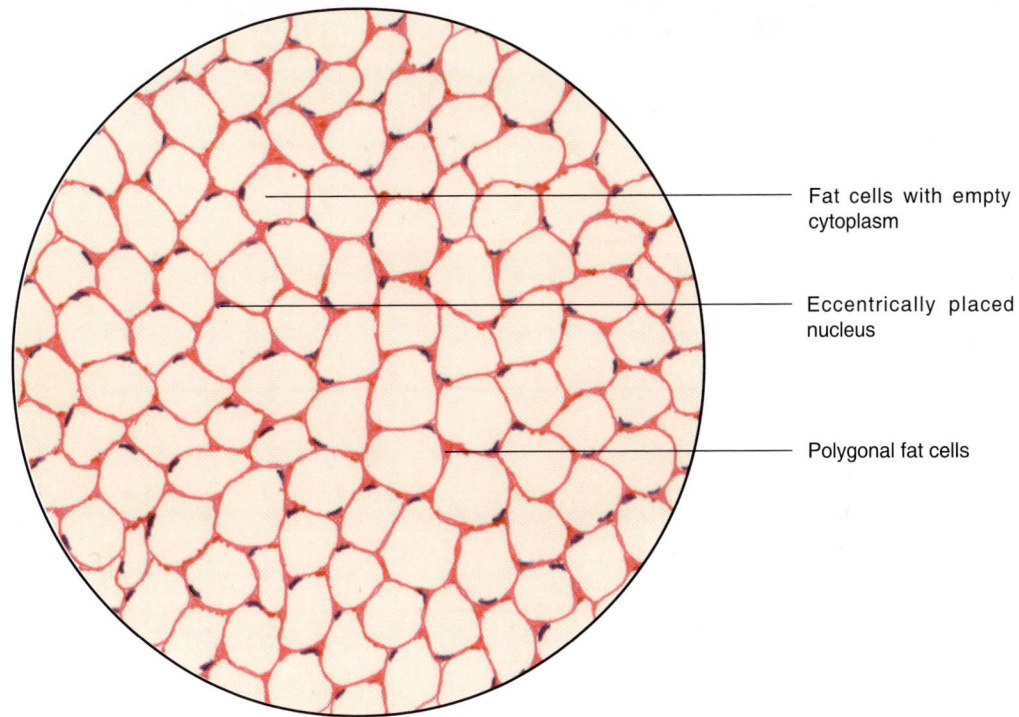

Fat cells with empty cytoplasm

Eccentrically placed nucleus

Polygonal fat cells

Fig. 2.4: Fat cells

Osteoblasts, Osteocytes and Osteoclasts (Fig. 2.5)

Osteoblasts are synthetic cells of bone that help in the formation of bone, by matrix deposition and mineralization. They are cuboidal or ovoid cells with centrally placed ovoid open face nucleus. Osteoblasts are arranged along the periphery of the bony trabeculae, forming a lining or rimming of the trabeculae.

Osteocytes are resting cells found entrapped in the bone. They occupy spaces called lacunae. Osteocytes have a cell body and processes called canaliculi. Cells are ovoid or flat with close faced nucleus and scanty cytoplasm.

Osteoclasts are the cells which resorb the bone. Osteoclasts are derived from circulating monocytes. They are large giant cells with multiple nuclei. These cells occupy irregular resorption bays called Howship's lacunae.

Chondroblasts and Chondrocytes (Fig. 2.6)

Chondroblasts are cartilage forming cells. They appear as flattened or elliptical cells and are located at the periphery of cartilage parallel to the surface.

Chondrocytes are the cells entrapped in the cartilaginous matrix. They are located in spaces called lacunae. Usually the chondrocytes are seen as groups of 2–4 cells and is described as 'cell nests'.

Endothelial Cells (Fig. 2.3)

Endothelial cells are the cells lining the blood capillaries. They form a single layer flattened cells having flattened nucleus resting on the basement membrane.

Striated Muscle (Fig. 2.7)

Striated muscle is seen as highly eosinophilic cylinder like structures in a hematoxylin and eosin stained sections. Each muscle fiber is

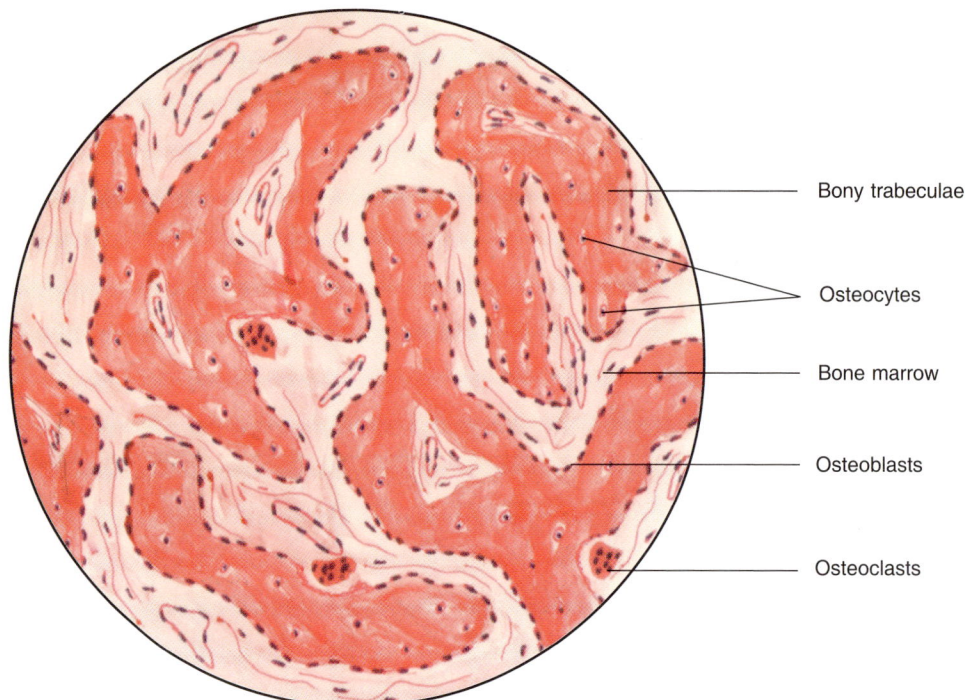

Fig. 2.5: Osteoblasts, osteocytes and osteoclasts

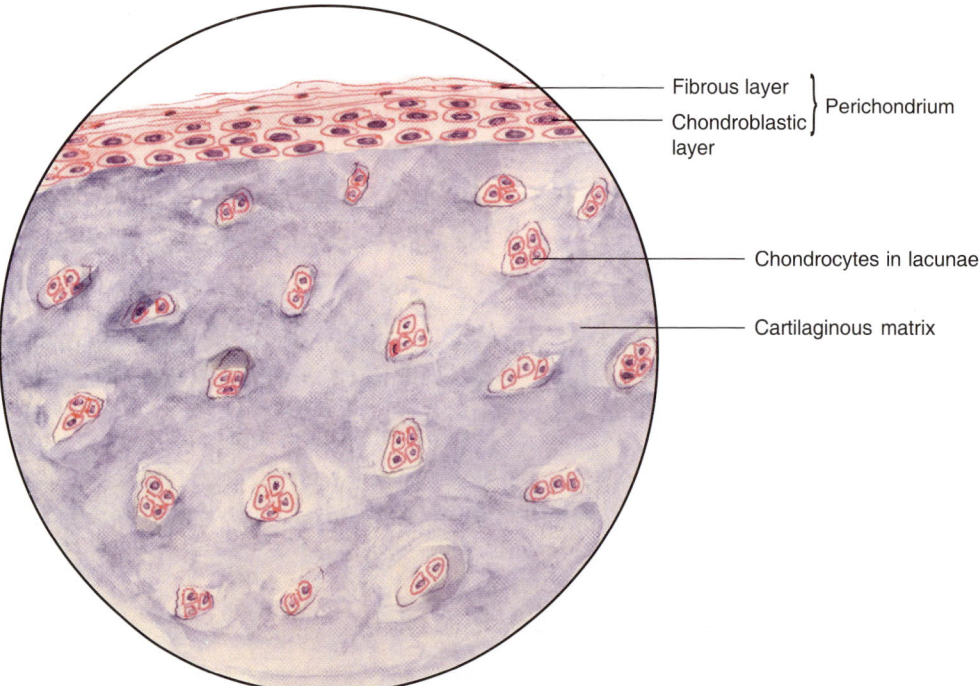

Fig. 2.6: Chondrocytes and chondroblasts

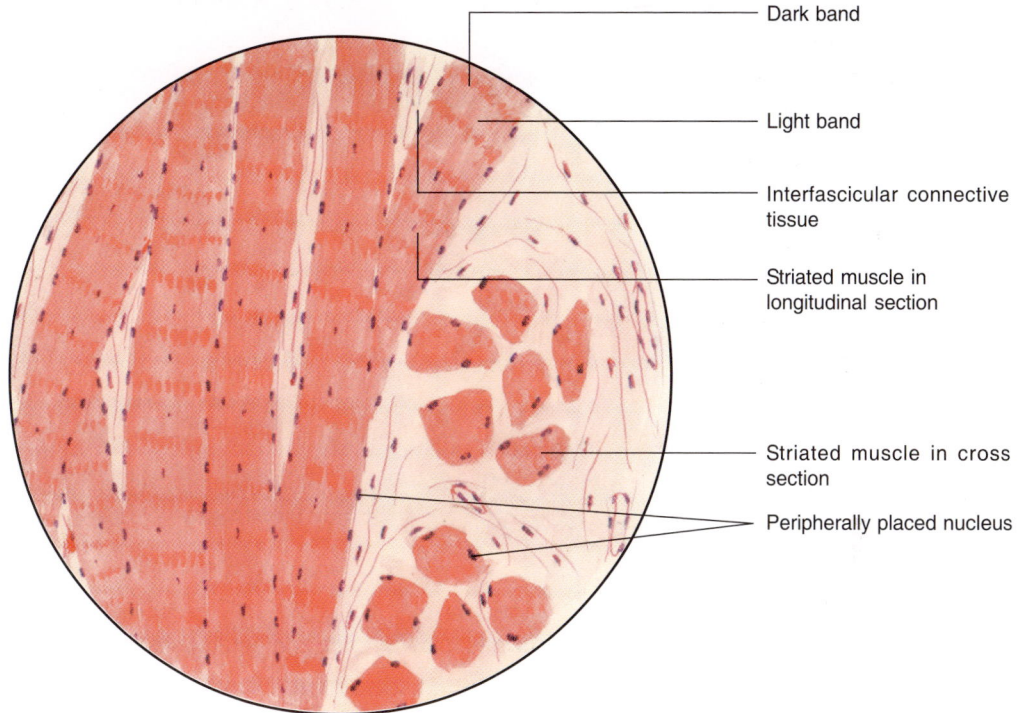

Dark band

Light band

Interfascicular connective tissue

Striated muscle in longitudinal section

Striated muscle in cross section

Peripherally placed nucleus

Fig. 2.7: Striated muscle

composed of many myofibrils. Fibers show characteristics transverse striations. The cytoplasm of muscle or sarcoplasm is rich in cytoplasmic organelles. Nuclei are flattened, multiple and are located at the periphery. The muscle as a whole is enclosed in connective tissue called epimysium. This connective tissue extends inwards dividing muscle into fasciculi. These extensions are called perimysium, from which again septa (endomysium) extend that invests individual muscle fibers.

Neutrophils (Fig. 2.8)

Neutrophils are defence cells of the body functioning as first line of defence against invading microorganisms. They are active in acute infections and thereby belong to the group of acute inflammatory cells. Neutrophils are 7 to 9 microns in diameter, have three to five lobes of nuclei and cytoplasmic granules, containing various enzymes.

Plasma Cells (Fig. 2.8)

Plasma cells are derived from B-lymphocytes and are specialized for the synthesis of antibodies (immunoglobulin) thereby imparting resistance to the body against diseases. They are ovoid in shape with basophilia of cytoplasm and eccentric, oval or round nucleus. The nucleus shows chromatin condensation in a radial pattern giving rise to a 'cartwheel' or 'clock face' appearance. Plasma cells are seen in connective tissue of the oral mucosa. These cells belong to the group of chronic inflammatory cells. Sometimes collection of immunoglobulin is seen as eosinophilic globules called Russel bodies in close proximity to groups of plasma cells.

Lymphocytes (Fig. 2.8)

These are defence cells of the body belonging to the group of chronic inflammatory cells. Lymphocytes can be large or small according to their size. Small lymphocytes are round cells

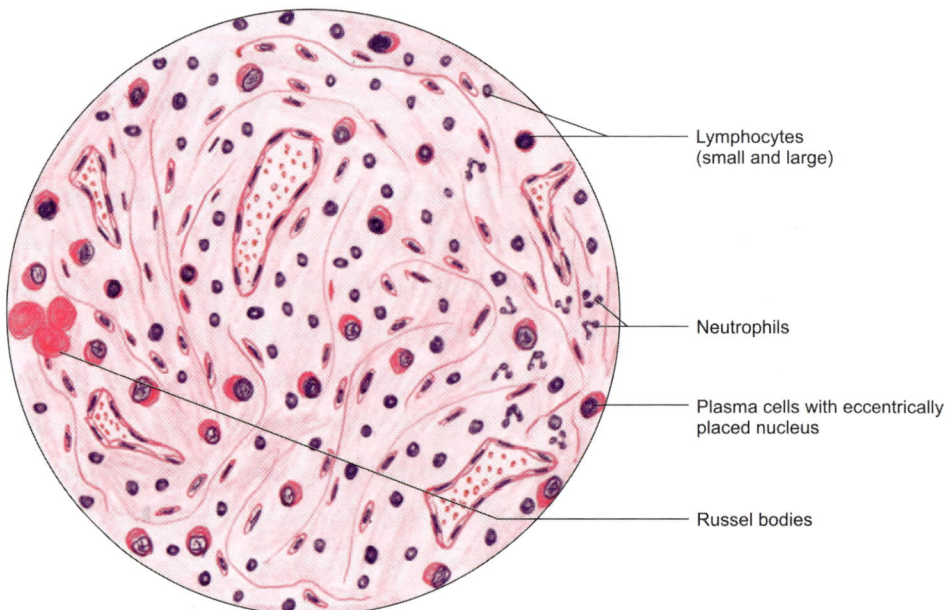

Fig. 2.8: Inflammatory cells (lymphocytes, plasma cells and neutrophils)

with 6–8 microns diameter. Nucleus is round occupying the major part of cytoplasm. Only a thin rim of cytoplasm is seen around the nucleus. Large lymphocytes are larger than small lymphocytes with greater amount of cytoplasm.

Mast Cells (Fig. 2.9)

These connective tissue cells are widely distributed in the oral mucosa. Mast cells are round or ovoid with small centrally placed nucleus. The cytoplasm contains granules rich in histamine, heparin and serotonin that have important role in allergic reaction. These cells can be seen in sections stained by toluidine blue as cells filled with purple/violet colored coarse granules. Mast cells are concerned with inflammation and immune response.

Giant Cells (Fig. 2.10)

Large and/or multinucleated cells are called giant cells. Giant cells can be seen in physiological or pathological conditions. Osteoclast is an example for giant cells seen in physiological conditions. Commonest giant cells in pathological conditions are foreign body giant cells.

They are seen in chronic inflammatory reactions in relation to a foreign body. These giant cells are large cells having multiple nuclei dispersed in the cytoplasm.

Cells of Odontogenic Apparatus

Ameloblasts are enamel forming cells which differentiate from the cells of inner enamel epithelium of enamel organ. They are columnar in shape with approximately 40 microns in length and diameter of 4 to 5 microns. Ameloblasts shows reversal of polarity with nucleus located at the proximal end (away from the basement membrane). During formative stage, ameloblasts develop a conical projection at the basal portion which is termed as Tomes' process.

Odontoblasts are the cells which form dentin. These cells differentiate from the dental papilla of the tooth germ. Odontoblasts are located in the pulp adjacent to the predentin with the cell body in the pulp and cell processes in the dentinal tubules. These cells are 5 to 7 microns in diameter and 25 to 40 microns in length. In the root region the odontoblasts are ovoid or spindle shaped.

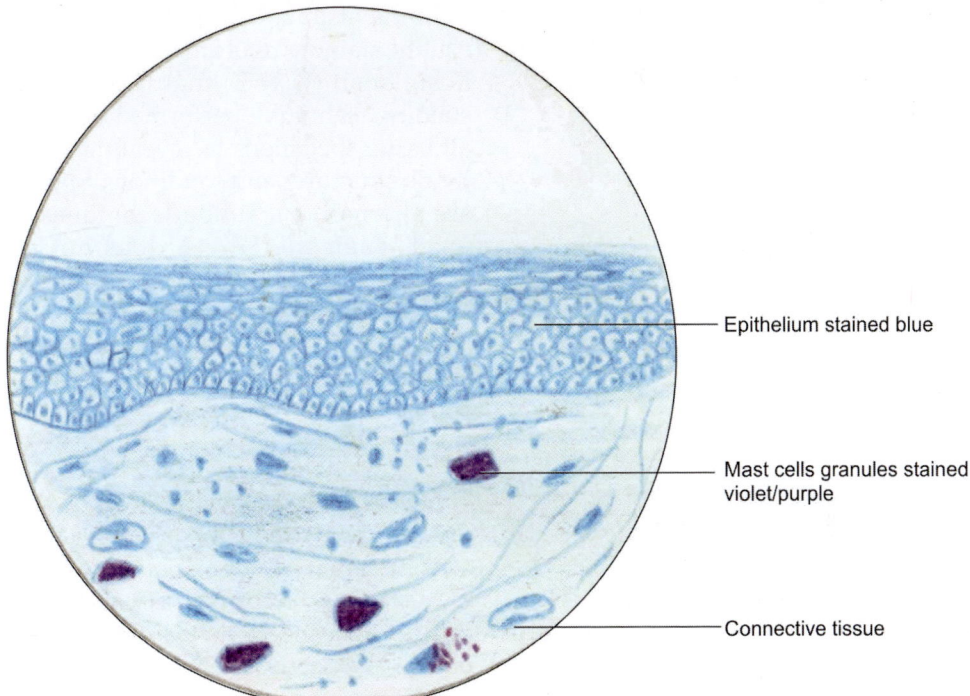

Epithelium stained blue

Mast cells granules stained violet/purple

Connective tissue

Fig. 2.9: Mast cells

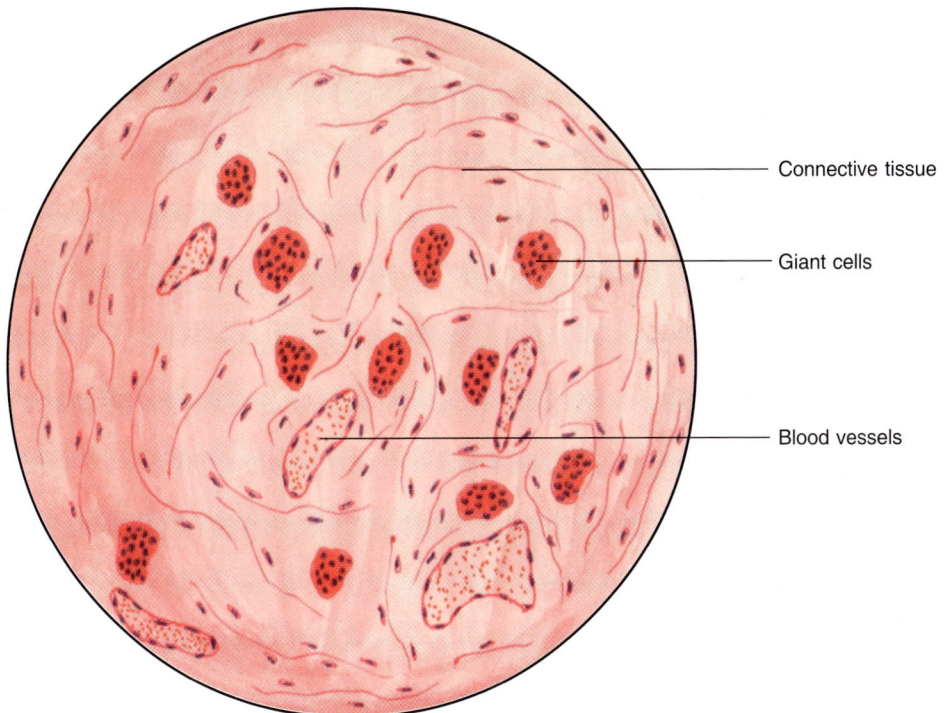

Connective tissue

Giant cells

Blood vessels

Fig. 2.10: Giant cells

Cementoblasts and Cementocytes

Cementoblasts are the cells forming cementum and are derived from dental follicle of the tooth germ. These cells are cuboidal in shape and line the outer surface (periodontal ligament surface) of cementum.

Cementocytes are the cells found entrapped in cellular cementum. They are spider shaped cells which lie in spaces called lacunae. These cells have a cell body and numerous processes or canaliculi radiating from it. The canaliculi are directed towards the periodontal ligament which is the source of their nutrition.

STAINS USED IN HISTOPATHOLOGY LABORATORIES

Staining of otherwise transparent tissue sections, is highly essential to demonstrate various cellular and tissue components and tissue structure and is a basic requirement for studying histologic structure of various tissues and also for making accurate diagnosis of a disease condition. Therefore routine and special stains have a critical role in histology and histopathology.

In the histopathology laboratory, the term routine staining refers to the Hematoxylin and Eosin stain (H & E) that is used as a basic staining technique performed routinely with all tissue specimens to reveal the underlying tissue structures and conditions. Special stains are alternative staining techniques that are used when the H & E does not provide adequate information. A pathologist or researcher requires special stains to obtain additional information for more detailed analysis, for differentiating two morphologically similar disease conditions.

Hematoxylin and Eosin (Fig. 2.11)

Hematoxylin and eosin (H & E) staining is used routinely in histopathology laboratories as it has ability to demonstrate a wide range of cell and tissue components and allows very detailed view of the tissue. As indicated in the name, this staining technique involves application of two different components: (i) A basic dye hematoxylin, which stain basophilic structures of the tissue mainly cell nuclei with blue color, (ii) eosin which stain eosinophilic structures (cytoplasm, organelles and extracellular components) pink or red.

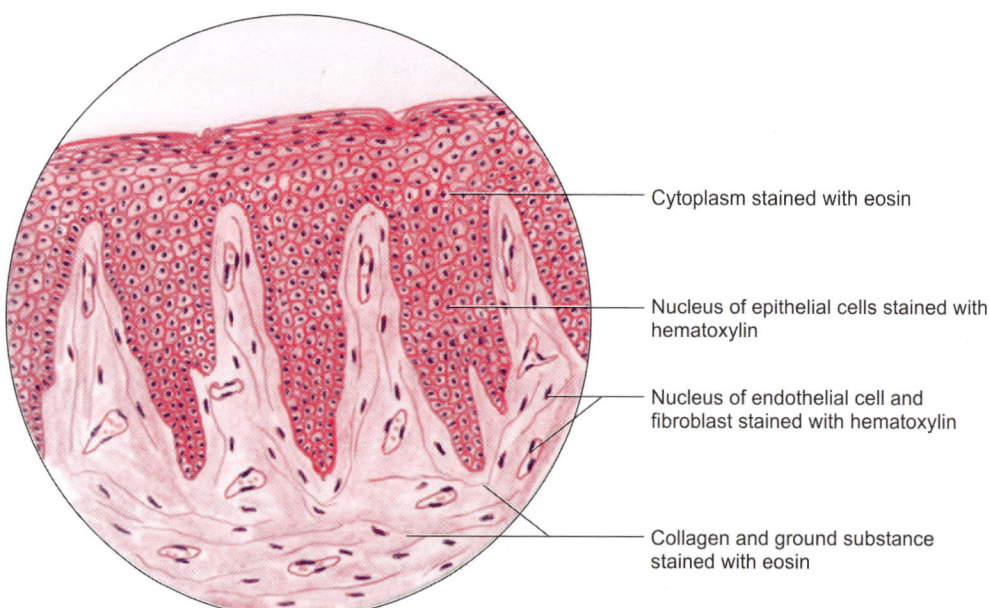

        — Cytoplasm stained with eosin

        — Nucleus of epithelial cells stained with hematoxylin

        — Nucleus of endothelial cell and fibroblast stained with hematoxylin

        — Collagen and ground substance stained with eosin

Fig. 2.11: Hematoxylin and eosin stain

This information obtained with H & E stain is often sufficient to observe basic histologic structures. As this staining technique reveals organization/disorganization of the cells and tissues and also abnormalities such as nuclear changes, it is widely used in medical diagnosis and still remains as the gold standard for diagnosis.

Special Stains

In a histopathology laboratory, special or advanced stains are ordered, subsequent to routine H & E stain, if additional information is needed for more detailed analysis.

Special Stains for Connective Tissue

Trichrome Stains

Trichrome stains are a group of staining techniques that can be used for differential demonstration of connective tissue components such as collagen fibers, muscle tissue, erythrocytes, etc. This is called trichrome stain as three dyes are used of which one may be nuclear stain.

The trichrome staining technique uses different dyes with varying molecular weight and the basic principle is that when used to stain a section, smaller molecules penetrate and stain various tissue elements. Further, when large dye molecules are allowed to penetrate the same tissue elements, larger ones replace the smaller one. This helps to selectively stain different tissue components.

a. **Van Gieson stain** (Fig. 2.12): This is one of the commonly used special stain to demonstrate collagen. When paraffin embedded tissue sections are stained using this staining technique: **collagen take up red colour; nucleus, blue/black and other tissues, yellow**

b. **Masson trichrome stain** (Fig. 2.13): This trichrome stain is used to differentially stain collagen and muscle. When this technique is employed: **cytoplasm, muscles and erythrocytes stain red while collagen take up blue colour and nuclei, blue/black.**

Special Stains for Demonstrating Carbohydrates

Demonstration of carbohydrate (CHO) is essential in many situations in a histopathology laboratory as it helps in differentiating and

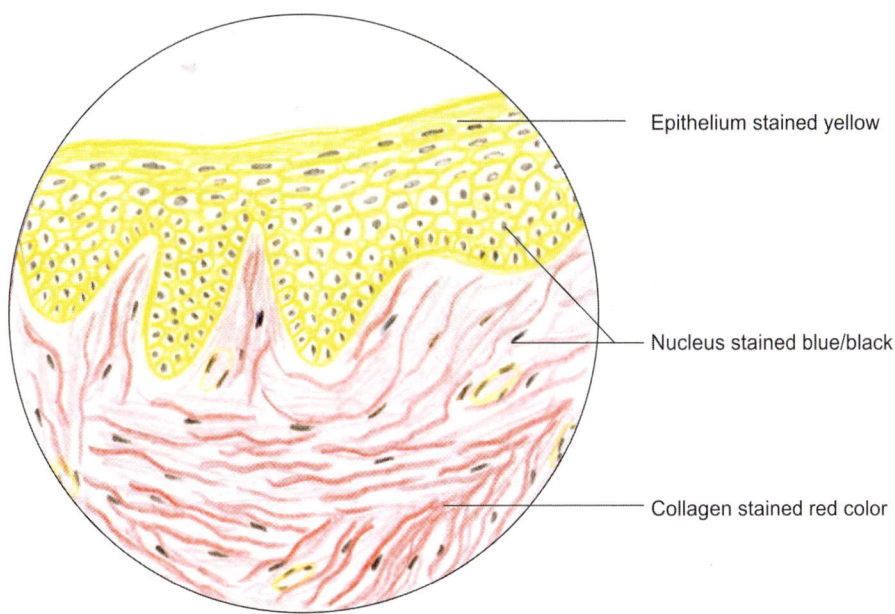

Epithelium stained yellow

Nucleus stained blue/black

Collagen stained red color

Fig. 2.12: Van Gieson stain

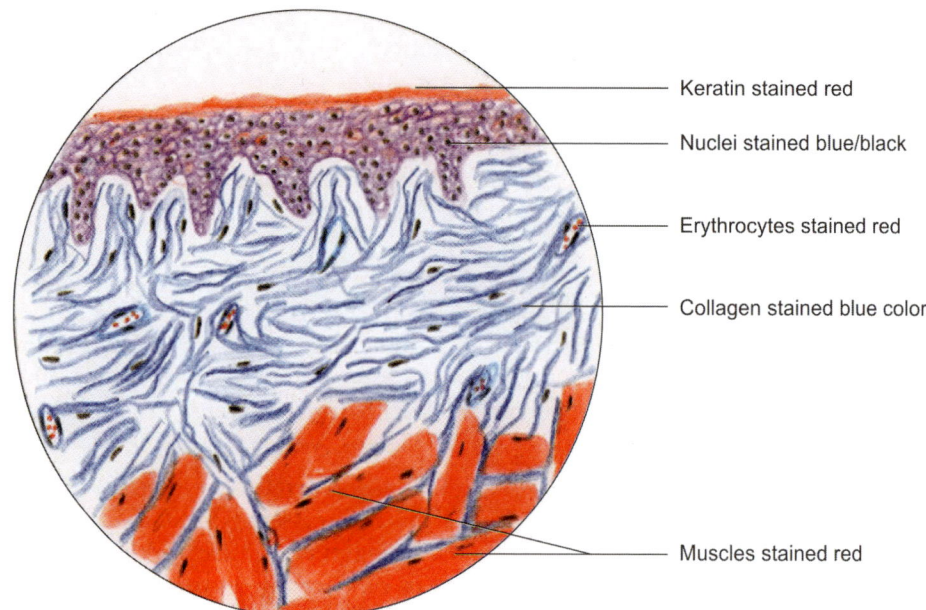

Keratin stained red

Nuclei stained blue/black

Erythrocytes stained red

Collagen stained blue color

Muscles stained red

Fig. 2.13: Masson trichrome stain

characterizing various pathological conditions. Pure CHO or CHO conjugated with other molecules such as proteins or lipids occur in cells and tissues and demonstration of CHO or glycol-conjugates such as glycogen or mucin help in confirming histopathology diagnosis. A number of staining techniques are used to demonstrate different types of mucopoly-saccharides components in tissue specimens in histopathology laboratory which include Periodic acid–Schiff (PAS) stain, Alcian blue, colloidal iron, mucicarmine, or metachromatic dyes.

a. **Periodic acid–Schiff (PAS) stain** (Figs 2.14 and 2.15): This is the most popular technique used in histopathology laboratories to demonstrate glycogen or mucin. This special stain is used to demonstrate basement membrane as Schiff reagent used in this technique react with glycoprotein present in basement membrane separating epithelial compartment from connective tissue. As the periodic acid, another component of this stain react with polysaccharides present in wall of fungi, this technique is also employed for demonstrating fungi such as *Candida*

albicans. When this stain is used **glycogen and various glycoproteins take up magenta colour and nuclei stain blue.**

b. **Mucicarmine stain:** This stain is used to demonstrate mucin, specific for acidic epithelial mucin and therefore of great importance in diagnosing salivary gland tumors, particularly adenocarcinomas. **Epithelial mucin appear deep rose or red in mucicarmine stained tissue sections while other tissue elements stain light yellow and nuclei, black** (Fig. 2.16).

Special Stains for Demonstrating Melanin (Fig. 2.17)

Melanin is a light brown to black pigment, produced by melanocytes, normally found in skin, hair, eyes and to some extent in oral mucosa. Melanin in protein bound form is present in cytoplasm of melanocytes as melanin granules and demonstration of it helps identifying melanin producing cells. Extensive melanin pigmentation resulting either from increased activity/proliferation of melanin producing cells is characteristic

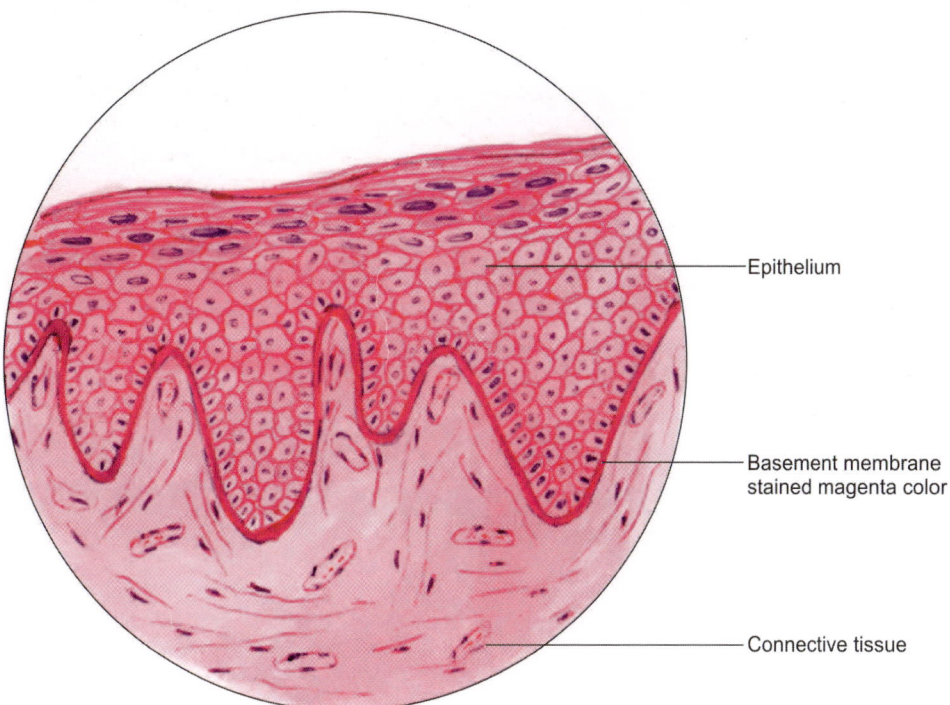

Fig. 2.14: PAS stain for basement membrane

Epithelium

Basement membrane stained magenta color

Connective tissue

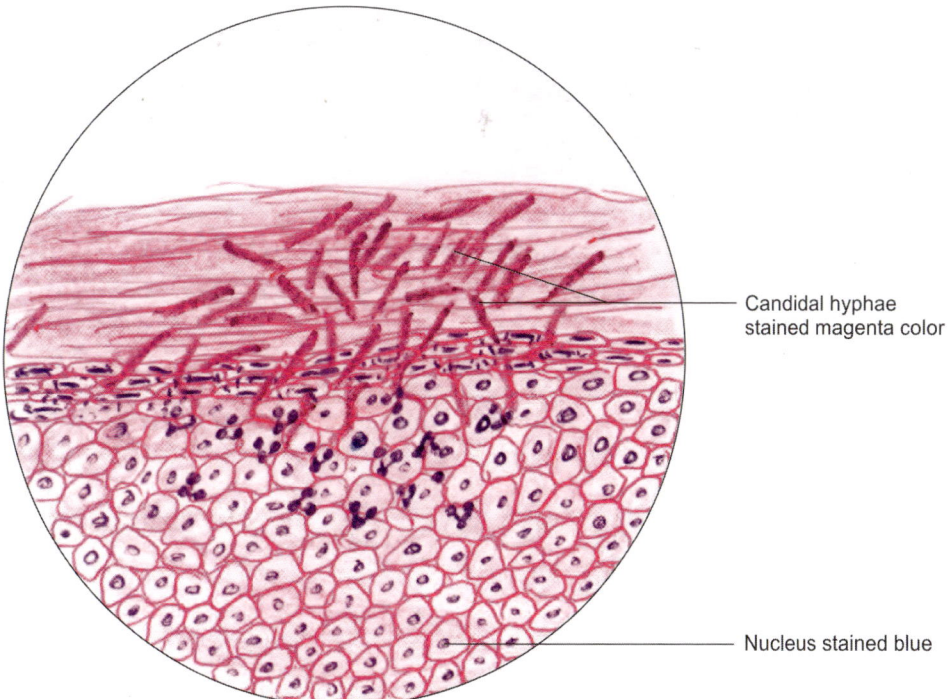

Fig. 2.15: PAS stain for Candida

Candidal hyphae stained magenta color

Nucleus stained blue

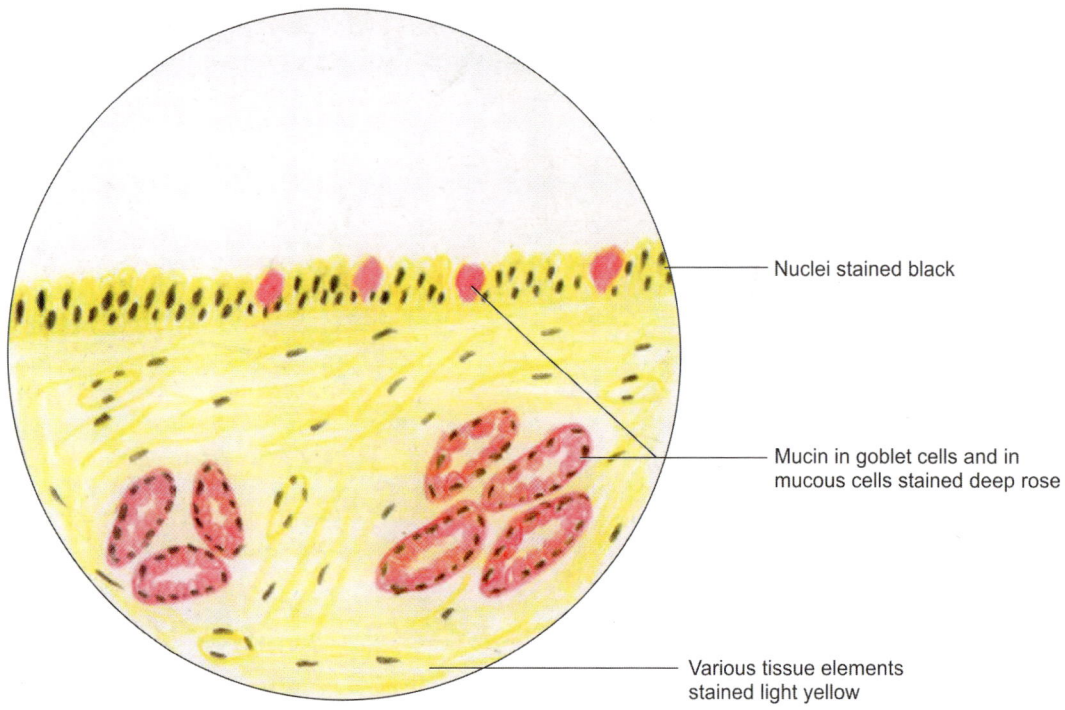

Nuclei stained black

Mucin in goblet cells and in mucous cells stained deep rose

Various tissue elements stained light yellow

Fig. 2.16: Mucicarmine stain

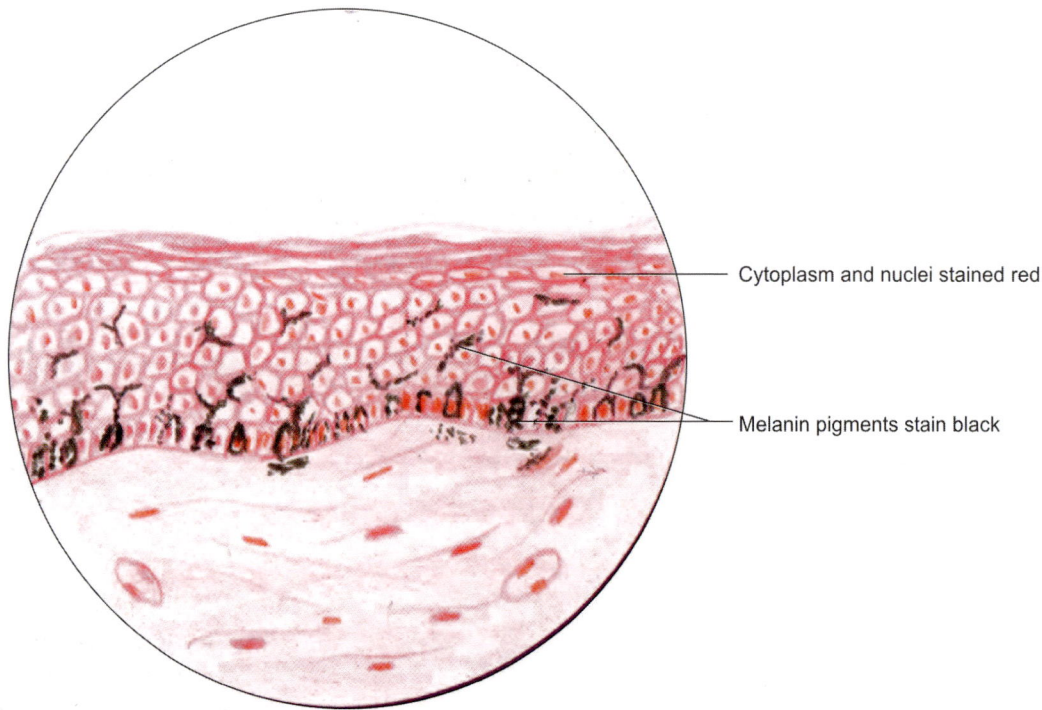

Cytoplasm and nuclei stained red

Melanin pigments stain black

Fig. 2.17: Masson-Fontana stain

feature of pigmented lesions. In inflammatory conditions, melanin is found in phagocytic cells referred to as melanophages.

Demonstration of melanin in a tissue section is of particular importance in diagnosis of benign conditions like nevus and malignant diseases like malignant melanoma. Melanin can be demonstrated using a number of techniques, which Masson-Fontana is a commonly used and reliable method. This method is based on capability of melanin to reduce silver solution. In this method formalin fixed tissue sections are treated with 10% silver nitrate solution and further counter stained with neutral red. **In Masson-Fontana stained sections, melanin pigments stain black and cytoplasm and nuclei of cells red.**

Special Stain for Mast Cells

Toluidine blue is special stain used to demonstrate mast cells. It is a polychromatic dye that stains tissues via the phenomenon known as metachromasia; which means a dye stains some tissue components, a different color from the dye solution and the rest of the tissue. When tissue sections are stained with toluidine blue, mast cell granules and polysaccharides will stain violet/purple, while the rest of the tissue stain blue (Fig. 2.18).

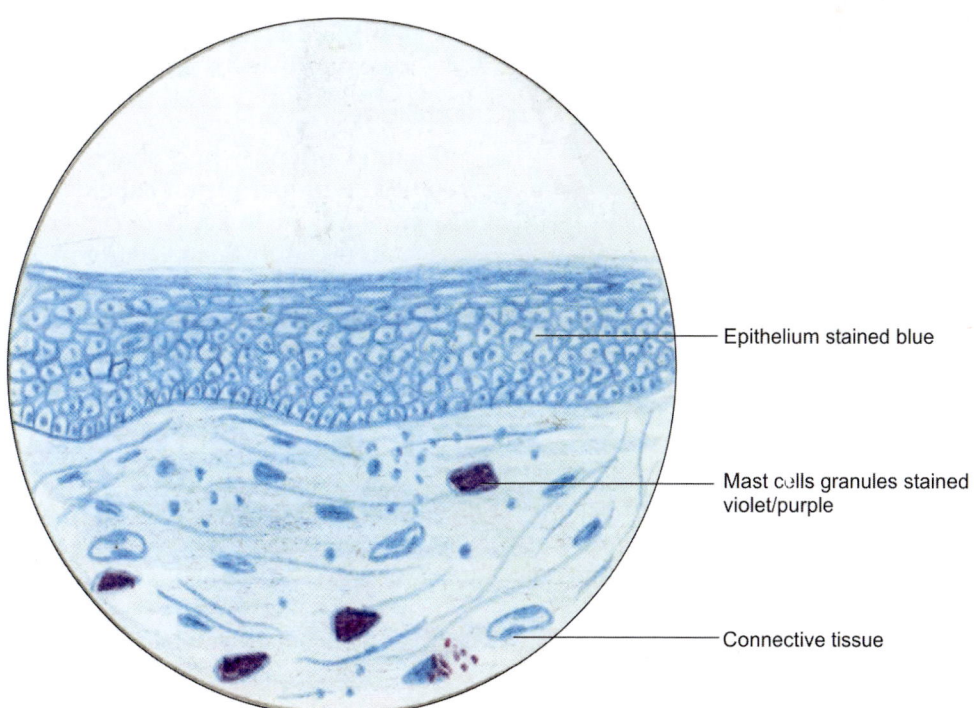

Epithelium stained blue

Mast cells granules stained violet/purple

Connective tissue

Fig. 2.18: Toluidine blue stain

3

Development of Teeth

- Stages of tooth development
  - Bud stage
  - Cap stage
  - Early bell stage
  - Advanced bell stage
- Development of root

Development of tooth is a complex process. The various tissues of the tooth and its supporting structures develop from tooth germ. The term tooth germ thus includes all the formative tissues for the entire tooth and its supporting structures. Tooth germ has three main components.

1. *Enamel organ:* The ectodermal component that gives rise to enamel.

2. *Dental papilla:* The ectomesenchymal component that gives rise to dentin and pulp.

3. *Dental follicle or dental sac:* The ectomesenchymal component giving rise to cementum, periodontal ligament, and part of the alveolar socket.

STAGES OF TOOTH DEVELOPMENT

Based on the shape of enamel organ during the development of tooth, developmental stages of the tooth are divided into three morphological stages.

1. Bud stage
2. Cap stage

3. Bell stage
   - Early
   - Late or advanced

Bud Stage (Fig. 3.1)

- **Enamel organ** is bud shaped (round or ovoid) with peripheral cuboidal cells and central polyhedral cells. Peripheral cells of enamel organ are separated from ectomesenchymal components by a basement membrane. All the cells are attached to each other by desmosomal junctions.
- Ectomesenchymal condensation adjacent to enamel organ forms the **dental papilla**.
- Marginal condensation of ectomesenchymal cells enclosing dental papilla and enamel organ is called **dental follicle or dental sac.**

Identification Points (Fig. 3.1)

Bud Stage
- Round or ovoid (bud shaped) enamel organ
- Peripheral cuboidal and central polyhedral cells
- Dental papilla adjacent to enamel organ
- Dental follicle surrounding dental papilla and enamel organ

Cap Stage (Fig. 3.2)

Enamel organ increases in size and attain the shape of a cap by invagination of the deep portion of the bud. Cells undergo change in

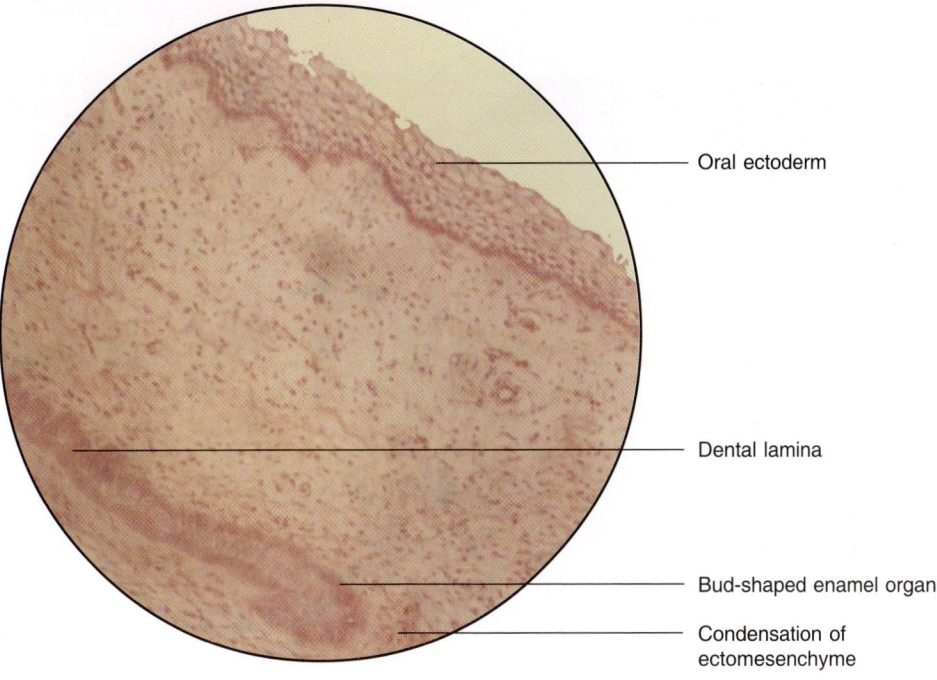

Oral ectoderm

Dental lamina

Bud-shaped enamel organ

Condensation of
ectomesenchyme

Bud stage of tooth development (photomicrograph 10X)

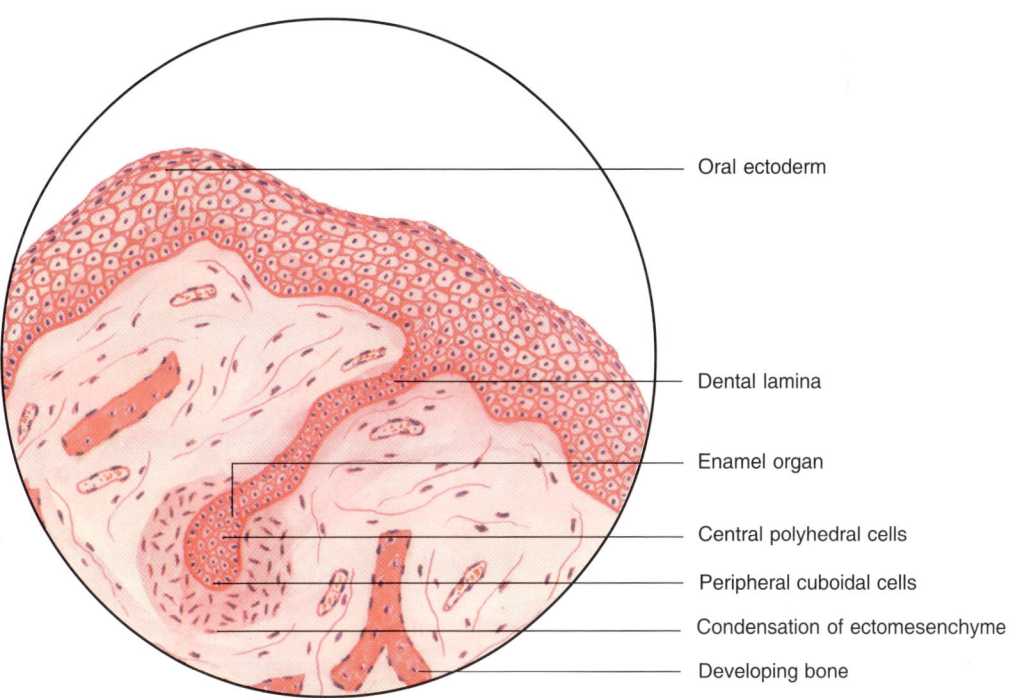

Oral ectoderm

Dental lamina

Enamel organ

Central polyhedral cells

Peripheral cuboidal cells

Condensation of ectomesenchyme

Developing bone

Fig. 3.1: Bud stage of tooth development

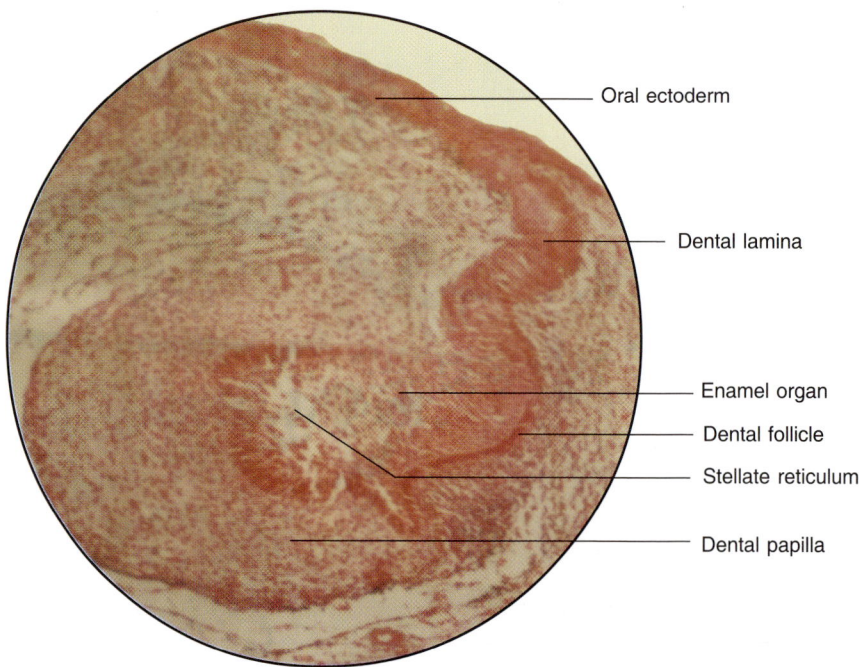

Cap stage of tooth development (photomicrograph 10X)

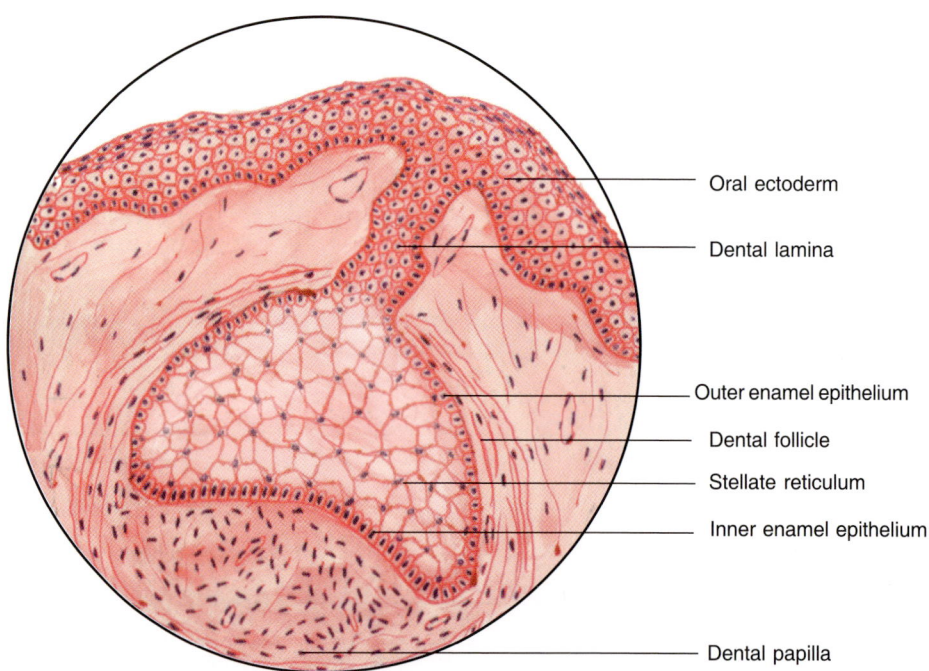

Fig. 3.2: Cap stage of tooth development

shape so that **three separate cell groups** can be identified. Cells lining the convexity or the periphery of the cap are cuboidal in shape and are called outer enamel epithelium. The cells lining the concave or invaginated portion change to columnar cells named as inner enamel epithelium. The central polyhedral cells transform into a network of star-shaped cells called stellate reticulum.

Dental papilla gets partially enclosed by the invaginated portion of enamel organ. Cells of dental papilla undergo proliferation and further condensation.

Dental follicle shows further condensation of ectomesenchymal cells. It becomes more fibrous and denser in cap stage.

Identification Points (Fig. 3.2)

Cap Stage
- Cap-shaped enamel organ
- Three layers in enamel organ—inner enamel epithelium, stellate reticulum and outer enamel epithelium
- Dental papilla with condensation of ectomesenchyme and budding capillaries
- Dense fibrous dental follicle

Bell Stage (Fig. 3.3)

Enamel organ enlarges further and invagination deepens changing the shape to that of a bell in a longitudinal section. In bell stage **four different layers** of cells are seen in the enamel organ.

Cells lining the invaginated portion, the inner enamel epithelium is composed of single layer of tall columnar cells that differentiate to ameloblasts (enamel forming cells). During bell stage a new layer appears which is called stratum intermedium. This layer is located between inner enamel epithelium and stellate reticulum and is composed of two to three layers of squamous cells. Stellate reticulum expands further in early bell stage. Cells of outer enamel epithelium lining the periphery of enamel organ flatten to low cuboidal cells. All the cells are attached to each other by desmosomal junctions. At the cervical region of the enamel organ outer enamel epithelium loops inward to join with inner enamel epithelium. This is called cervical loop.

During early bell stage enamel organ loses its connection to oral ectoderm due to degeneration of dental lamina. Remnants of the dental lamina are called cell rests of Serres. Successional lamina develops at this stage which is the primordium for the permanent successor.

Dental papilla: The dental papilla is fully enclosed in the invaginated portion of the enamel organ in this stage. Peripheral cells of dental papilla differentiate into odontoblasts (dentin forming cells) under the organizing influence of inner enamel epithelial cells.

Dental follicle becomes more fibrous, with three layers, i.e. inner cellular, outer fibrous layer and middle loose connective tissue.

Identification Points (Fig. 3.3)

Early Bell Stage
- Enamel organ having bell shape
- Four layers in enamel organ—inner enamel epithelium, stratum intermedium, stellate reticulum and outer enamel epithelium
- Dental papilla with peripheral cells differentiating to odontoblasts
- Distinct dental follicle

Advanced Bell Stage (Fig. 3.4)

Differentiating feature between early and advanced bell stage is formation of hard tissues.

Enamel organ shows four different layers, inner enamel epithelium (ameloblasts), stratum intermedium, stellate reticulum and outer enamel epithelium.

Histological differences from early bell stage are
- Hard tissue (enamel and dentin) formation.
- Collapsed stellate reticulum and folding of outer enamel epithelium bringing capillaries of the dental follicle nearer to the ameloblasts.

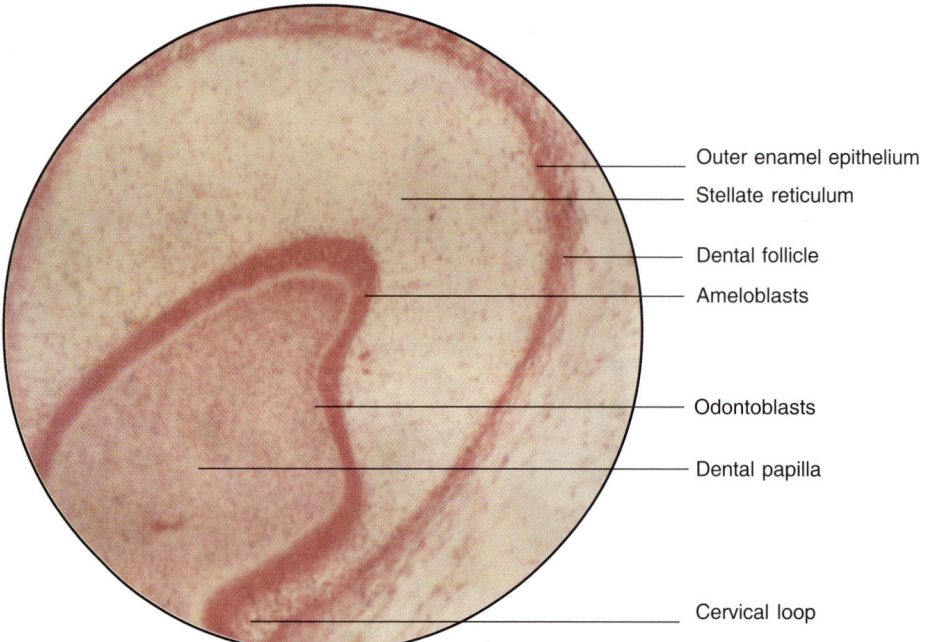

Early bell stage of tooth development (photomicrograph 10X)

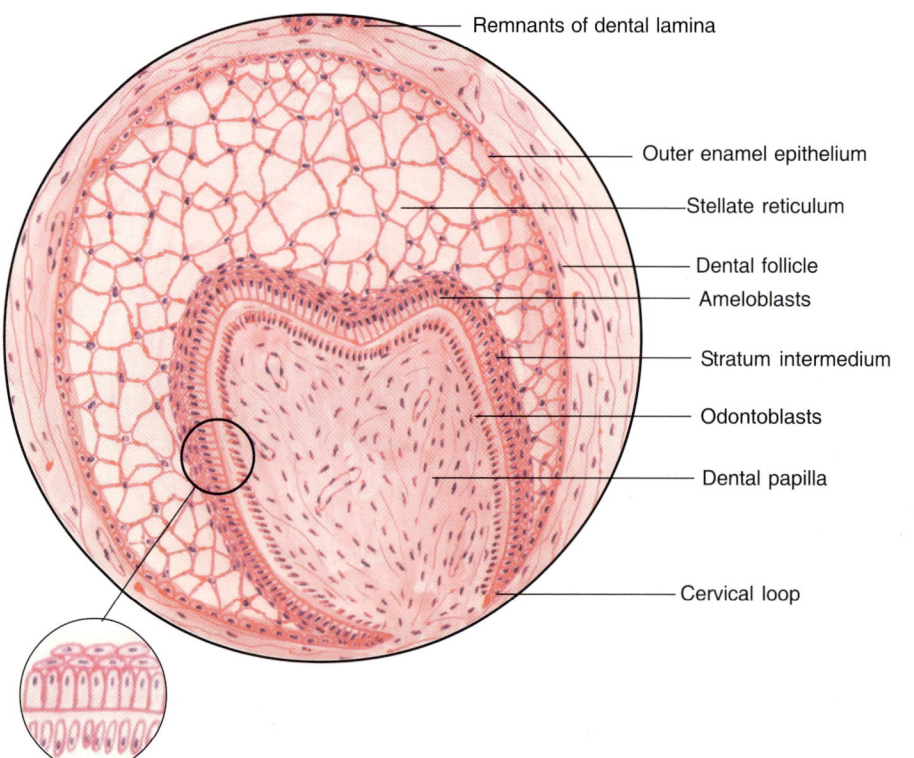

Fig. 3.3: Early bell stage of tooth development

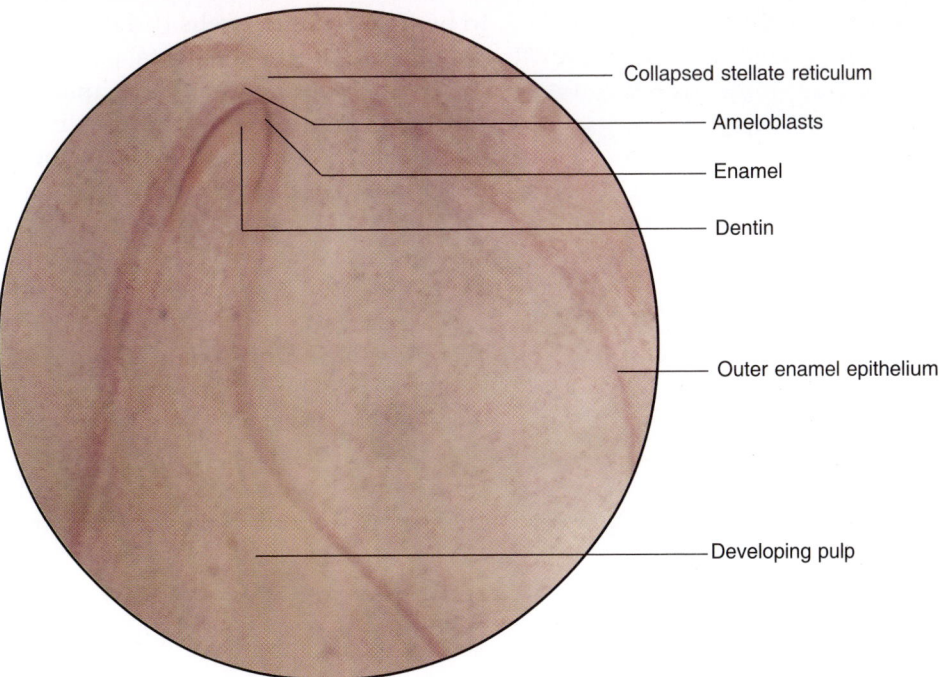

Collapsed stellate reticulum
Ameloblasts
Enamel
Dentin
Outer enamel epithelium
Developing pulp

Advanced bell stage of tooth development (photomicrograph 4X)

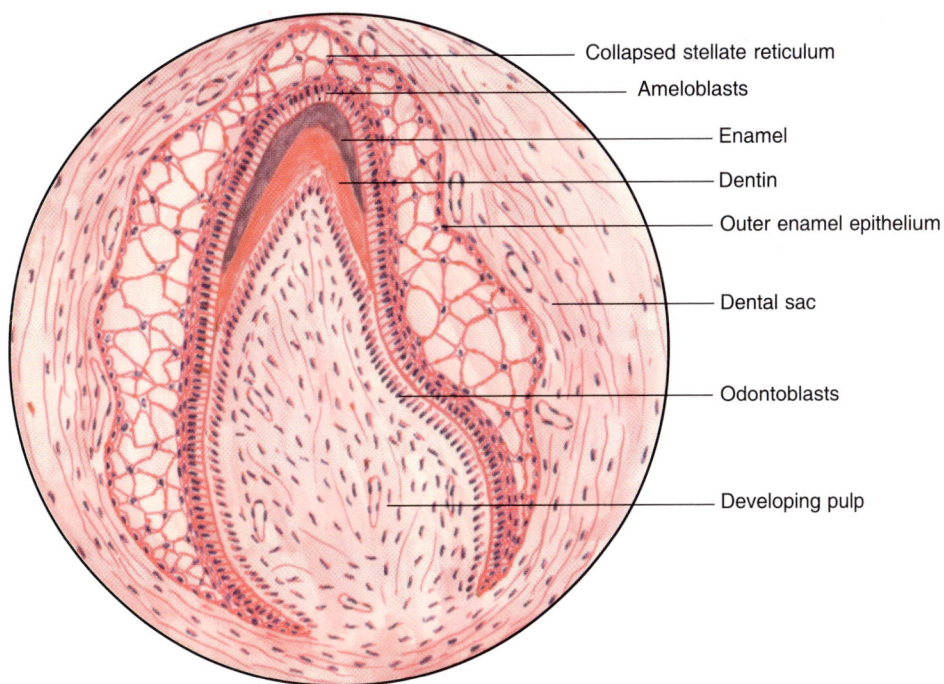

Collapsed stellate reticulum
Ameloblasts
Enamel
Dentin
Outer enamel epithelium
Dental sac
Odontoblasts
Developing pulp

Fig. 3.4: Advanced bell stage of tooth development

Ameloblasts are brought closer to the dental follicle which now becomes their source of nutrition.

Dental papilla shows differentiated odontoblast at the periphery.

Dental follicle is distinct enclosing enamel organ and dental papilla.

Identification Points (Fig. 3.4)

Advanced Bell Stage
- Dentin and enamel formation
- Four distinct layers of enamel organ, collapse of stellate reticulum
- Distinct layer of odontoblasts
- Distinct dental follicle

Development of Root (Fig. 3.5)

Root development occurs in advanced bell stage after the enamel and dentin formation reaches the cervical region of tooth. The cervical loop which is composed of outer and inner enamel epithelium, proliferates to form Hertwig's epithelial root sheath (HERS) which determines the size, shape and number of roots to be formed. Inner cells of HERS exert an organizing influence on dental papilla cells to differentiate into odontoblasts that deposit radicular dentin. Once the root dentin is formed HERS degenerates allowing the dental follicle cells to come in contact with dentin. The cells of dental follicle differentiate to form cementoblasts and lays down cementum over the root dentin. As the cementum formation progresses, the rest of the dental follicle becomes more fibrous and develops into periodontal ligament. The remnants of HERS remain in periodontal ligament and are called 'cell rests of Malassez'. Under pathological conditions these cell rests may proliferate giving rise to odontogenic cysts or tumors.

Identification Points (Fig. 3.5)

Development of Root
- Formation of Hertwig's epithelial root sheath
- Formation of radicular dentin
- Degeneration of Hertwig's epithelial root sheath
- Formation of radicular cementum
- Orientation of periodontal ligament fibers

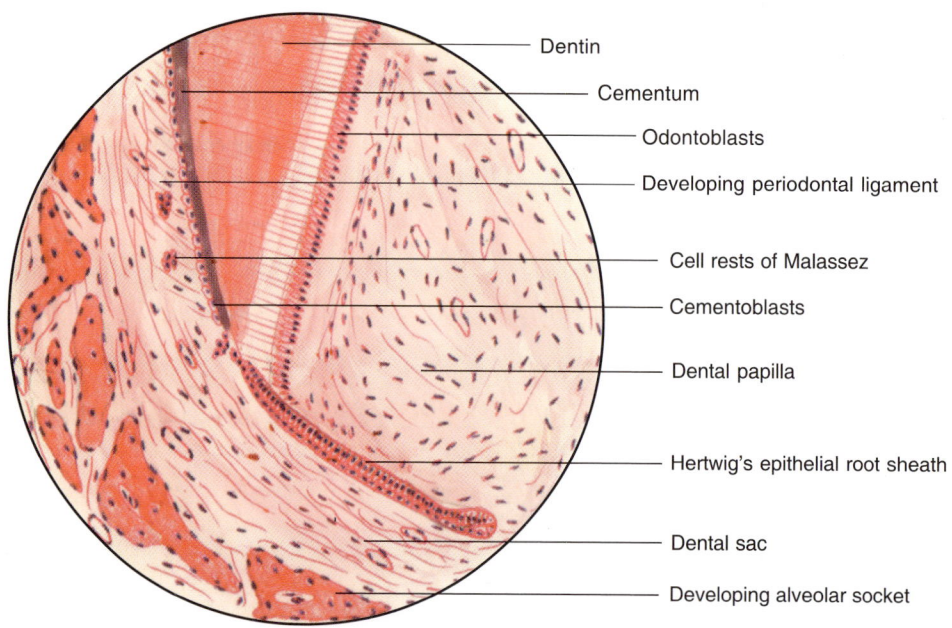

Dentin
Cementum
Odontoblasts
Developing periodontal ligament
Cell rests of Malassez
Cementoblasts
Dental papilla
Hertwig's epithelial root sheath
Dental sac
Developing alveolar socket

Fig. 3.5: Development of root

4

Enamel

- Structure of enamel rod
- Striae of Retzius
- Neonatal line
- Enamel lamellae
- Enamel tufts
- Enamel spindle
- Hunter-Schreger bands
- Gnarled enamel

Identification Points (Figs 4.1 and 4.2)

Enamel Rods
- Basic structural units of enamel
- Rod-shaped in longitudinal sections
- Resemble fish scale or keyhole in cross section

Enamel is the hardest calcified tissue of the body covering the anatomic crown of the tooth. Enamel, in contrast to other calcified structures of the body, is ectodermal in origin, has 96% inorganic component, and unique organic constituent which do not contain collagen. Structure of enamel is studied using ground sections. Decalcified sections are not of much use because enamel is lost during decalcification due to its high mineral content.

Enamel Rods (Figs 4.1 and 4.2)

Enamel rods are the basic structural units of enamel. They run from the dentinoenamel junction to the outer surface of enamel and follow somewhat tortuous course. In a longitudinal section (Fig. 4.1) enamel rods appears to be divided into segments by dark lines. These dark lines across the enamel rods are called cross striations. These cross striations are separated by a distance of 4 microns making each segment 4 microns which is the increment of enamel deposited daily.

In cross section (Fig. 4.2) enamel rods may resemble a fish scale or keyhole pattern with a head and a tail. Head represents the rods and tail represents the inter rod region. The head portion is directed towards the occlusal aspect and tail to the cervical region of the tooth.

Striae of Retzius (Fig. 4.3)

Striae of Retzius are the incremental lines of enamel representing the successive apposition of enamel. These structural lines appear as brownish bands in ground sections. In the region of incisal edge and cusps they surround the dentin while in cervical region they are seen as oblique lines extending from DEJ towards the outer surface deviating in an occlusal direction. In transverse sections of teeth incremental lines are seen as concentric rings. These lines are hypocalcified and reflects variation in structure and mineralization.

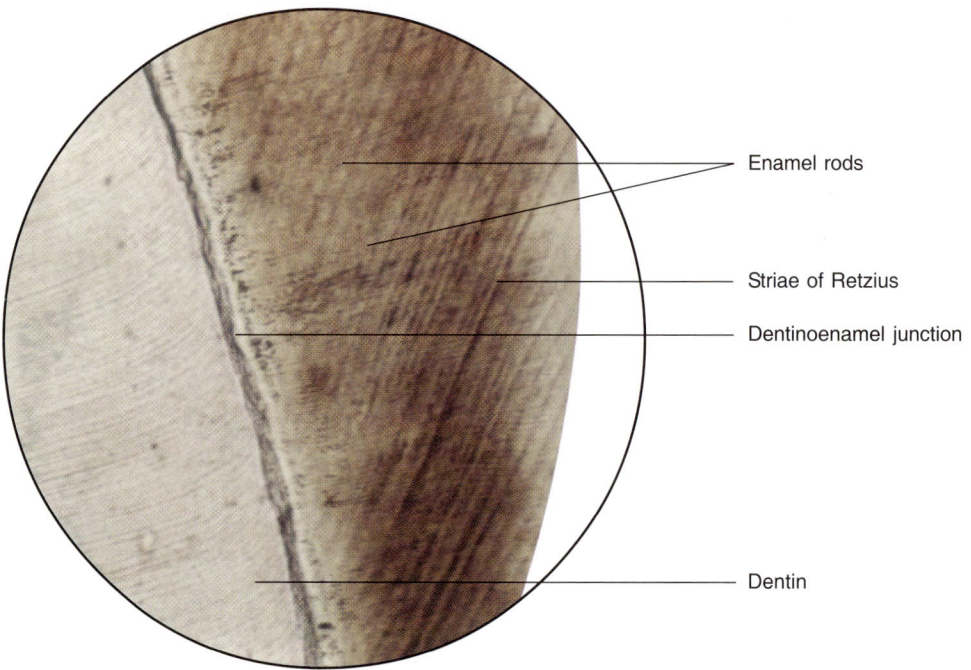

Enamel rods

Striae of Retzius

Dentinoenamel junction

Dentin

Enamel rods: Longitudinal section (photomicrograph 10X)

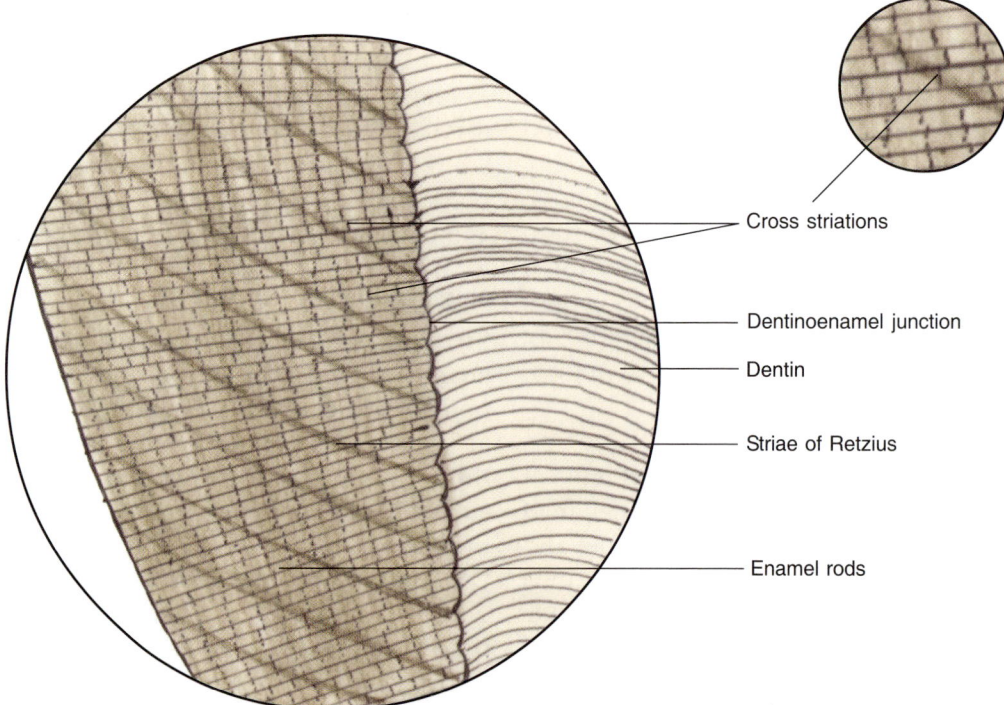

Cross striations

Dentinoenamel junction

Dentin

Striae of Retzius

Enamel rods

Fig. 4.1: Enamel rods: Longitudinal section

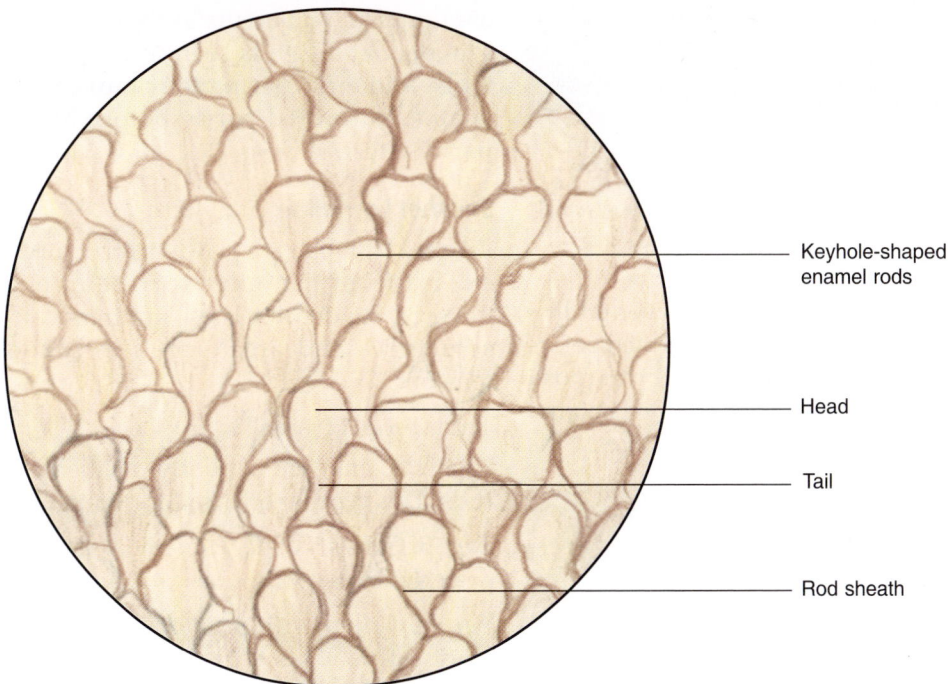

Keyhole-shaped enamel rods

Head

Tail

Rod sheath

Fig. 4.2: Enamel rods—transverse section

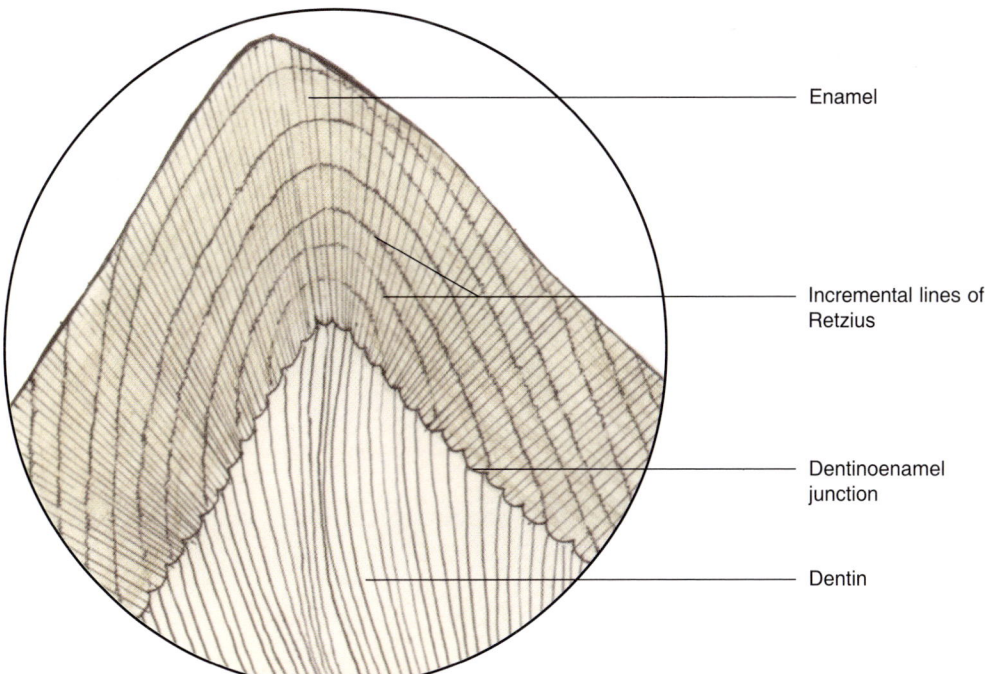

Enamel

Incremental lines of Retzius

Dentinoenamel junction

Dentin

Fig. 4.3: Striae of Retzius

Identification Points (Fig. 4.3)

Stage of Retzius
- Incremental lines of enamel
- Appears as brownish bands in ground section
- Hypocalcified structures

Neonatal Line (Fig. 4.4)

Neonatal line is prominent incremental line that separates the enamel that is formed before birth (prenatal enamel) and after birth (post-natal enamel). The incremental line becomes prominent because of abrupt change in the

Identification Points (Fig. 4.4)

Neonatal Line
- Accentuated incremental line
- Separates pre- and postnatal enamel
- Seen in all deciduous teeth and first permanent molars

environment that occurs at the time of birth. The neonatal line is seen in all deciduous teeth and first permanent molars where enamel is formed partly before birth and partly after.

Enamel Lamellae (Fig. 4.5)

Enamel lamellae are leaf-like structures that extend from the outer surface of enamel towards the dentin. These are hypocalcified structures and are formed in planes of tension.

Three types of lamellae are seen.

Type A: Composed of poorly calcified enamel rods. This type is restricted to enamel.

Type B: Consists of degenerated cells and may extend into dentin.

Type C: Filled with organic matter derived from saliva. This type is formed after the eruption of the tooth and may be extended into the dentin.

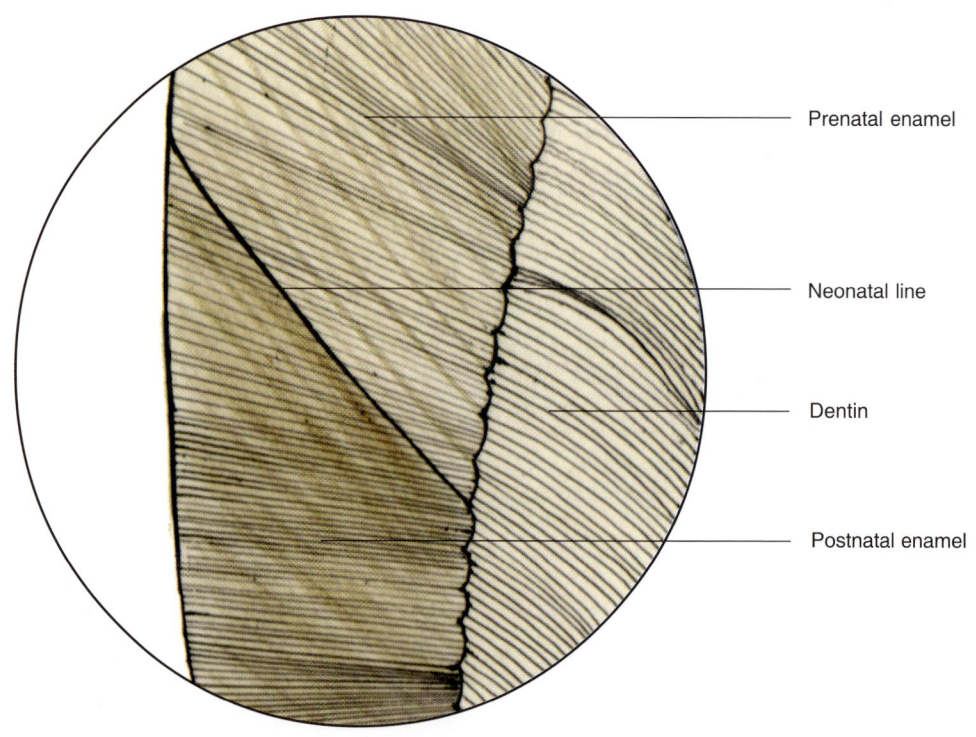

Prenatal enamel

Neonatal line

Dentin

Postnatal enamel

Fig. 4.4: Neonatal line

Identification Points (Fig. 4.5)

Enamel Lamellae
- Hypocalcified structures of enamel
- Extend from outer surface of enamel towards the dentin
- Types A, B, or C can be seen

Enamel Tufts
- Hypocalcified structure of enamel
- Ribbon-like structures extending from DEJ to enamel to a distance of one-third to one-fifth of enamel thickness
- Resemble tufts of grass in ground section

Enamel Tufts (Fig. 4.5)

Enamel tufts are ribbon-like structures extending from dentinoenamel junction into enamel to a distance of one-third to one-fifth of enamel thickness. In thick sections these ribbon-like structures arising from different planes are projected to one plane giving the appearance of tuft of grass. These are hypocalcified structures containing greater concentration of organic components. Enamel tufts are better visualized in transverse sections.

Enamel Spindle (Fig. 4.6)

The enamel spindles are the odontoblastic processes crossing the dentinoenamel junction and extending to the enamel. These are spindle-shaped structures extending from dentinoenamel junction to enamel to a distance of approximately 10 microns. They appear dark in a ground section under transmitted light because the organic content of spindle is lost and is replaced by air.

Identification Points (Fig. 4.6)

Enamel Spindles
- Odontoblast processes extending to enamel
- Appears as dark spindle-shaped structure
- Found more in the cuspal region

Enamel spindles are seen more in the region of cusp tip.

Hunter-Schreger Bands (Fig. 4.7)

Hunter-Schreger bands (HS bands) are alternate dark and light bands of varying width observed in enamel when a longitudinal section is viewed under reflected light. These bands arise from the dentinoenamel junction and pass outward till the inner two-thirds of enamel thickness. These bands are slightly curved with convexity directed to the cervical region. HS bands are not seen in outer one-third of enamel, because the enamel rods are straight in this region.

HS bands are optical effect created due to variation in course of adjacent groups of enamel rods; each group consists of 10–13 enamel rods. Because of this change in direction, when a longitudinal section is made some prisms are cut longitudinally and some transversely. When viewed under reflected light those prisms lying parallel to the light beam would reflect the light away from microscope and appear as dark bands. The prisms lying less parallel to the light would reflect the light through the microscope and appear bright. There is also an opinion that the dark and light bands of Hunter-Schreger bands may be composed of zones having altered permeability, difference in organic component or an area with variation in calcification.

Identification Points (Fig. 4.7)

Hunter-Schreger Band
- Appear as alternate light and dark bands.
- Seen under reflected light.
- Occur due to abrupt change in direction of enamel rods.

Gnarled Enamel (Fig. 4.8)

Enamel rods follow a wavy course as they extend from dentinoenamel junction towards the outer surface. In the region of the cusps and incisal edges the arrangement of enamel rods

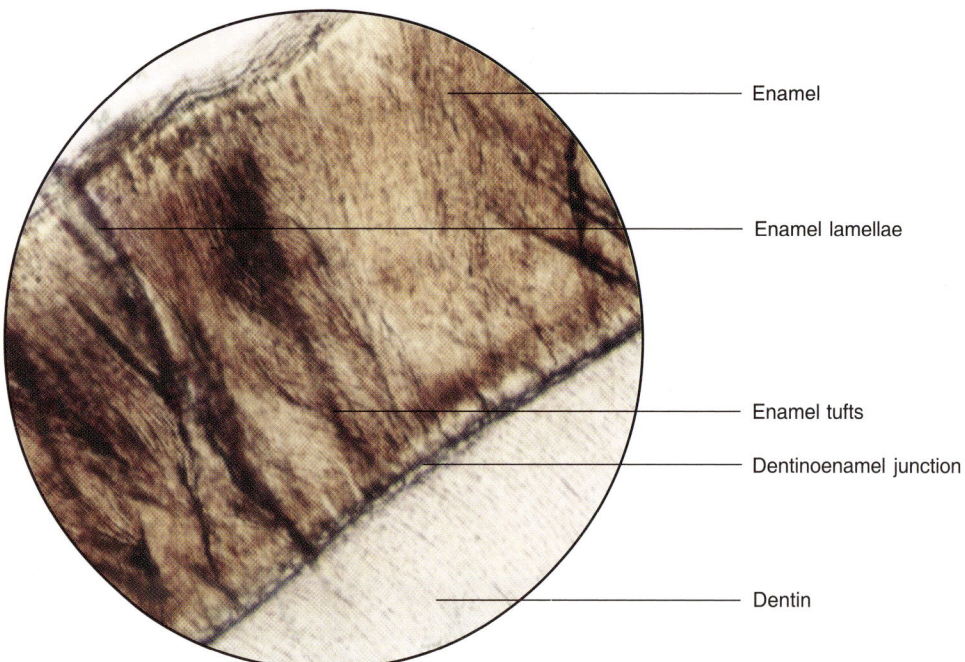

Enamel

Enamel lamellae

Enamel tufts

Dentinoenamel junction

Dentin

Enamel lamellae and enamel tufts (photomicrograph 4X)

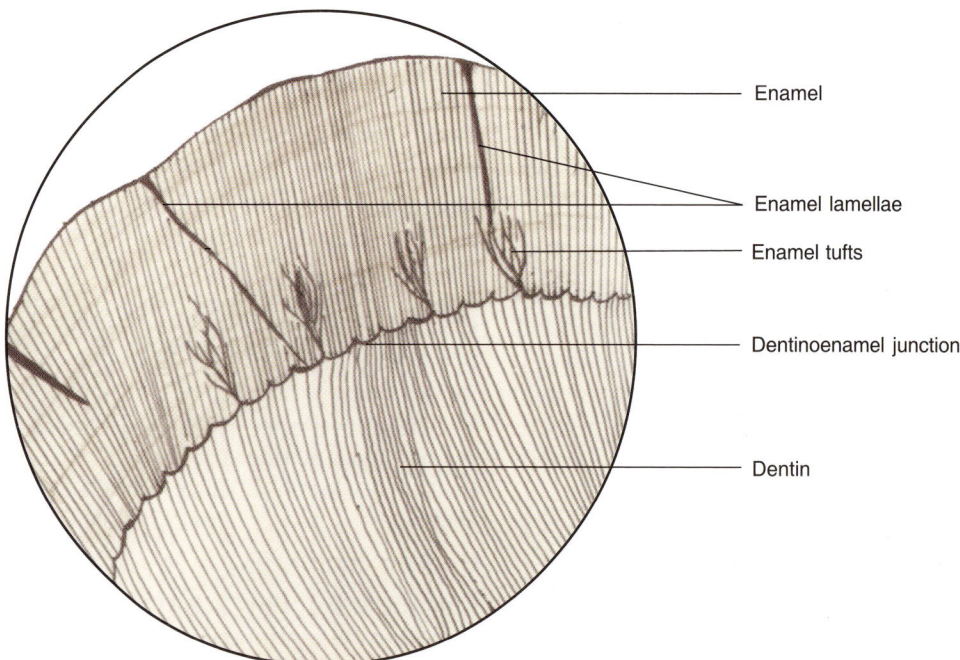

Enamel

Enamel lamellae

Enamel tufts

Dentinoenamel junction

Dentin

Fig. 4.5: Enamel lamellae and enamel tufts

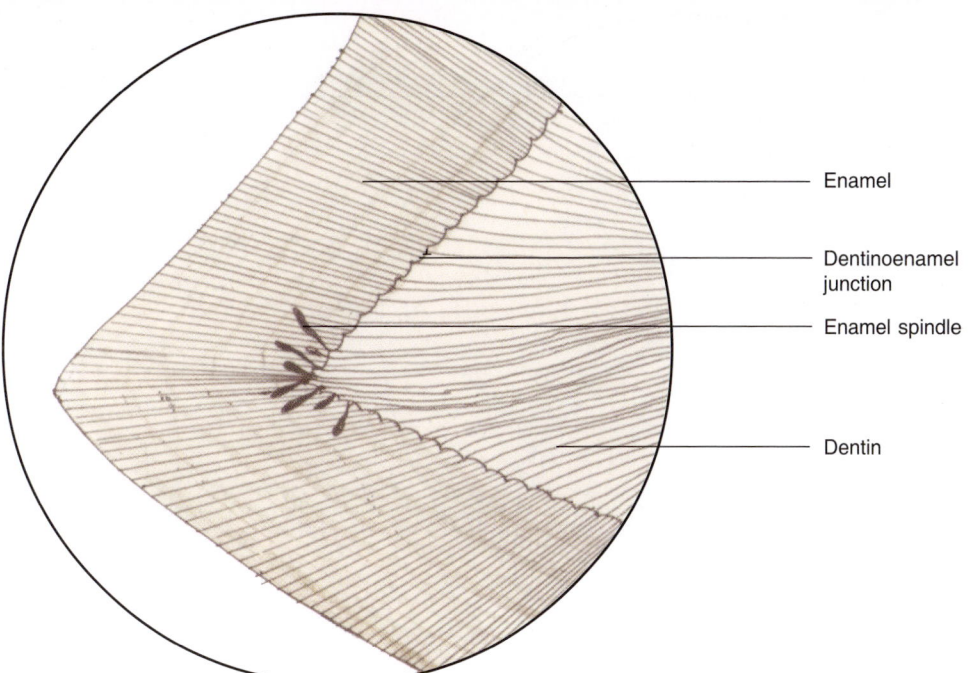

Fig. 4.6: Enamel spindles

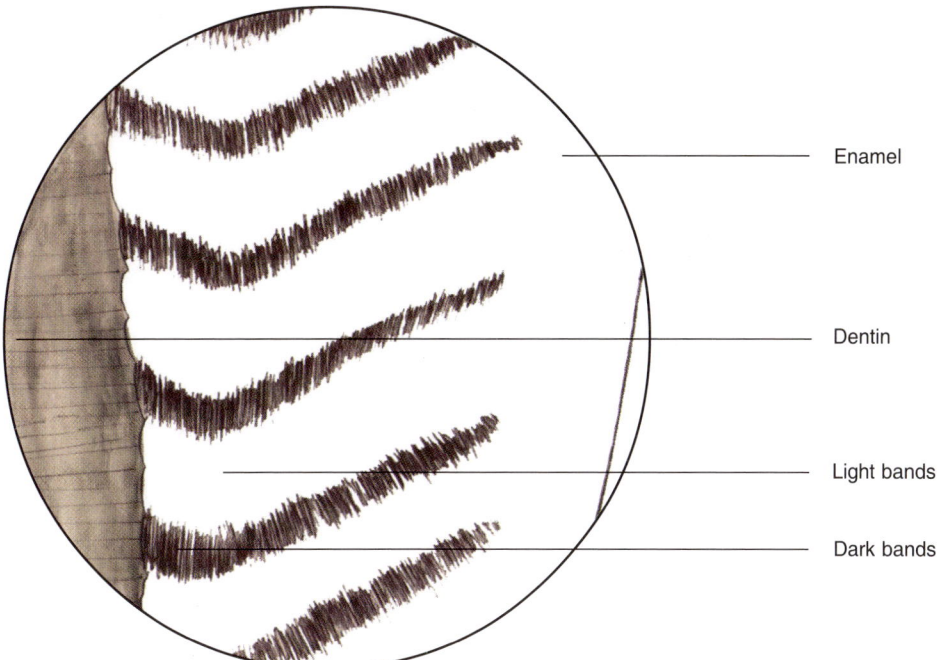

Fig. 4.7: Hunter-Schreger bands

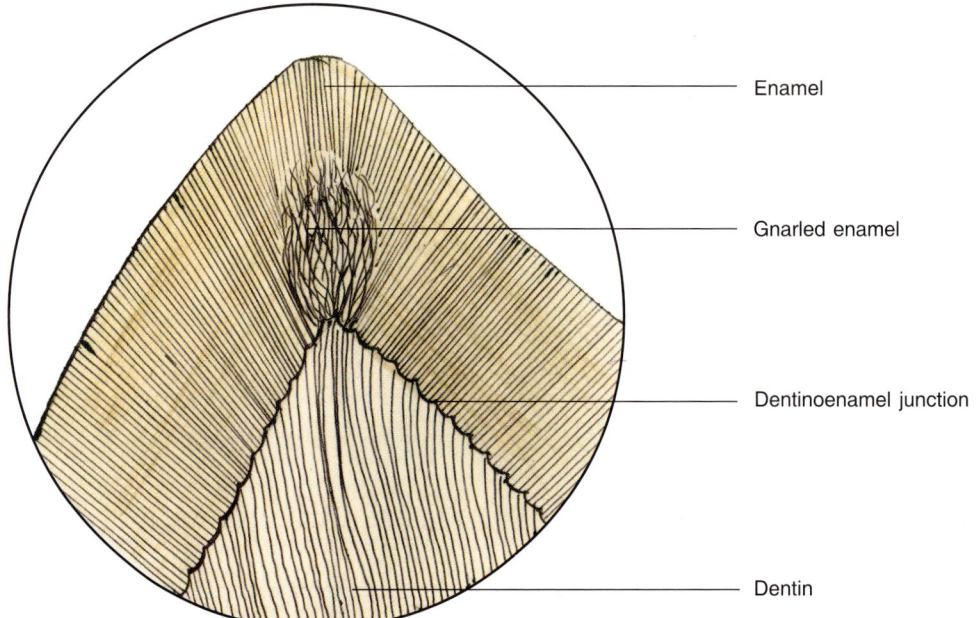

Enamel

Gnarled enamel

Dentinoenamel junction

Dentin

Fig.4.8: Gnarled enamel

are more complicated. The enamel rods are more wavy and irregular and intertwine with each other in this region especially near DEJ. This arrangement creates an optical appearance referred to as Gnarled enamel. This particular arrangement of rods in cuspal and incisal regions makes enamel stronger to withstand masticatory stress.

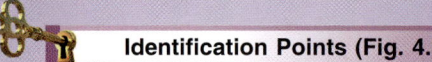

Identification Points (Fig. 4.8)

Gnarled Enamel
- Optical appearance seen in the incisal or cuspal region
- Occur due to wavy intertwining enamel rods
- This arrangement makes enamel stronger

5

Dentin

- Structure of dentinal tubules
  - S-shaped dentinal tubules
  - Y-shaped terminal branching
  - Transverse section of dentin
- Dentinoenamel junction
- Incremental lines of dentin
- Interglobular dentin
- Tomes' granular layer
- Dead tracts

Dentin is the hard tissue component that makes up the bulk of the tooth. The structure of dentine can be studied using ground sections or decalcified sections under light microscope. The structural features seen under light microscope are dentinal tubules, which are the basic structural units of dentin, peritubular or intratubular dentin, intertubular dentin, incremental lines, interglobular dentin and Tomes' granular layer. Functional changes may be evident like dead tracts, reparative dentin and sclerotic dentin.

S-shaped Dentinal Tubules (Fig. 5.1)

Dentinal tubules extend from pulpal surface to dentinoenamel or dentinocemental junction. Dentinal tubules are S-shaped or doubly curved structures and is described as primary curvature of dentinal tubules. The first convexity from the pulpal side is directed towards the root of tooth and second convexity towards the crown. These tubules are perpendicular to

pulpal surface and dentinoenamel junction. Along the length of primary curvature small oscillations will be found at intervals and are referred to as secondary curvatures.

Identification Points (Fig. 5.1)

S-shaped Dentinal Tubules
- First convexity from pulpal side directed towards the root
- Second convexity directed towards the crown
- All along the course secondary curvatures are seen

Y-shaped Terminal Branches and Lateral Branches of Dentinal Tubules (Fig. 5.2)

The terminal end of dentinal tubule near dentinoenamel junction fork off from the main tubule at 45 degree to form Y-shaped terminal branching. Some of the odontoblastic processes may cross the dentinoenamel junction to form enamel spindles.

Also all along the course, the tubules have lateral branches at every 1 micrometer distance. These lateral branches are somewhat perpendicular to the main tubule and may contain odontoblast processes. Lateral branches may communicate with those of adjacent tubules or blindly end at intertubular dentin.

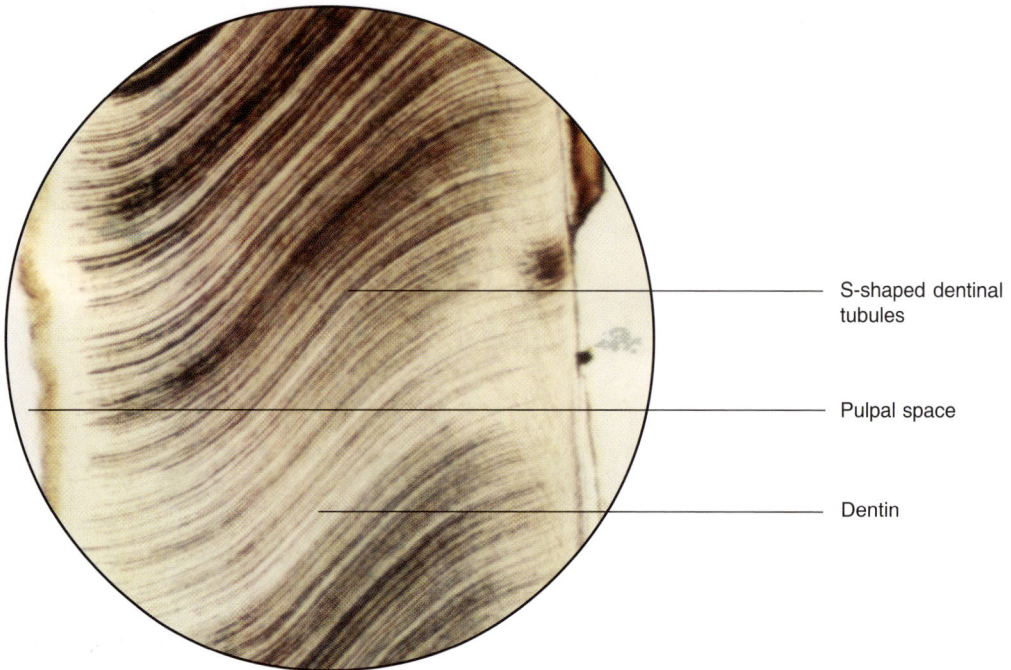

S-shaped dentinal tubules (photomicrograph 4X)

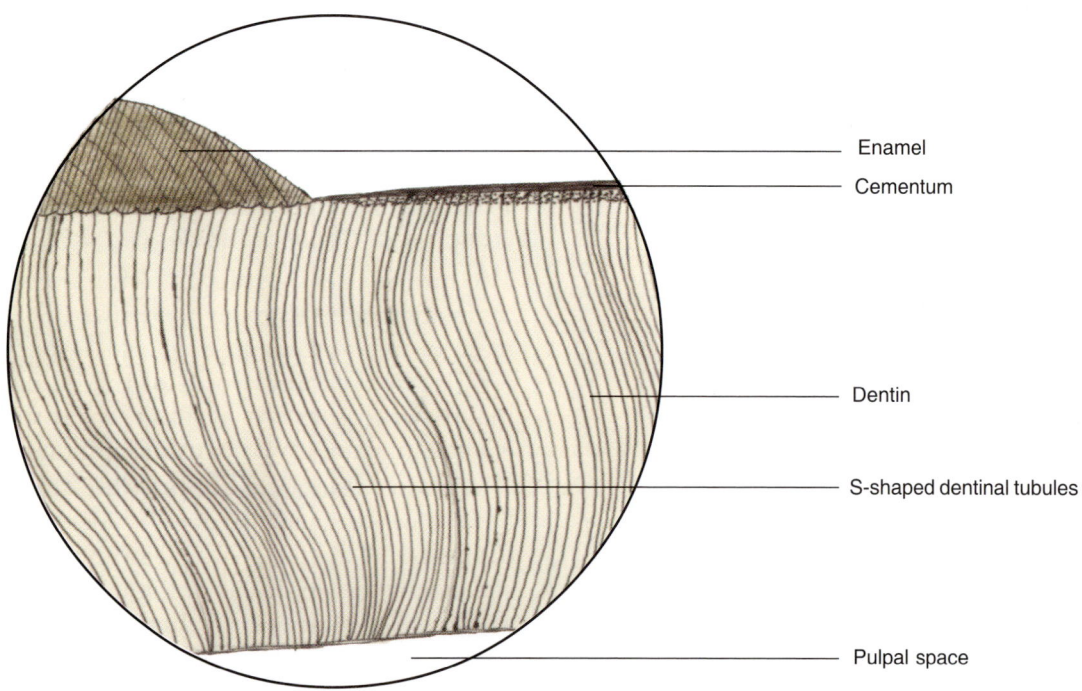

Fig. 5.1: S-shaped dentinal tubules

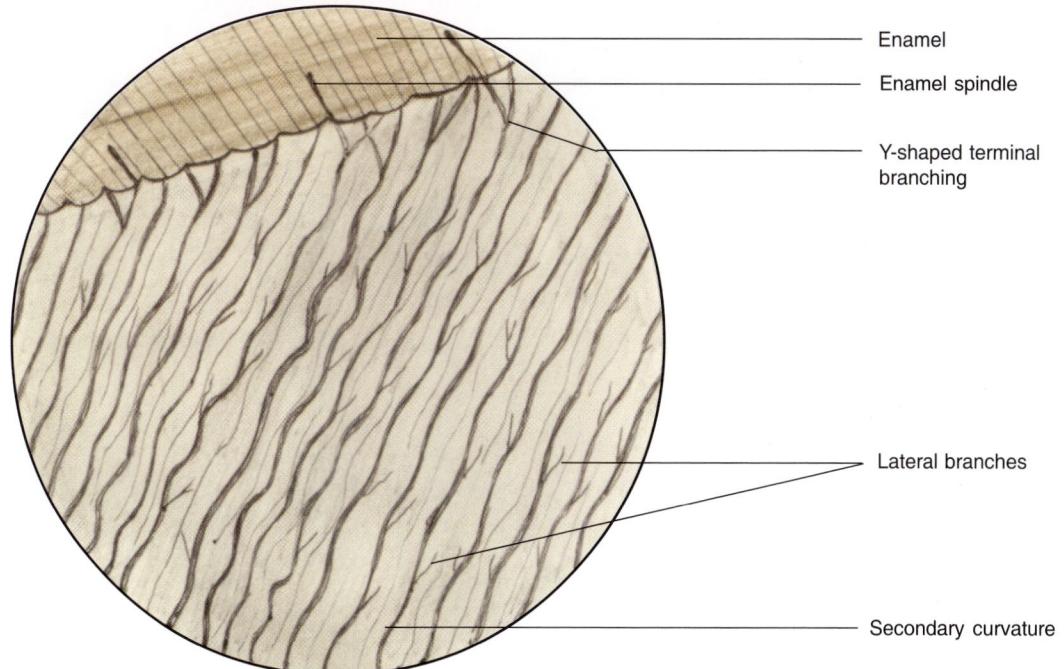

Fig. 5.2: Terminal branches and lateral branches of dentinal tubules

 Identification Points (Fig. 5.2)

Terminal and Lateral Branches of Dentinal Tubules
- Near DEJ, terminal end of dentinal tubules show Y-shaped branching
- Lateral branches are seen along the course
- Lateral branches may contain odontoblast process

 Identification Points (Fig. 5.3)

TS of Dentin
- Dentinal tubules appear as circular structures
- Within the tubules odontoblast process is seen
- Around the tubule peritubular dentin and in between intertubular dentin are seen

Transverse Section of Dentin (Fig. 5.3)

Transverse or cross section of dentin shows numerous dentinal tubules appearing as circular structures. These tubules have odontoblast processes at the center that appear as dark spot with periodontoblast space surrounding it. The periodontoblast space contains tissue fluid named as dental lymph. The inner aspect of the tubule is thought to be lined by an organic membrane called lamina limitans. The dentinal tubules are surrounded by peritubular or intra-tubular dentin. In between the dentinal tubules the bulk of dentin is made of intertubular dentin.

Dentinoenamel Junction (Fig. 5.4)

DEJ is scalloped with the convexity facing the dentin. This scalloped shape increases the adherence between enamel and dentin and also helps to prevent shearing of enamel during function.

 Identification Points (Fig. 5.4)

Dentinoenamel Junction
- Scalloped with convexity facing dentin
- Increases adherence between enamel and dentin
- Prevents shearing of enamel

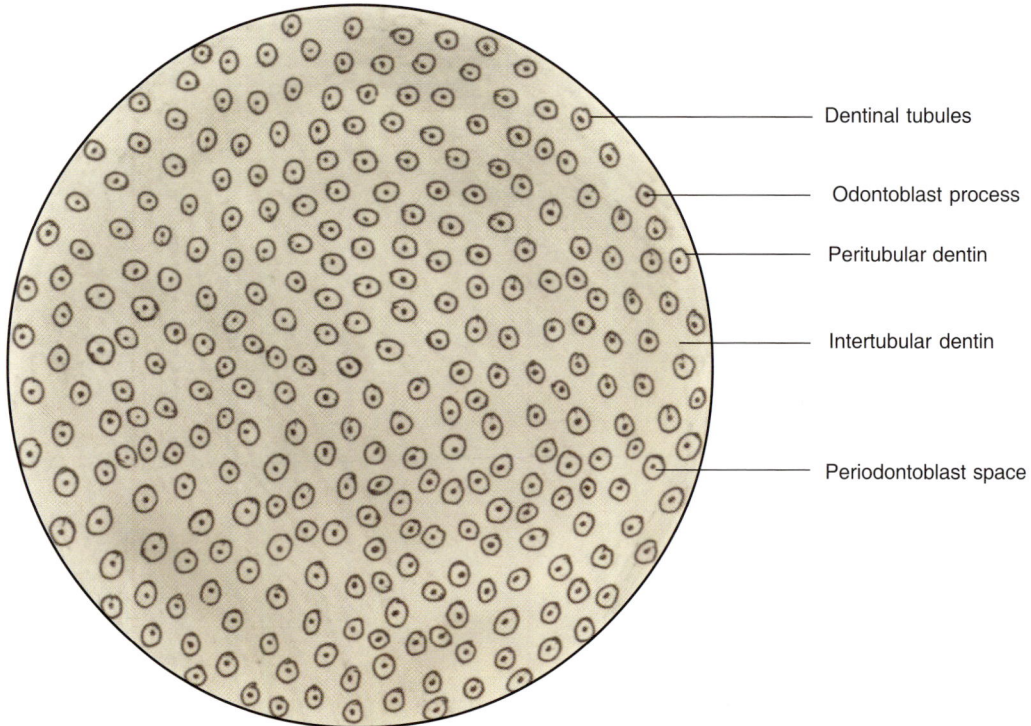

Dentinal tubules

Odontoblast process

Peritubular dentin

Intertubular dentin

Periodontoblast space

Fig. 5.3: Transverse section of dentin

Incremental Lines of Dentin (Fig. 5.5)

Formation of dentin is a rhythmic process with alternating phases of activity and quiescence. This rhythmic deposition is indicated by incremental lines. The incremental lines of dentin are called 'lines of von Ebner' which run perpendicular to the dentinal tubules. The distance between these incremental lines are 4–6 microns and much less in radicular dentin. Sometimes due to disturbance in either matrix deposition or mineralization these incremental lines may become accentuated and are called 'contour lines of Owen'. The accentuated incremental line formed due to the change in environment at the time of birth is called neonatal line, and this line separates prenatal dentin from postnatal dentin.

Interglobular Dentin (Fig. 5.6)

Interglobular dentin is a hypocalcified area seen in coronal circumpulpal dentin immediately below mantle dentin. These areas

 Identification Points (Fig. 5.5)

Incremental Lines of Dentin

- Incremental lines run perpendicular to the dentinal tubules
- Lines of von Ebner represent the rhythmic deposition
- Contour lines of Owen are accentuated incremental lines

 Identification Points (Fig. 5.6)

Interglobular Dentin

- Hypocalcified structure of dentin
- Appears as star-shaped structure in circumpulpal dentin
- Develop due to lack of fusion of globules of mineralization

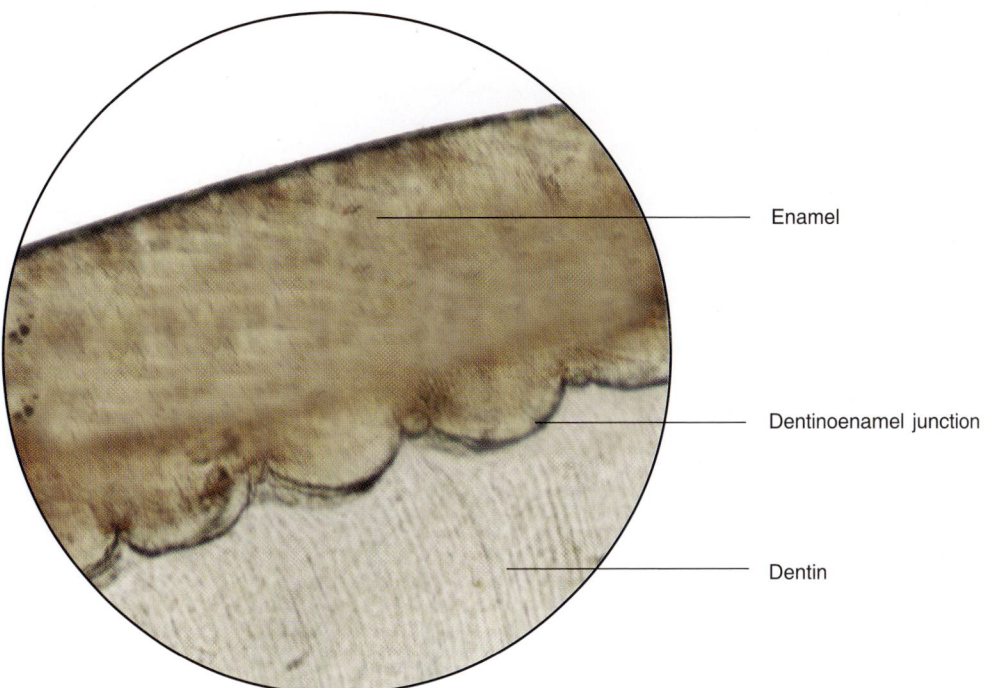

Enamel

Dentinoenamel junction

Dentin

Dentinoenamel junction (photomicrograph 4X)

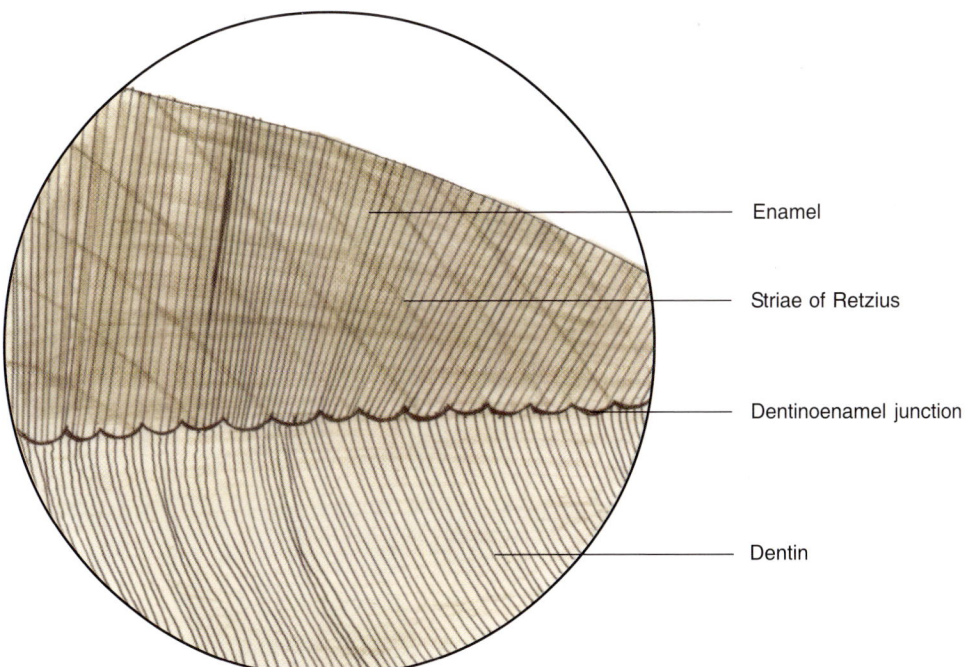

Enamel

Striae of Retzius

Dentinoenamel junction

Dentin

Fig. 5.4: Dentinoenamel junction

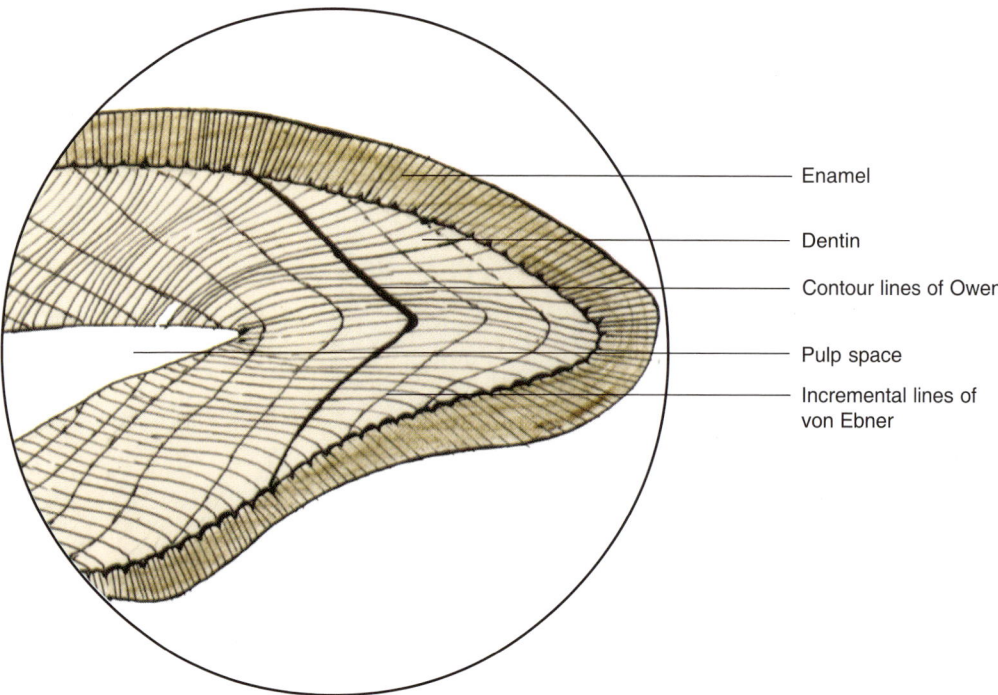

- Enamel
- Dentin
- Contour lines of Owen
- Pulp space
- Incremental lines of von Ebner

Fig. 5.5: Incremental lines of dentin

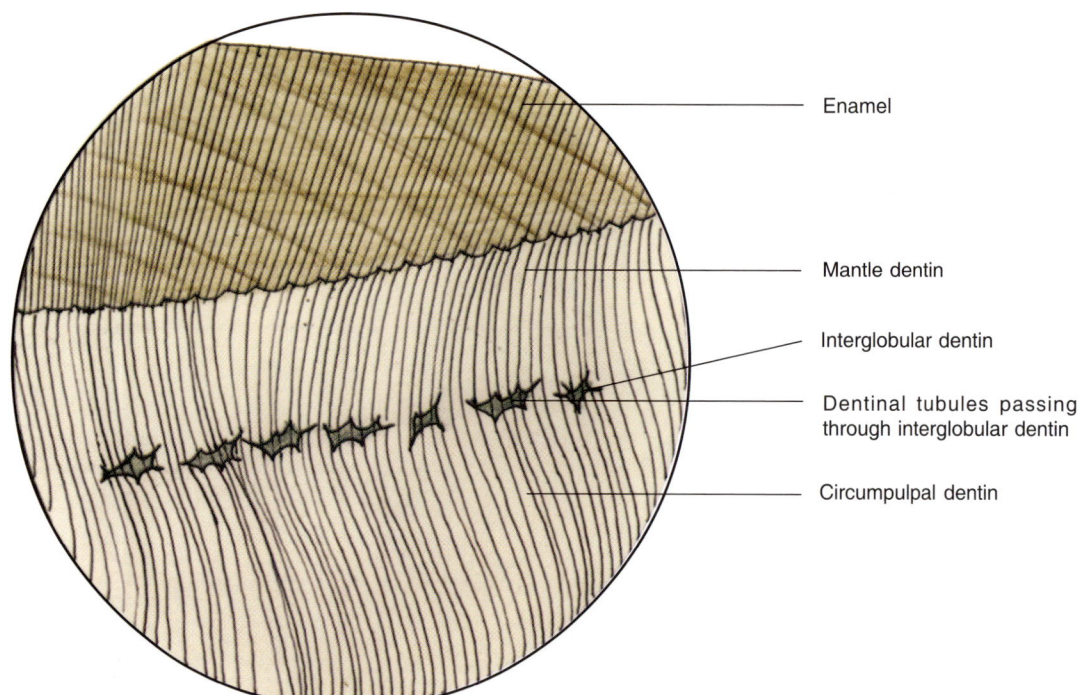

- Enamel
- Mantle dentin
- Interglobular dentin
- Dentinal tubules passing through interglobular dentin
- Circumpulpal dentin

Fig. 5.6: Interglobular dentin

appear slightly dark in a ground section under transmitted light. Dentin calcification occurs in the form of globules. Failures of fusion of these globules into a homogenous mass result in the formation of interglobular dentin. They appear star-shaped with curved outline of adjacent globules. The dentinal tubules passes uninterruptedly through interglobular dentin suggesting that this area results from defect in mineralization, and not matrix deposition.

Granular Layer of Tomes (Fig. 5.7)

It is a structure seen only in radicular dentin adjacent to cementodentinal junction. This layer appears in a ground section as dark granular structure, gradually increasing in thickness from CEJ till the apex. Tomes' granular layer is thought to be formed because of looping and coalescing of dentinal tubules near the dentinocemental junction.

Identification Points (Fig. 5.7)

Granular Layer of Tomes
- Seen in radicular dentin adjacent to DCJ
- Appear as dark granular structure
- Formed due to looping and coalescing of dentinal tubules

Dead Tracts (Fig. 5.8)

Dead tracts are empty dentinal tubules those appear dark in ground section of dentin under transmitted light and white under reflected light. These dead tracts are formed due to degeneration of odontoblast processes in the dentinal tubules. This occurs due to exposure of dentin following attrition, abrasion or erosion. These empty dentinal tubules are filled with air; and hence appear dark under transmitted light. Dead tracts may also develop in the region of cusp or incisal edges due to death of odontoblasts occurring as a result of over-crowding. True dead tracts can be identified by the presence of reparative dentin at their pulpal end.

Identification Points (Fig. 5.8)

Dead Tracts
- Appear dark under transmitted light and white under reflected light
- Formed due to degeneration of odontoblast processes in the tubules
- Presence of reparative dentin at the pupal end of dead tracts

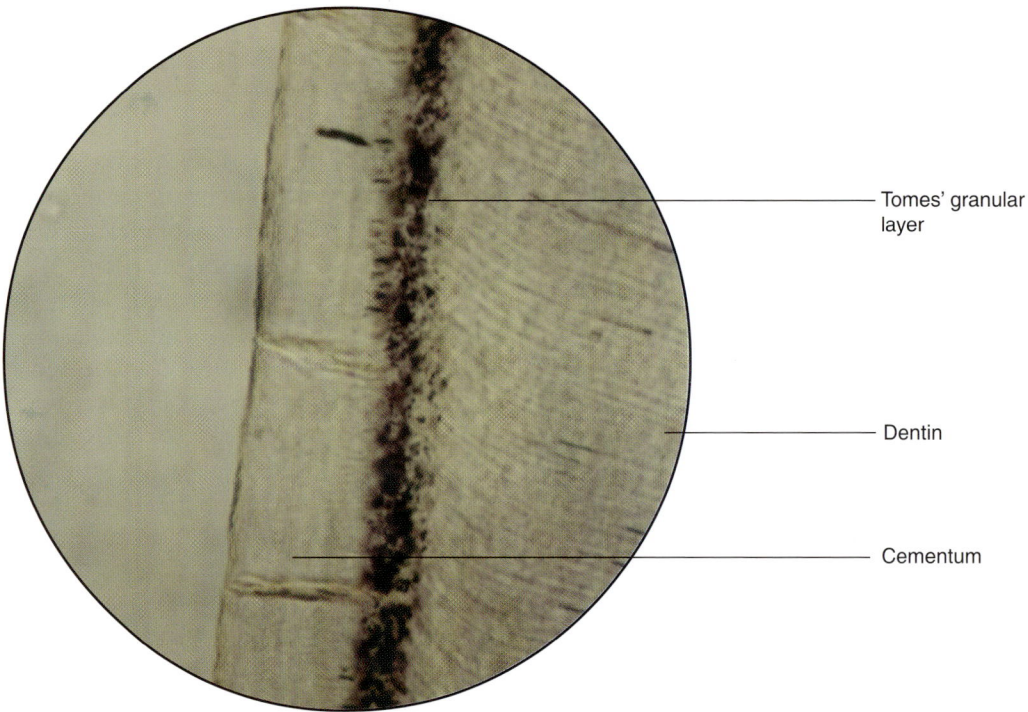

Tomes' granular layer (photomicrograph 10X)

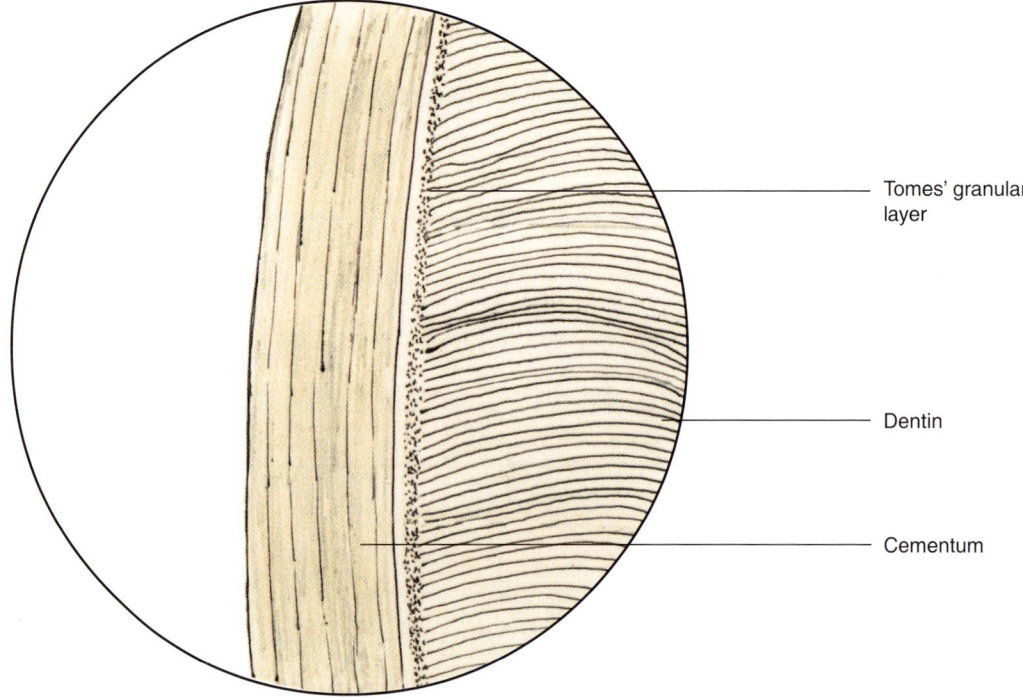

Fig. 5.7: Tomes' granular layer

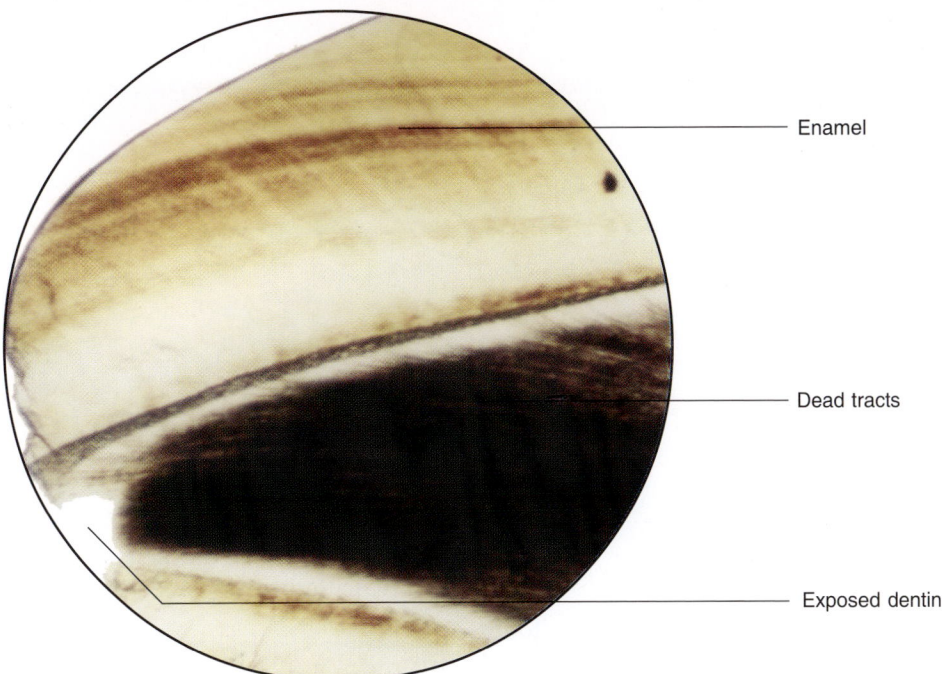

Enamel

Dead tracts

Exposed dentin

Dead tracts (photomicrograph 4X)

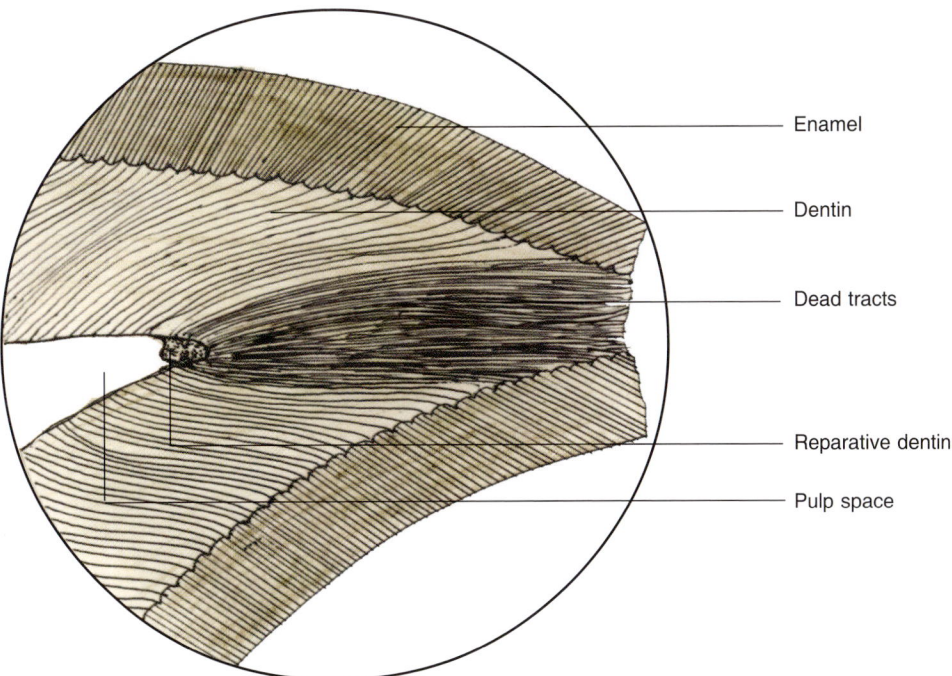

Enamel

Dentin

Dead tracts

Reparative dentin

Pulp space

Fig. 5.8: Dead tracts

6

Pulp

- Histology of pulp
- Pulp stones

Pulp is the soft tissue component of the tooth that is situated in the pulpal cavity located at the center of the tooth. Pulp is basically a connective tissue that contains formative cells of dentin, defense cells for protection, undifferentiated mesenchymal cells, and also blood vessels and nerves. Since the pulp is a soft tissue enclosed within calcified components, the structure can be studied only with the help of decalcified sections.

HISTOLOGY OF NORMAL PULP (Fig. 6.1)

In the pulp **four** distinct zones are seen microscopically.

Odontoblastic zone: This is the most peripheral zone of pulp seen adjacent to the predentin

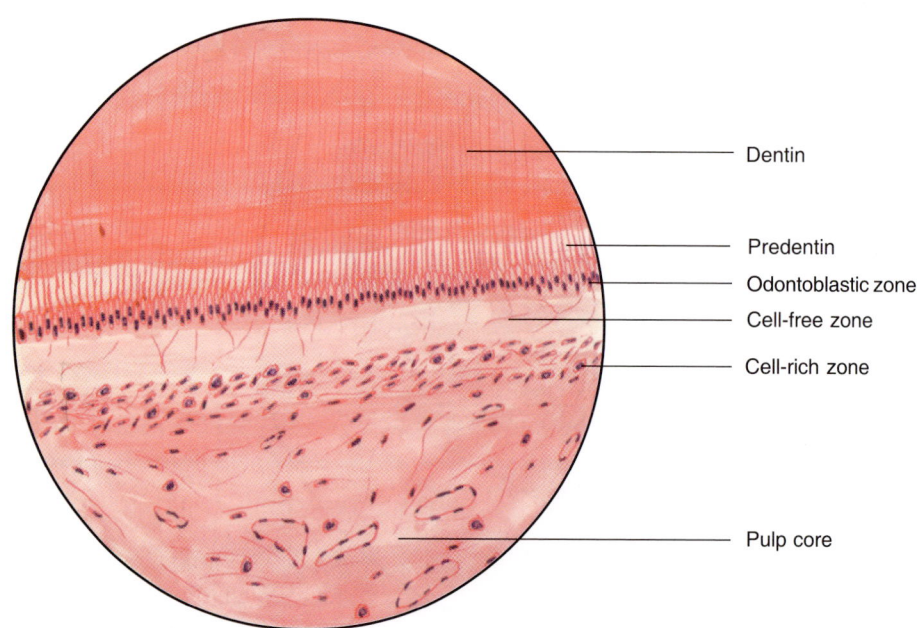

Dentin

Predentin
Odontoblastic zone
Cell-free zone
Cell-rich zone

Pulp core

Fig. 6.1: Histology of pulp

Identification Points (Fig. 6.1)

Pulp
- Four zones are seen
- Zones are odontoblast zone, cell-free zone, cell-rich zone and pulp core
- Pulp core contains large vessels and nerves

layer. Odontoblast cells are columnar in the crown and flattened in the root. They have process at their apical portion extending into the dentinal tubules. Cells in the coronal pulp shows a pseudo-stratified arrangement due to cell crowding.

Cell-free zone: Beneath the odontoblast layer is cell-free zone of Weil which is devoid of cells, but has fibers and nerves.

Cell-rich zone: This zone is seen beneath the cell-free zone and is rich in cells. The cells present are mainly fibroblasts and progenitor cells.

Pulp core: The central portion of pulp is called pulp core that contains cells, large blood vessels and nerves, etc. distributed in the ground substance.

PULP STONES (Fig. 6.2)

Pulp stones are calcifications seen in the pulp. They can be true or false depending on structure. True pulp stones have a tubular structure resembling dentin while false pulp stones are concentric rings of calcified material not resembling dentin. Pulp stones are also classified into:

1. **Free pulp stones:** Lying free in the pulp without being attached to the dentin.

2. **Attached pulp stones:** These are attached to the dentin.

3. **Embedded pulp stones:** When pulp stones are completely surrounded by dentin.

Identification Points (Fig. 6.2)

Pulp Stones
- Calcifications seen in pulp.
- May be true or false pulp stones
- Can be free, attached or embedded.

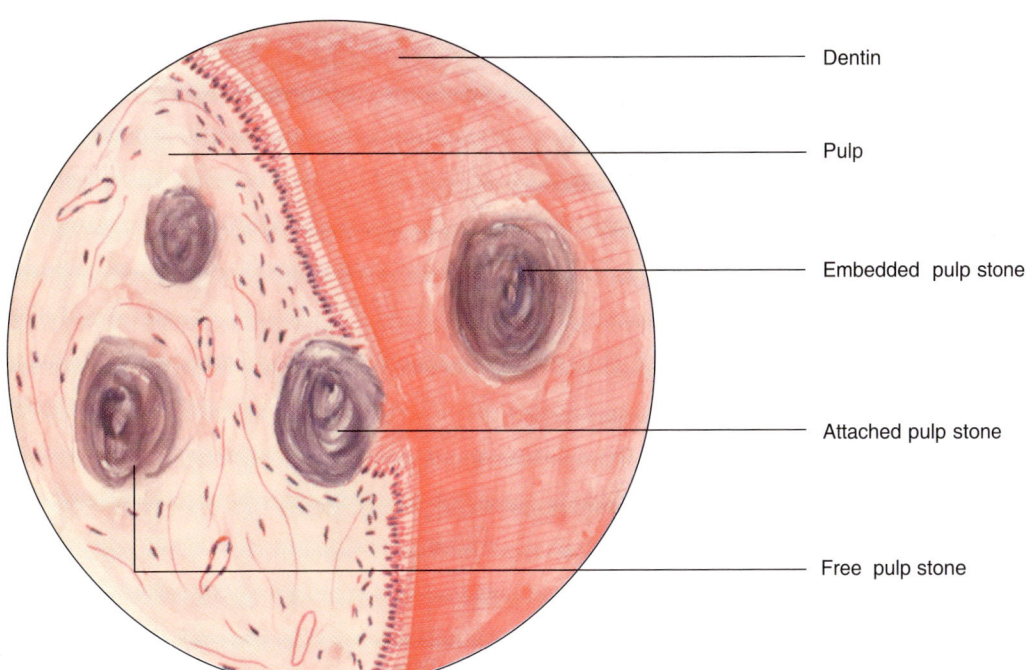

Dentin

Pulp

Embedded pulp stone

Attached pulp stone

Free pulp stone

Fig. 6.2: Pulp stones

7

Cementum

- Structure of cementum
  - Cellular cementum
  - Acellular cementum
- Cementoenamel junctions

Cementum is a calcified structure that forms the outer covering of the root of the tooth. Cementum forms a part of attachment apparatus into which periodontal ligament is inserted to hold the tooth in the alveolar socket. The structure of cementum can be studied using a ground sections or decalcified sections.

STRUCTURE OF CEMENTUM

Based on histological structure cementum is classified into acellular and cellular cementum.

Cellular Cementum (Fig. 7.1)

Cellular cementum is the cementum in which cementocytes are entrapped. In a ground section of cellular cementum, cementocytes can be easily identified as spider-shaped cells. These cells have a cell body and numerous processes or canaliculi radiating from it. The canaliculi are directed towards the periodontal ligament which is the source of nutrition. Sharpey's fibers are the inserted portion of the periodontal ligament and are seen as black faint lines at an angle to the root surface. Incremental lines of Salter appear as dark lines

parallel to root surface. Cellular cementum is located at apical one-third of roots and the furcation areas of multi-rooted teeth.

Identification Points (Fig. 7.1)

Cellular Cementum
- Entrapped cementocytes are seen
- Cementocytes are spider-shaped with canaliculi directed to the periodontal ligament
- Located at the apical one-third

Acellular Cementum (Fig. 7.2)

Acellular cementum is the type of cementum that do not contain any cells. In a ground section under transmitted light acellular cementum is seen as a structureless layer. Incremental lines of cementum referred to as lines of Salter are seen as dark lines parallel to the root surface representing rhythmic deposition of cementum. Sharpey's fibers are not distinct because they are fully mineralized. Acellular cementum is generally located at the cervical two-thirds of the root.

Identification Points (Fig. 7.2)

Acellular Cementum
- Appear as structureless layer
- No entrapped cells
- Located at the cervical two-thirds

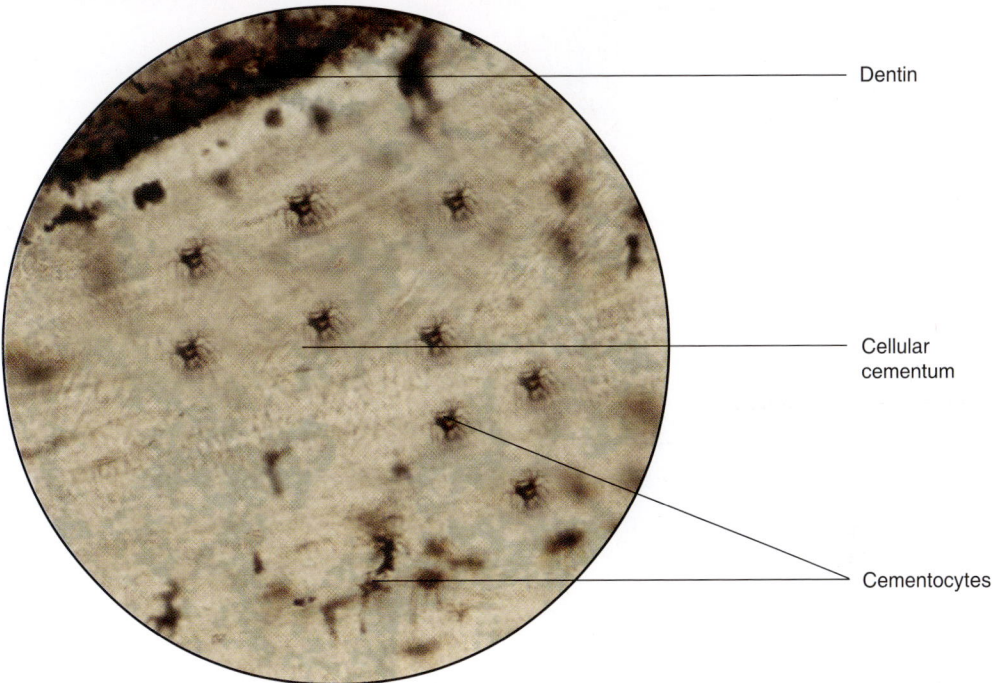

Dentin

Cellular cementum

Cementocytes

Cellular cementum (photomicrograph 10X)

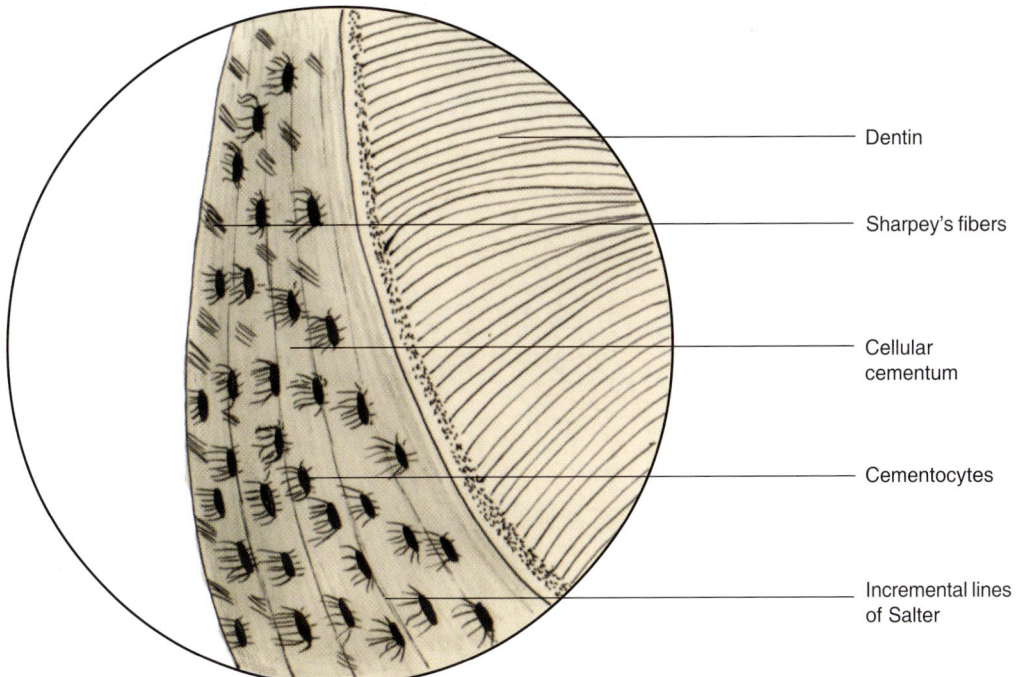

Dentin

Sharpey's fibers

Cellular cementum

Cementocytes

Incremental lines of Salter

Fig. 7.1: Cellular cementum

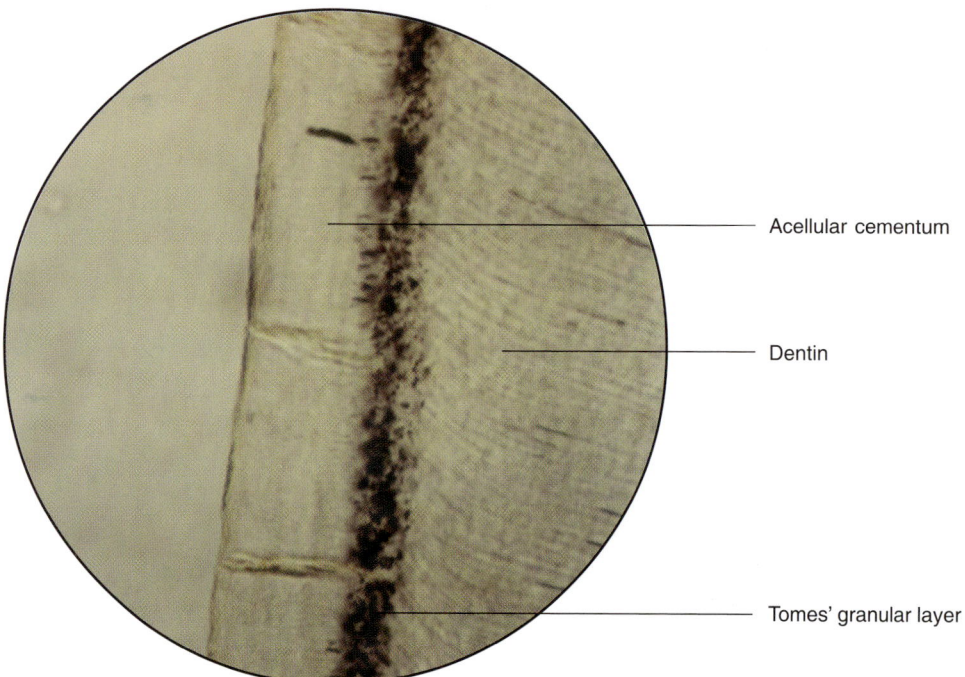

Acellular cementum (photomicrograph 10X)

Acellular cementum

Dentin

Tomes' granular layer

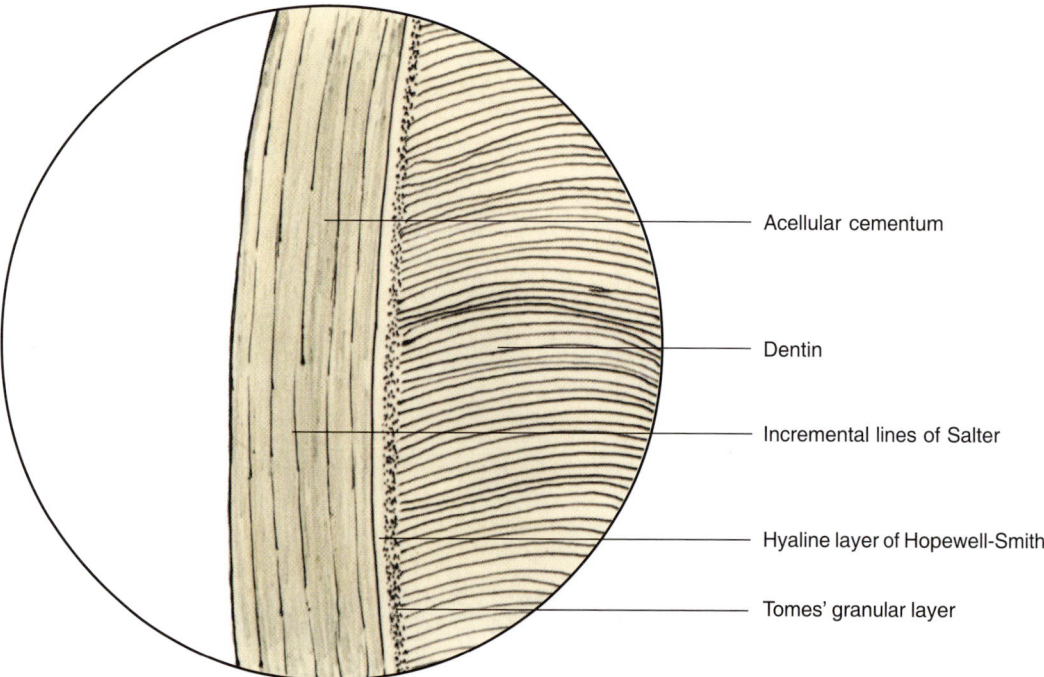

Acellular cementum

Dentin

Incremental lines of Salter

Hyaline layer of Hopewell-Smith

Tomes' granular layer

Fig. 7.2: Acellular cementum

CEMENTOENAMEL JUNCTIONS

Cementoenamel junction (CEJ) is the junction between enamel and cementum that occur at cervical region of tooth.

There are three types of CEJs

Sharp Junction (Fig. 7.3)

Enamel and cementum meet edge to edge. This type of junction is seen in 30% of teeth.

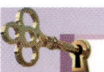

Identification Points (Fig. 7.3)

Cementoenamel Junction—Sharp
- Cementum and enamel meet at sharp point
- Seen in 30% of teeth

Gap Type (Fig. 7.4)

In this type there is no junction, instead a zone of root devoid of cementum is seen. This occurs due to lack of degeneration of

Identification Points (Fig. 7.4)

Cementoenamel Junction—Gap
- A gap is present between enamel and cementum
- Occur due to lack of degeneration of HERS
- Seen in 15% of teeth

Hertwig's epithelial root sheath preventing the differentiation of cementoblasts and therefore cementum formation. In this type of junction, a portion of radicular dentin is exposed causing sensitivity if root is exposed due to gingival recession. This type is seen in 15% of teeth.

Overlap Type (Fig. 7.5)

Cementum overlaps the cervical region of enamel in this type of cementoenamel junction. The type of cementum seen overlapping enamel is acellular afibrillar

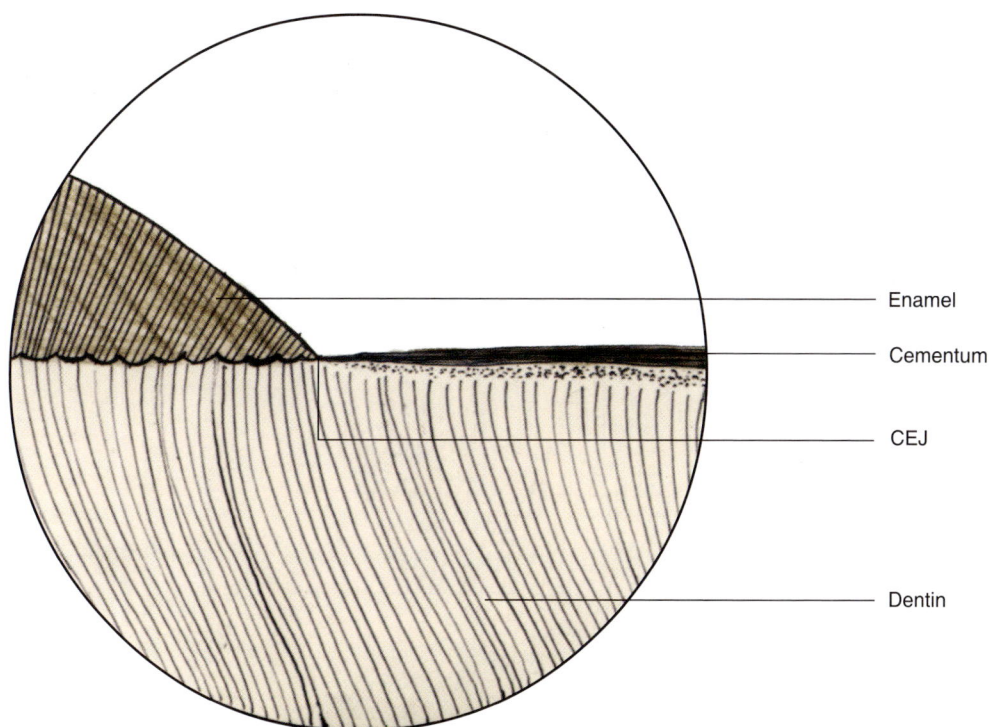

Fig. 7.3: Cementoenamel junction—sharp junction

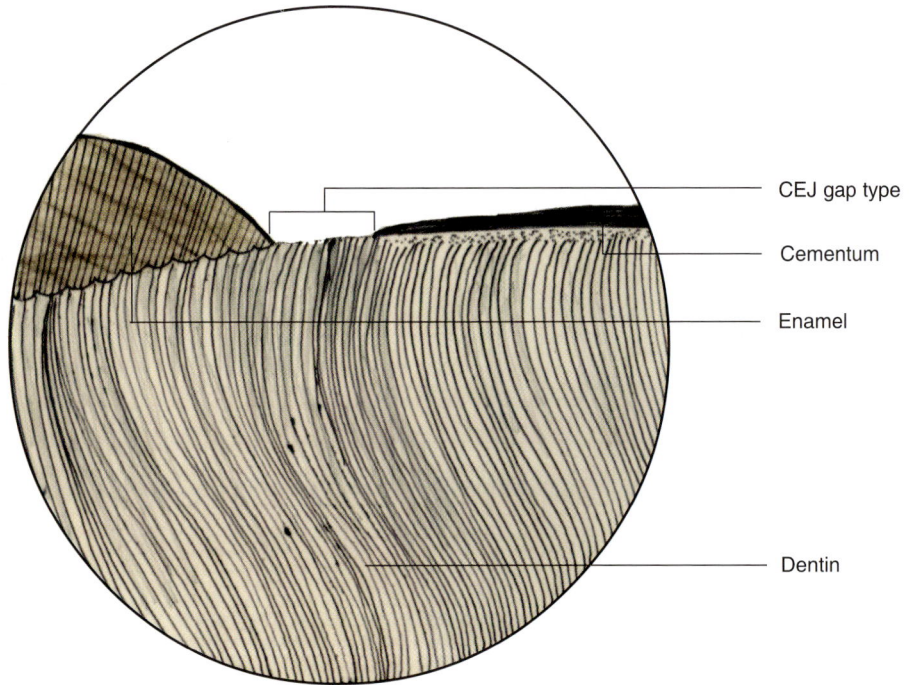

CEJ gap type

Cementum

Enamel

Dentin

Fig. 7.4: Cementoenamel junction—gap type

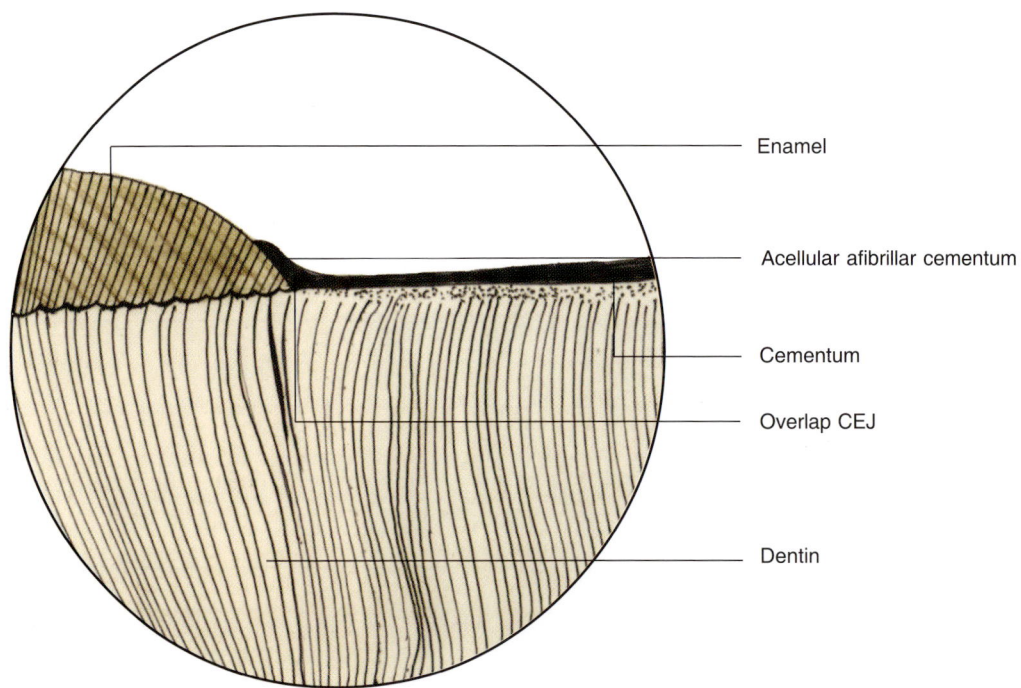

Enamel

Acellular afibrillar cementum

Cementum

Overlap CEJ

Dentin

Fig. 7.5: Cementoenamel junction—overlap type

cementum. This occurs due to degeneration of reduced enamel epithelium which allows the dental follicle cells to come in contact with newly formed enamel. Then these cells differentiate into cementoblasts and lay down cementum. This type of junction is seen in 60% of teeth.

Identification Points (Fig. 7.5)

Cementoenamel Junction—Overlap
- Cementum overlap cervical portion of enamel
- Acellular afibrillar cementum is seen in the region of overlap
- Seen in 60% of teeth

8

Periodontal Ligament

- Principal fibers of periodontal ligament
- Gingival group of fibers

Periodontal ligament is a connective tissue structure that attaches the tooth to the alveolar bone. It is a part of attachment apparatus of the tooth. The attachment apparatus of the tooth has two hard tissue components, cementum and alveolar bone and two soft tissue components, periodontal ligament and lamina propria of the gingiva. These four components are together called periodontium.

PRINCIPAL FIBERS OF PERIODONTAL LIGAMENT (Fig. 8.1)

Periodontal ligament comprises bundles of collagen fibers attached to cementum on one side and alveolar socket on the other side. The portion of fibers inserted into the bone and cementum are called Sharpey's fibers. These groups of fibers, having specific orientation are called principal fibers of periodontal ligament. They are:

- **Alveolar crest group of fibers:** Extending from the crest of alveolar bone to the cervical part of the cementum.
- **Horizontal group:** Running horizontally between cementum and alveolar bone and arranged perpendicular to the long axis of the tooth.

Identification Points (Figs 8.1 and 8.2)

Principal Fibers
- Fiber groups having specific orientation
- Five groups are seen, helping to attach the tooth to alveolar bone
- Principal fibers are alveolar crest, horizontal, oblique, apical and inter-radicular fibers

- **Oblique group:** These are arranged obliquely from cementum to alveolar bone and insertion in cementum is more apical than insertion in bone. These constitute the major group of fibers.
- **Apical group (Fig. 8.2):** These are located in the apical region of the tooth, radiating from the apex of the root to the base of the alveolar socket.
- **Inter-radicular fibers:** These are seen only in multi-rooted teeth. These fibers radiate from the furcation area to the crest of inter-radicular septum.

GINGIVAL GROUP OF FIBERS (Fig. 8.3)

These are the secondary fibers of periodontal ligament seen in the lamina propria of the gingiva and supplement the principal fibers in maintaining the functional integrity of the teeth. These include:

Dentogingival: Extending from the cervical portion of the cementum to the lamina propria of gingiva.

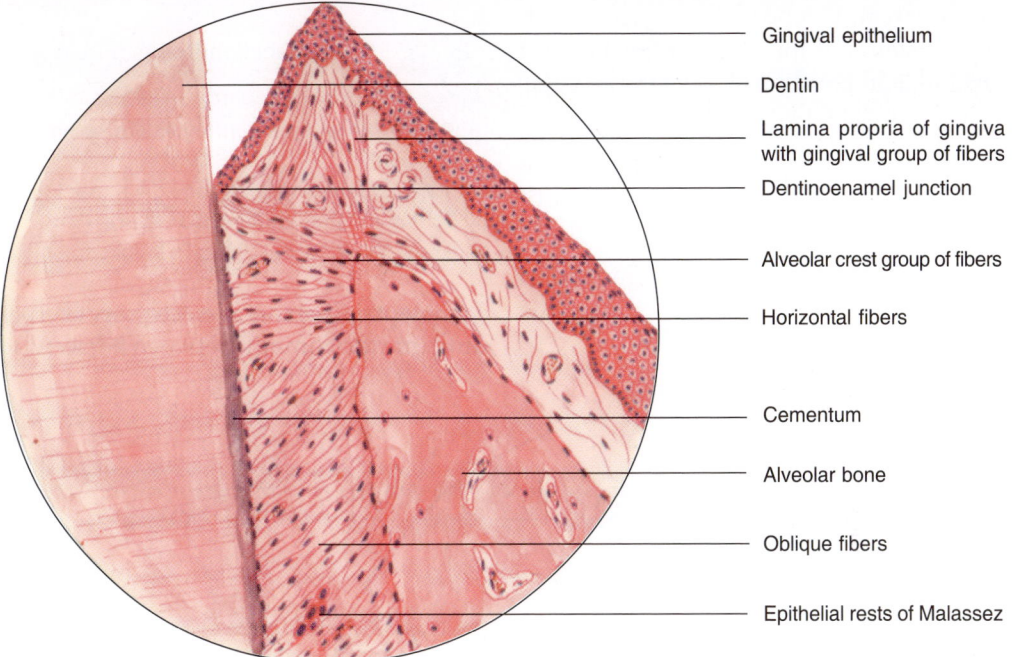

Gingival epithelium

Dentin

Lamina propria of gingiva with gingival group of fibers

Dentinoenamel junction

Alveolar crest group of fibers

Horizontal fibers

Cementum

Alveolar bone

Oblique fibers

Epithelial rests of Malassez

Fig. 8.1: Principal fibers of periodontal ligament

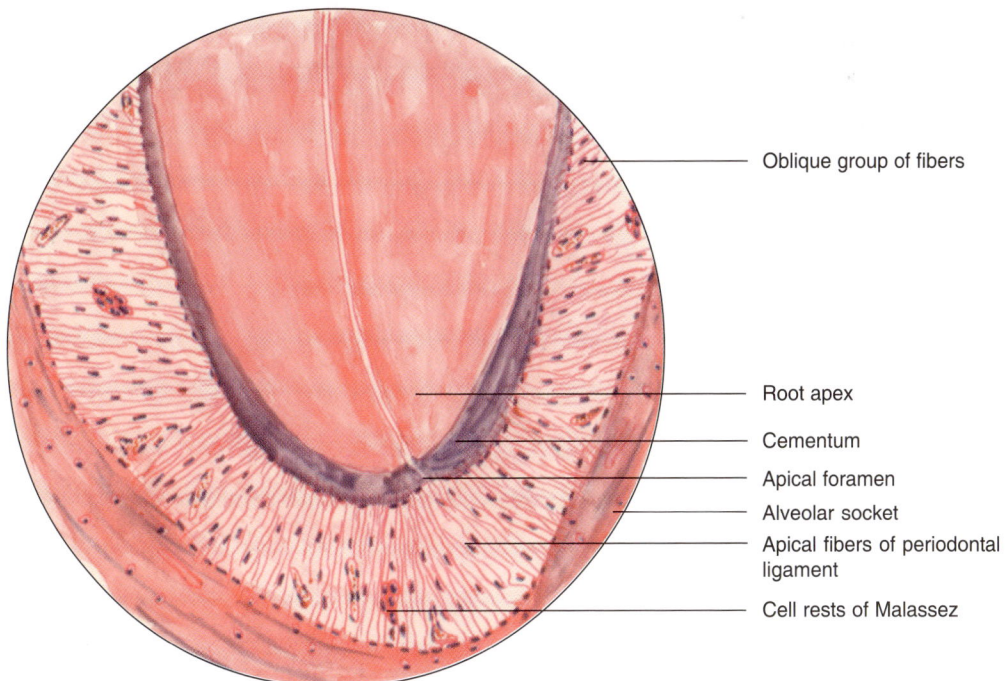

Oblique group of fibers

Root apex

Cementum

Apical foramen

Alveolar socket

Apical fibers of periodontal ligament

Cell rests of Malassez

Fig. 8.2: Apical group of fibers

Dentoperiosteal: Extending from cementum to the periosteum of the alveolar crest and of the vestibular and oral surfaces of the alveolar bone.

Alveologingival: Extending from the crest of the alveolar bone to the lamina propria of gingiva.

Circular fibers: These fibers are arranged in the gingival connective tissue, encircling the tooth like a collar.

Identification Points (Fig. 8.3)

Gingival Group of Fibers
- These are supplementary fibers of periodontal ligament
- Major groups are alveologingival, dentogingival, dentoperiosteal and circular fibers
- Assist the principal fibers in function

Transseptal fibers are also accessory fibers extending interproximally between adjacent teeth.

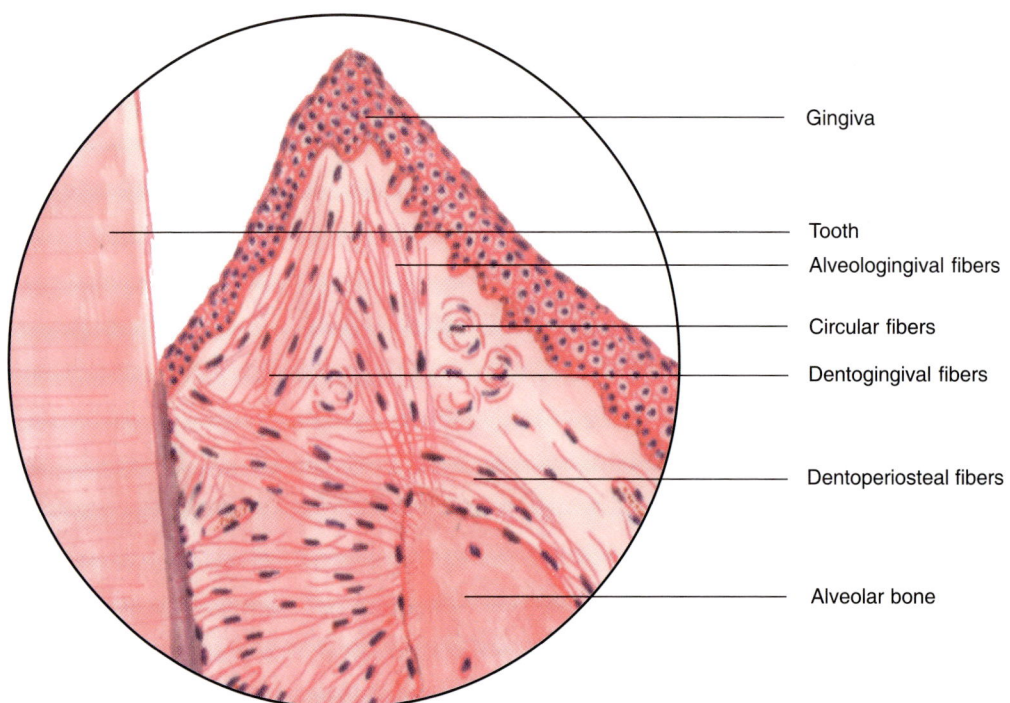

Gingiva

Tooth
Alveologingival fibers

Circular fibers

Dentogingival fibers

Dentoperiosteal fibers

Alveolar bone

Fig. 8.3: Gingival group of fibers

9

Maxillary Sinus

- Microscopic features

Maxillary sinus is a paranasal sinus located in the body of the maxilla. Maxillary sinus is also called antrum of Highmore.

MICROSCOPIC FEATURES (Fig. 9.1)

Maxillary sinus is lined by pseudostratified ciliated columnar epithelium. This epithelial layer is mainly composed of ciliated columnar cells. Along with these, there are non-ciliated columnar cells, basal cells and goblet cells. Goblet cells are unicellular secretory organ which are goblet-shaped with a basally placed nucleus and apical cytoplasm filled with secretory products. In a hematoxylin and eosin stained section cytoplasm of goblet cells appear empty. Cilia of the lining epithelium help to move the secretions.

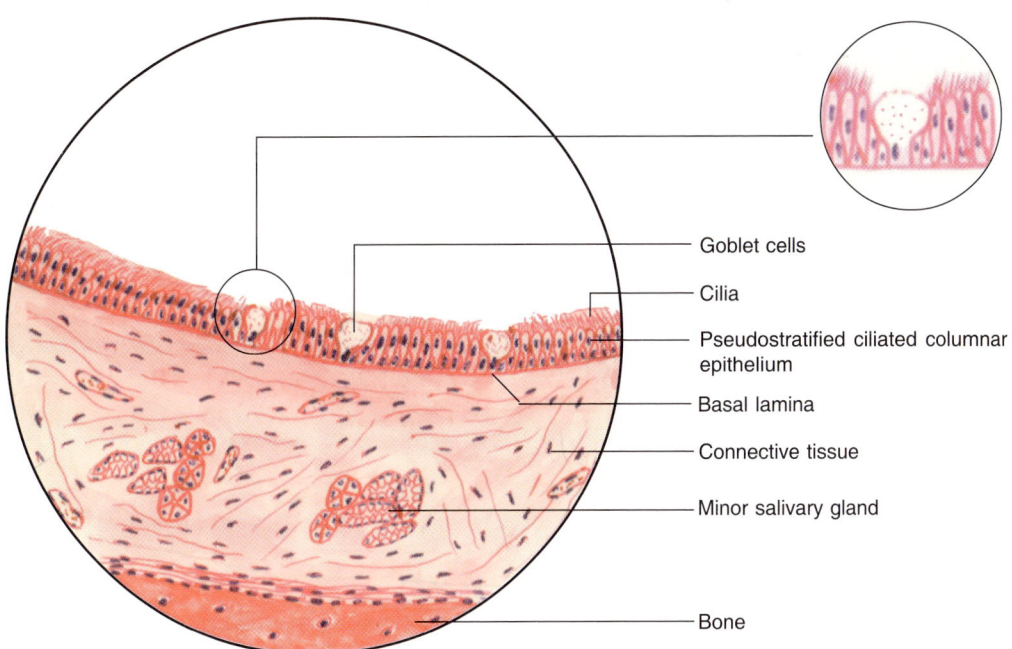

Goblet cells

Cilia

Pseudostratified ciliated columnar epithelium

Basal lamina

Connective tissue

Minor salivary gland

Bone

Fig. 9.1: Histology of maxillary sinus

This epithelium is separated from sub-epithelial connective tissue by a basal lamina. Subepithelial connective tissue layer has collagen fibers and fibroblasts and also minor salivary glands which include both serous and mucous glands. This layer is attached to the periosteum of the bone of the maxilla.

Identification Points (Fig. 9.1)

Maxillary Sinus

- Lined by pseudostratified ciliated columnar epithelium
- Goblet cells are present
- Connective tissue contains mixed salivary gland

10

Oral Mucosa

- Structure of oral mucosa
  - Buccal mucosa
  - Gingiva
  - Hard palate
  - Vermilion border of lip
  - Tongue

STRUCTURE OF ORAL MUCOSA

Oral mucosa is the moist lining of the oral cavity, which is lined by stratified squamous epithelium. The connective tissue beneath is called lamina propria and is composed of collagen fibers, along with the various cells of connective tissue in a ground substance. The interface between epithelium and connective tissue is irregular with projections of epithelium interdigitating with those of connective tissue. The projections of epithelium are called epithelial ridges or rete ridges and of connective tissue are called connective tissue papillae. Epithelium is separated from lamina propria by a distinct basement membrane. Below the mucosa is submucosa containing large vessels and nerves, fat tissue, minor salivary gland and muscle in certain regions of oral mucosa. Based on the histological structure oral mucosa is classified into keratinized and nonkeratinized mucosa. Nonkeratinized mucosa lines the cheek, lip, soft palate, alveolar mucosa, floor of the mouth, ventral aspect of the tongue, etc.

Keratinized mucosa is seen in gingiva and hard palate.

Buccal Mucosa
(Nonkeratinized Mucosa) (Fig. 10.1)

Histologically buccal mucosa shows two parts, overlying epithelium and lamina propria. The epithelium is thick and is non-keratinized stratified squamous. Epithelium has three distinct layers, **stratum basale, stratum intermedium and stratum superficiale.**

Stratum basale is composed of a single layer of cuboidal cells arranged on basement membrane. Above this a suprabasal layer resembling basal layer may be seen. Above the basal layer is stratum intermedium made up of a few layers of polyhedral cells with centrally placed nucleus. The stratum superficiale is made up of a few layers of flattened cells with flattened nuclei. Epithelial ridges of nonkeratinized epithelium are short

Identification Points (Fig. 10.1)

Nonkeratinized Mucosa

- Lined by stratified squamous epithelium
- Epithelium has three layers—stratum basale, stratum intermedium and stratum superficiale
- Lamina propria merges with submucosa

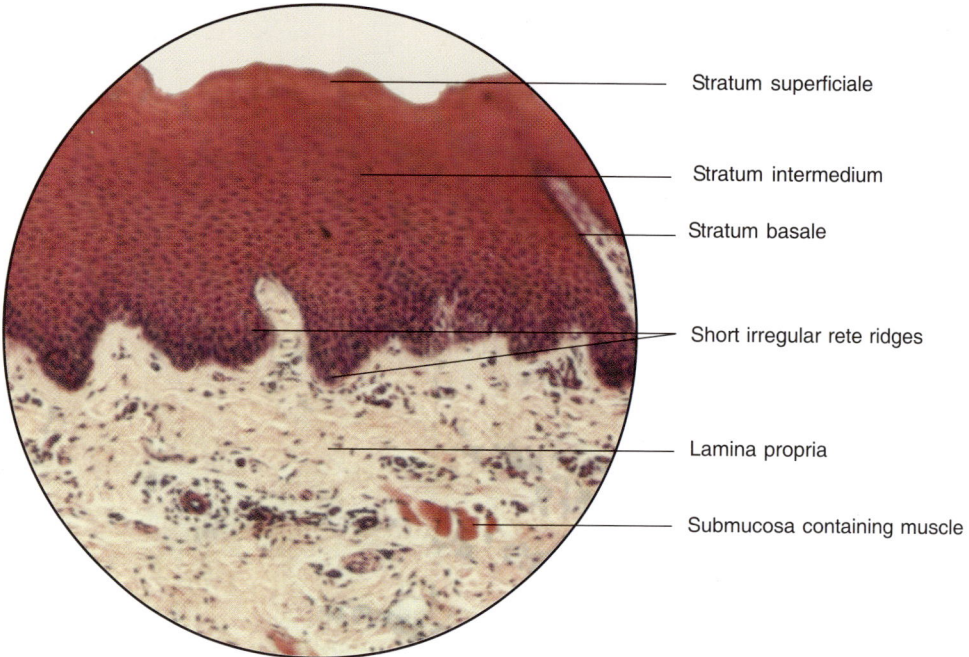

Stratum superficiale

Stratum intermedium

Stratum basale

Short irregular rete ridges

Lamina propria

Submucosa containing muscle

Buccal mucosa (photomicrograph 10X)

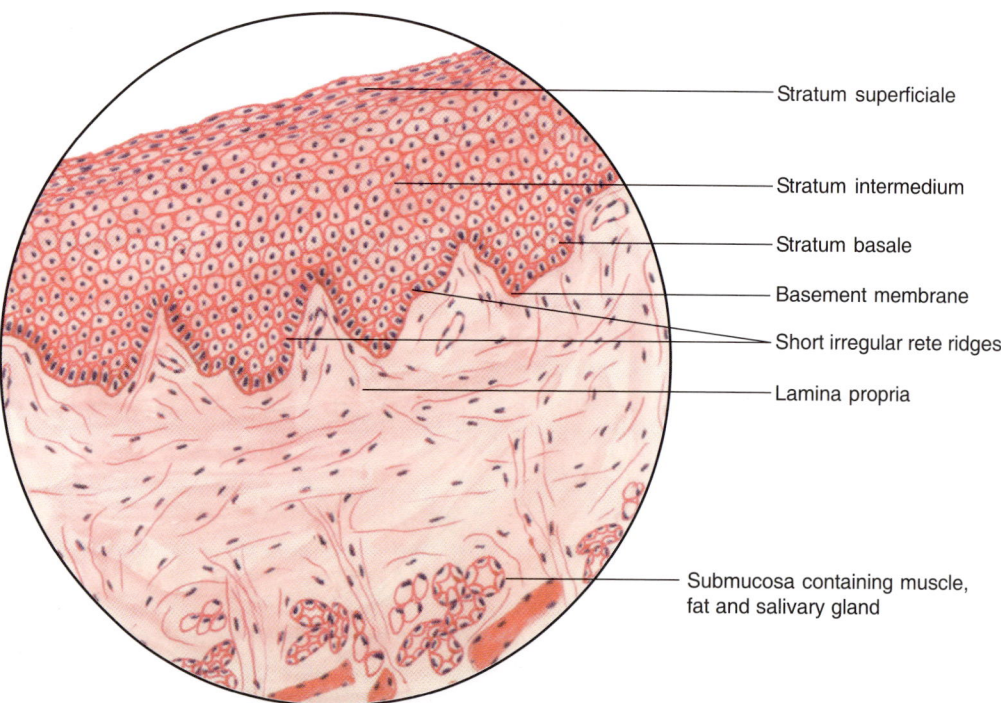

Stratum superficiale

Stratum intermedium

Stratum basale

Basement membrane

Short irregular rete ridges

Lamina propria

Submucosa containing muscle, fat and salivary gland

Fig.10.1: Buccal mucosa

and irregular, interdigitating with connective tissue papillae.

- Lamina propria is less dense compared to keratinized mucosa, and shows collagen fibers fibroblasts and blood vessels.
- The lamina propria of the buccal mucosa merges with underlying submucosa which contain large blood vessels, nerves, fat cells, muscle and minor salivary gland. This submucosa attaches the mucosa to the underlying muscle tissue.

Generally all the nonkeratinized mucosa histologically appear similar to the buccal mucosa except for slight structural variations.

Soft palate is lined by thin nonkeratinized stratified squamous epithelium which may show taste buds. Lamina propria is thick with numerous short papillae. Submucosa contains many minor salivary glands.

Ventral surface of the tongue has a thin nonkeratinized epithelial lining. Lamina propria is thin having numerous short papillae. Submucosa is thin and irregular with abundant blood vessels. In areas where submucosa is absent mucosa is directly attached to the muscles of the tongue.

Floor of the mouth is lined by very thin nonkeratinized epithelium. Lamina propria shows short papillae and is rich in vascular supply. Submucosa is loose fibrous tissue with fat and minor salivary glands.

In **alveolar mucosa** lining epithelium is thin and nonkeratinized with short rete ridges. Lamina propria has many capillary loops. Submucosa comprises loose connective tissue containing minor salivary glands. The submucosa attaches alveolar mucosa to the periosteum of alveolar bone.

Keratinized Mucosa—Gingiva (Fig. 10.2)

In a histological section gingiva shows two portions, epithelium and lamina propria.

Identification Points (Fig. 10.2)

Gingiva
- Lined by keratinized stratified squamous epithelium
- Epithelium has four layers—stratum basale, spinosum, granulosum and corneum
- Dense lamina propria is directly attached to the periosteum of alveolar bone

The overlying epithelium is keratinized and stratified squamous with four distinct layers. The first layer adjacent to the basement membrane is stratum basale composed of a single layer of cuboidal cells with nucleus arranged perpendicular to the basement membrane. The layer above is stratum spinosum or prickle cell layer composed of a few layers of polyhedral cells. Cells have a prickly appearance because they shrink while tissue processing retaining the intercellular attachment. The next layer is stratum granulosum made up of a few layers of flattened cells, cytoplasm of which contain hematoxyphilic keratohyaline granules. The most superficial layer is stratum corneum composed of many layers of flattened cells filled with keratin. These cells are devoid of nucleus and cytoplasmic organelles. Gingival epithelium predominantly shows parakeratinized surface layer which is characterized by the presence of retained pyknotic nucleus in the corneal layer (in case of orthokeratinization nuclei are absent).

The interface between epithelium and connective tissue is irregular with long irregular epithelial ridges. Lamina propria shows dense bundles of collagen fibers.

Submucosa is absent and lamina propria is directly attached to periosteum of alveolar bone. This type of attachment is called mucoperiosteal attachment which makes the attachment between epithelium and connective tissue firm and immobile.

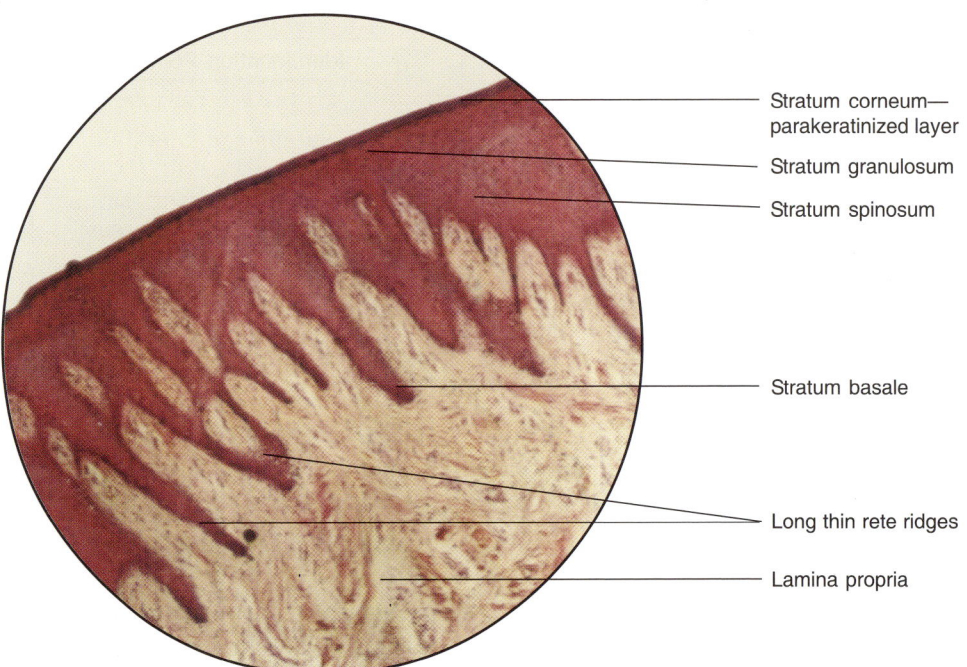

Stratum corneum—
parakeratinized layer

Stratum granulosum

Stratum spinosum

Stratum basale

Long thin rete ridges

Lamina propria

Gingiva (photomicrograph 4X)

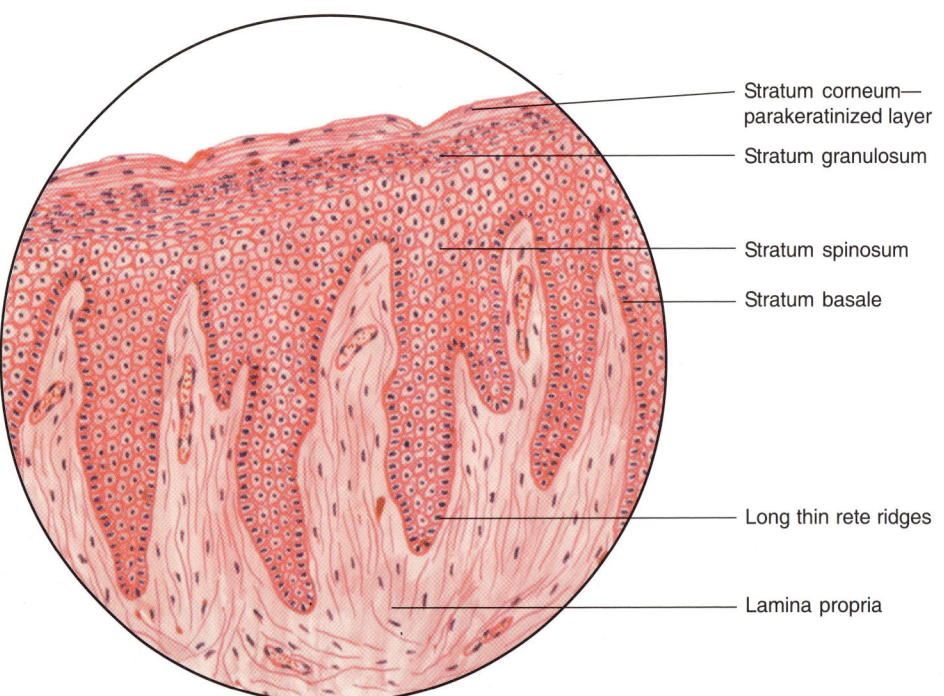

Stratum corneum—
parakeratinized layer

Stratum granulosum

Stratum spinosum

Stratum basale

Long thin rete ridges

Lamina propria

Fig. 10.2: Gingiva

Hard Palate—Anterolateral Region (Fatty Zone) (Fig. 10.3)

Hard palate is lined by masticatory mucosa and therefore structurally somewhat similar to gingiva. The anterolateral region of the palate is lined by keratinized stratified squamous epithelium with four distinct layers, i.e. stratum basale, stratum spinosum, stratum granulosum, stratum corneum. The epithelial ridges are long and regular interdigitating with connective tissue papillae. Lamina propria is dense and is more thicker than in the posterior region of hard palate. In contrast to gingiva this region has submucosa filled with fat tissue. The zone of fat tissue is divided into compartments by vertical band of dense connective tissue which attaches mucosa firmly to the periosteum of palatal bone.

Identification Points (Fig. 10.3)

Fatty Zone of Hard Palate

- Lined by keratinized stratified squamous epithelium
- Epithelium has four layers—stratum basale, spinosum, granulosum and corneum
- Submucosa is present containing fat tissue

Hard Palate—Posterolateral Region (Glandular Zone) (Fig. 10.4)

Glandular zone is structurally similar to fatty zone with overlying keratinized stratified squamous epithelium having four distinct layers, i.e. stratum basale, stratum spinosum, stratum granulosum and stratum corneum. The rete ridges are long and regular interdigitating with connective tissue papilla. Lamina

Identification Points (Fig. 10.4)

Glandular Zone of Hard Palate

- Lined by keratinized stratified squamous epithelium
- Epithelium has four layers—stratum basale, spinosum, granulosum and corneum
- Submucosa is present containing glandular tissue

propria is dense and is less thicker than in the anterior region of palate. In contrast to anterolateral region submucosa contains minor salivary gland tissue. The zone of submucosa is divided into compartments by vertical band of dense connective tissue which attaches mucosa firmly to the periosteum of palatal bone.

Vermilion Border of Lip (Transitional Zone) (Fig. 10.5)

This zone is the transitional zone between the skin lining the outer surface of the lip and the labial mucosa lining the inner aspect. The skin is composed of keratinized stratified squamous epithelium with all appendages like hair follicles, sweat glands and sebaceous glands. The labial mucosa is lined by nonkeratinized stratified squamous epithelium. The connective tissue beneath shows minor salivary gland tissue. The central portion of lip shows orbicularis oris muscle. The transitional zone has a thin lining epithelium with thin keratinization on the surface. There are many long papillae reaching high into epithelium carrying many capillary loops. This makes it more red compared to labial mucosa. Underlying connective tissue is characteristically devoid of glands.

Identification Points (Fig. 10.5)

Vermilion Border of Lip

- Transitional zone of lip
- Lined by thin parakeratinized epithelium
- Long thin connective tissue papillae containing many capillary loops

Papillae of the Tongue

Filiform Papillae (Fig. 10.6)

Filiform (hair-like) papillae are seen as hair-like or thread-like projection on the dorsal aspect of the tongue. Filiform papilla in a histological section is seen as cone-shaped structure lined by stratified squamous epithelium with thick keratin on the surface.

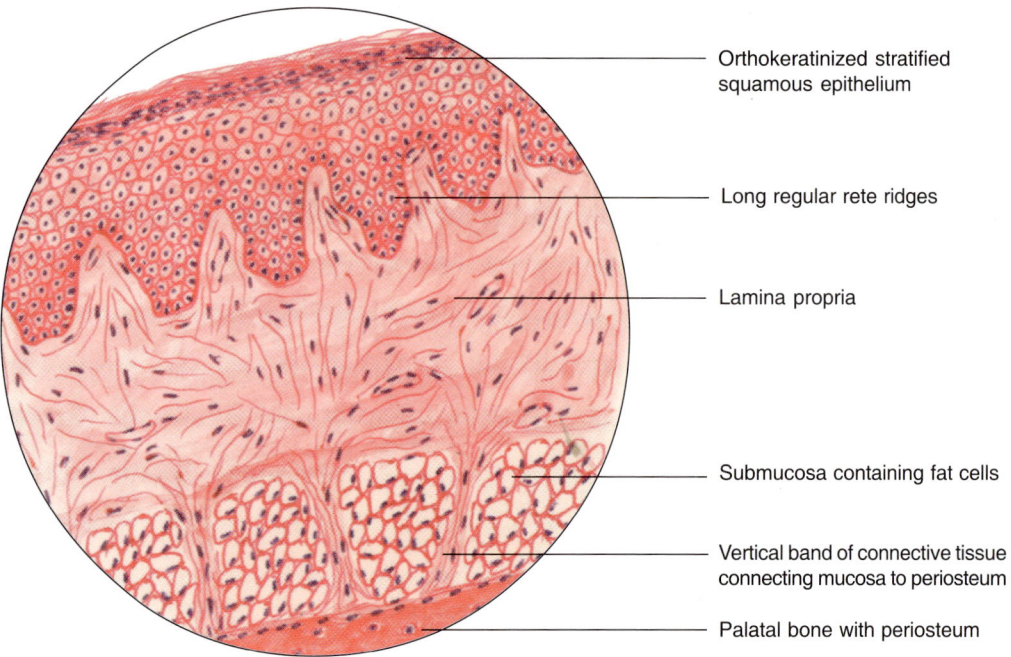

Orthokeratinized stratified squamous epithelium

Long regular rete ridges

Lamina propria

Submucosa containing fat cells

Vertical band of connective tissue connecting mucosa to periosteum

Palatal bone with periosteum

Fig. 10.3: Anterolateral area of palate (fatty zone)

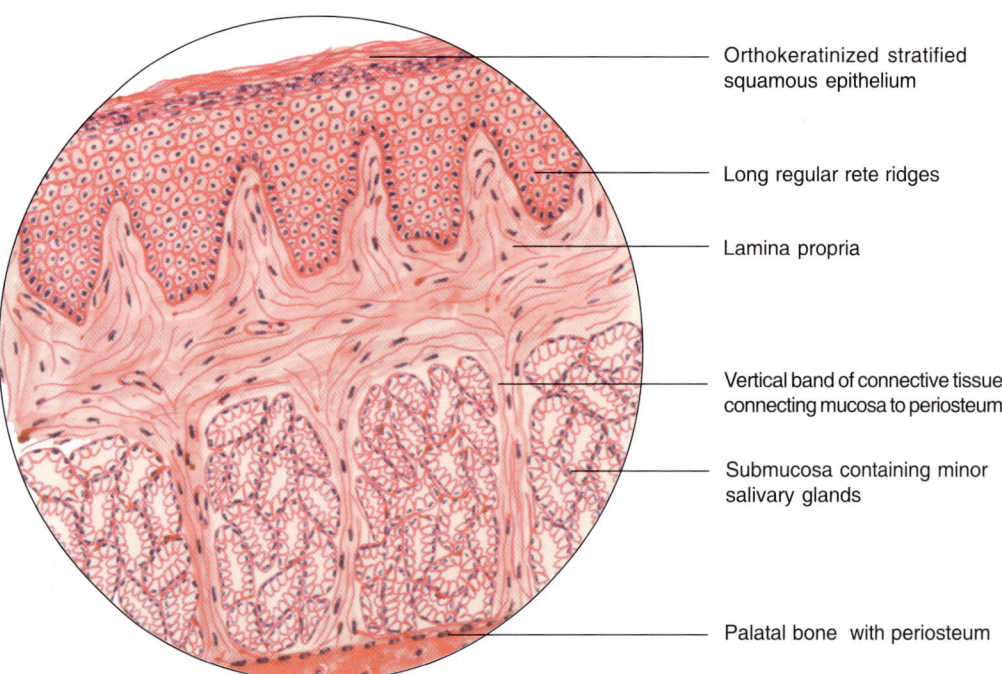

Orthokeratinized stratified squamous epithelium

Long regular rete ridges

Lamina propria

Vertical band of connective tissue connecting mucosa to periosteum

Submucosa containing minor salivary glands

Palatal bone with periosteum

Fig. 10.4: Posterolateral region of palate (glandular zone)

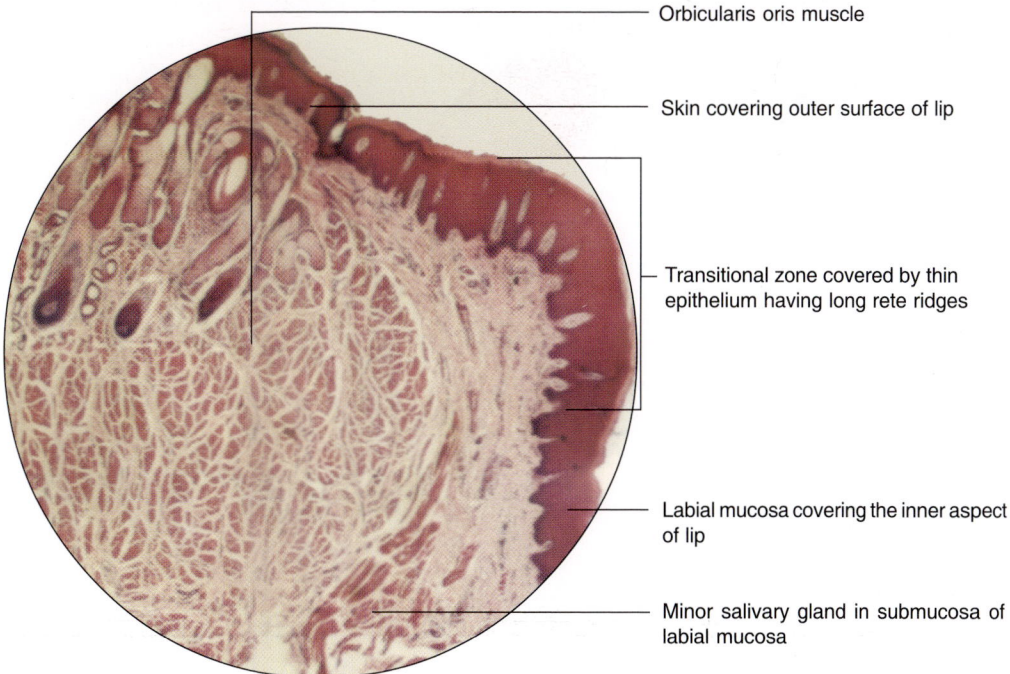

Orbicularis oris muscle

Skin covering outer surface of lip

Transitional zone covered by thin epithelium having long rete ridges

Labial mucosa covering the inner aspect of lip

Minor salivary gland in submucosa of labial mucosa

Vermilion zone of lip (photomicrograph 4X)

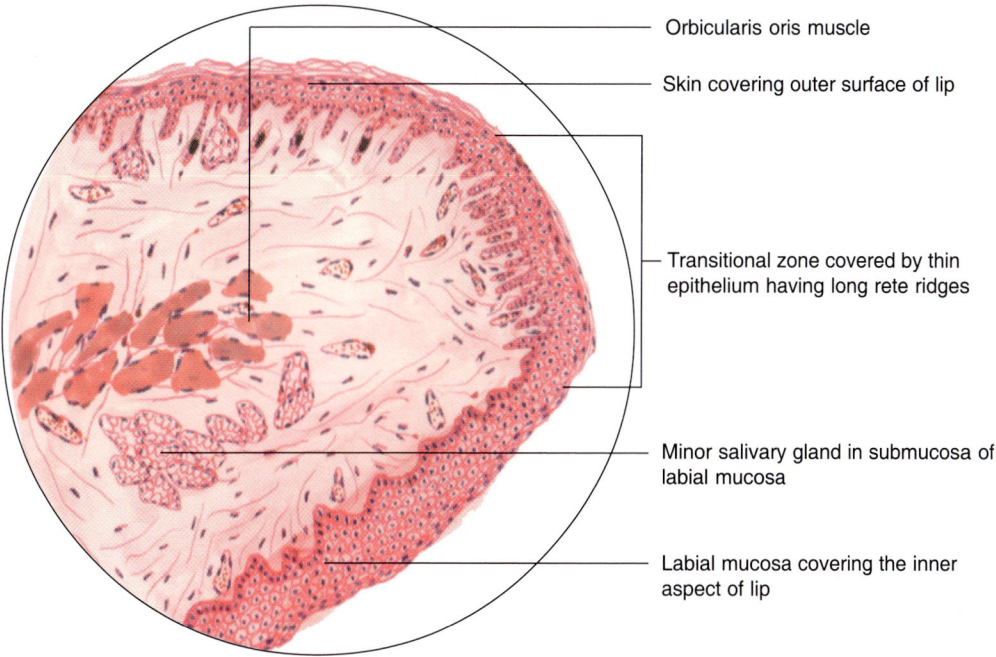

Orbicularis oris muscle

Skin covering outer surface of lip

Transitional zone covered by thin epithelium having long rete ridges

Minor salivary gland in submucosa of labial mucosa

Labial mucosa covering the inner aspect of lip

Fig. 10.5: Vermilion zone of lip

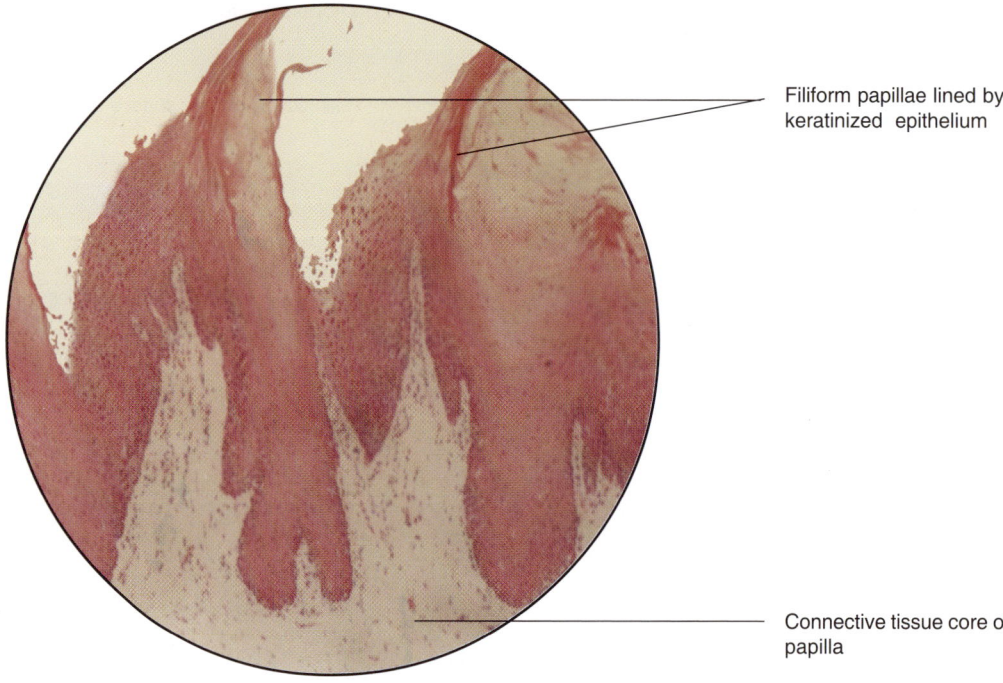

Filiform papillae lined by keratinized epithelium

Connective tissue core of papilla

Filiform papillae of tongue (photomicrograph 4X)

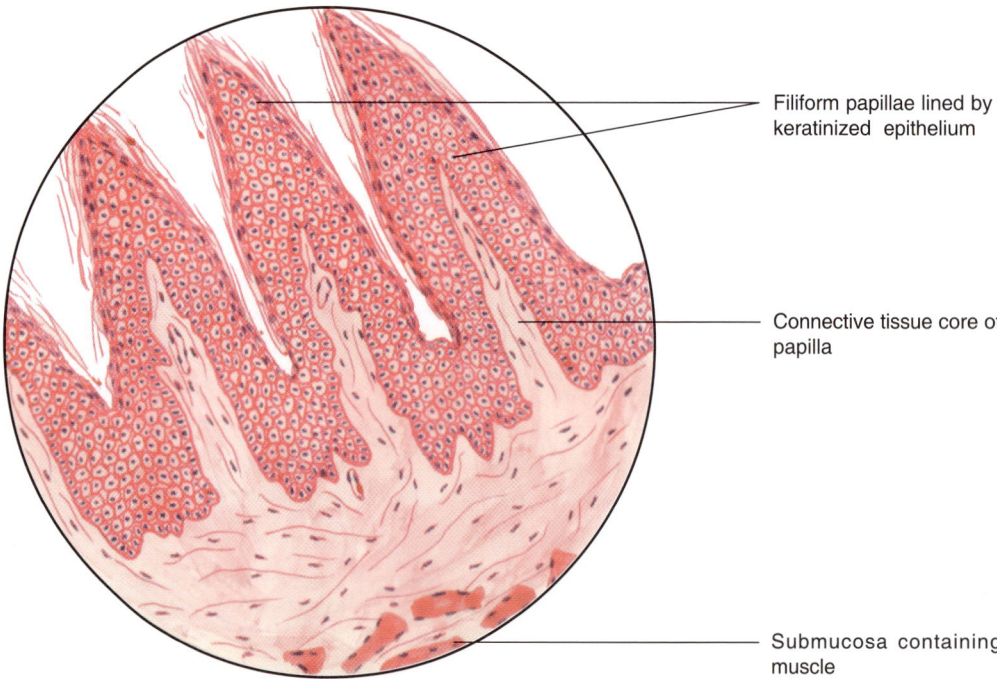

Filiform papillae lined by keratinized epithelium

Connective tissue core of papilla

Submucosa containing muscle

Fig. 10.6: Filiform papillae of tongue

Central core of connective tissue supports the blood vessels. *Taste buds are not seen* in these papillae.

Circumvallate Papillae *(Fig. 10.7)*

The circumvallate (walled) papillae are seen in the anterior two-thirds of the tongue just anterior to sulcus terminalis. These are 10–12 in number. The superficial surface of these papillae is at the level of surface of tongue and a V-shaped sulcus is present all around the papillae separating them from the adjacent portion of tongue. The lining epithelium is keratinized stratified squamous epithelium at the superficial surface and nonkeratinized on the lateral surface of circumvallate papillae. Taste buds are seen only on the lateral surface. Central portion is occupied by the connective tissue. The characteristic feature of this papilla is presence of serous minor salivary glands (von Ebner's gland) in the connective tissue beneath it. These glands secretes watery saliva into the V-shaped trough around the papillae to flush out the food debris.

Fungiform Papillae *(Fig. 10.8)*

Fungiform (fungus-like) papillae are dome-shaped structures projecting above the surface of the tongue and located between the filiform papillae. The epithelium covering the fungiform papillae is thin nonkeratinized stratified squamous epithelium making this papilla reddish in color. The superficial surface of the papillae contain few taste buds. The supporting connective tissue shows collagen fibers, fibroblasts and blood vessels.

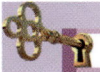

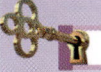

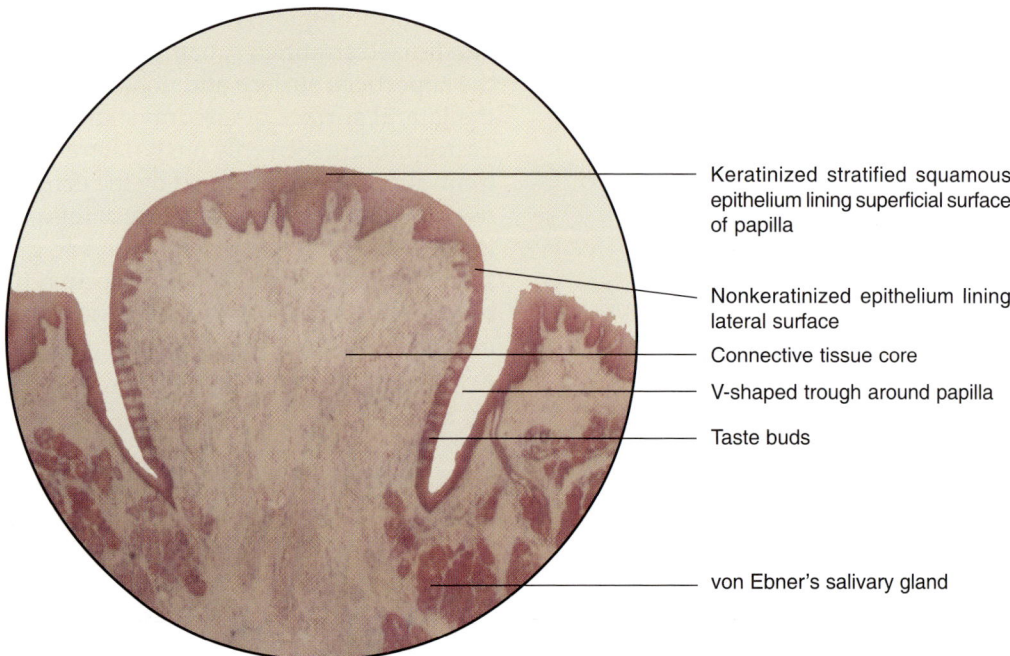

Keratinized stratified squamous epithelium lining superficial surface of papilla

Nonkeratinized epithelium lining lateral surface

Connective tissue core

V-shaped trough around papilla

Taste buds

von Ebner's salivary gland

Circumvallate papilla of tongue (photomicrograph 4X)

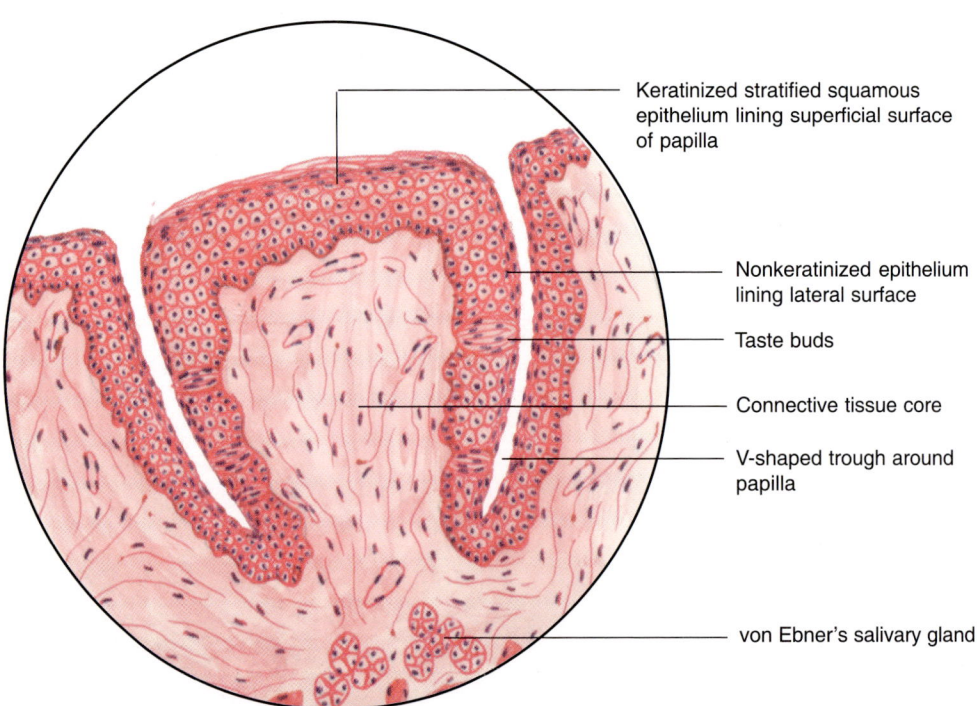

Keratinized stratified squamous epithelium lining superficial surface of papilla

Nonkeratinized epithelium lining lateral surface

Taste buds

Connective tissue core

V-shaped trough around papilla

von Ebner's salivary gland

Fig. 10.7: Circumvallate papilla of tongue

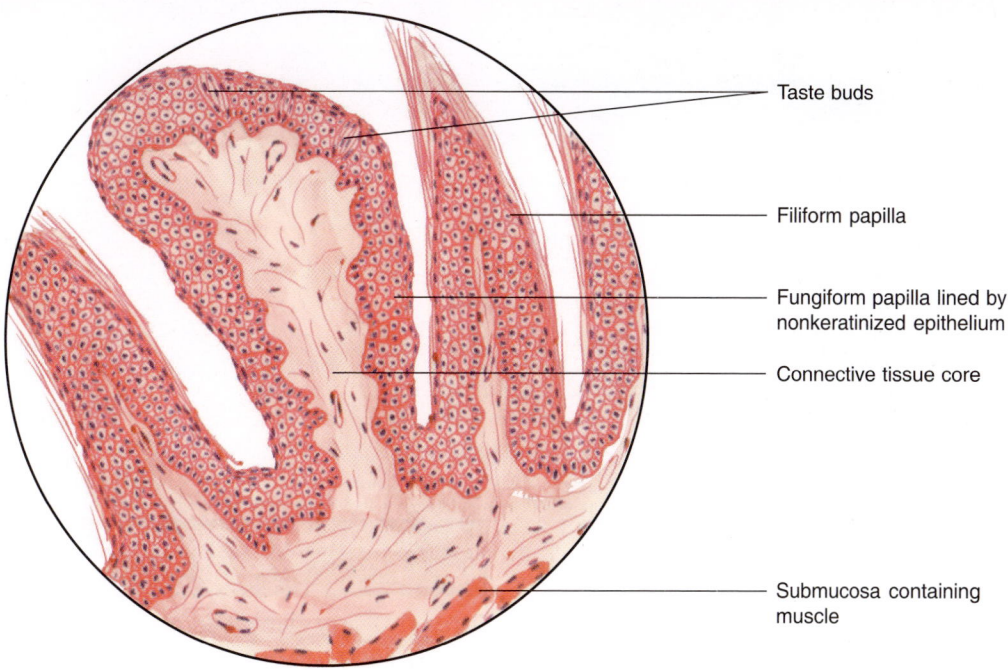

Taste buds

Filiform papilla

Fungiform papilla lined by
nonkeratinized epithelium

Connective tissue core

Submucosa containing
muscle

Fig. 10.8: Fungiform papillae of tongue

11

Salivary Gland

- Structure of salivary glands
  - Serous gland
  - Mucous gland
  - Mixed gland

Salivary glands are exocrine glands which secrete saliva that reaches the oral cavity through their ducts. There are three pairs of major salivary glands located extra orally and numerous minor salivary glands situated intra orally. Based on the type of secretion salivary glands are divided into:

- **Serous gland:** Parotid and von Ebner's gland.

- **Mucous glands:** Sublingual gland and all the minor salivary glands except for von Ebner's glands.

- **Mixed gland:** Submandibular salivary gland.

Both major and minor salivary glands are composed of parenchymal components supported by the connective tissue. Parenchymal component includes secretory acini and ductal system. Connective tissue forms a capsule around the gland and extends in between the acini to divide the gland into lobes and lobules. Connective tissue carries the blood vessels and nerves.

SEROUS SALIVARY GLAND—PAROTID GLAND (Fig. 11.1)

Serous salivary gland is composed of numerous serous secretory units called serous acini. Serous acinus is a collection of many serous cells. Serous cells are the secretory cells and are pyramidal in shape with a broad base resting on a basement membrane and a narrow apex facing towards the lumen. Nucleus is round and located at the basal one-third of the cell. Apical part of the cytoplasm is filled with zymogen granules and appears eosinophilic in a hematoxylin and eosin stained section. Serous cells are arranged to form an acinus. Serous acinus is round or circular in shape, has fewer cells and a small lumen. Salivary gland is divided into lobes by connective tissue septa that carry blood vessels. Intralobular and interlobular ducts are seen.

Identification Points (Fig. 11.1)

Serous Salivary Gland

- Composed of round acini with small lumen
- Nucleus of cells is ovoid and present at basal one-third
- Apical cytoplasm stain eosinophilic because of secretory granules

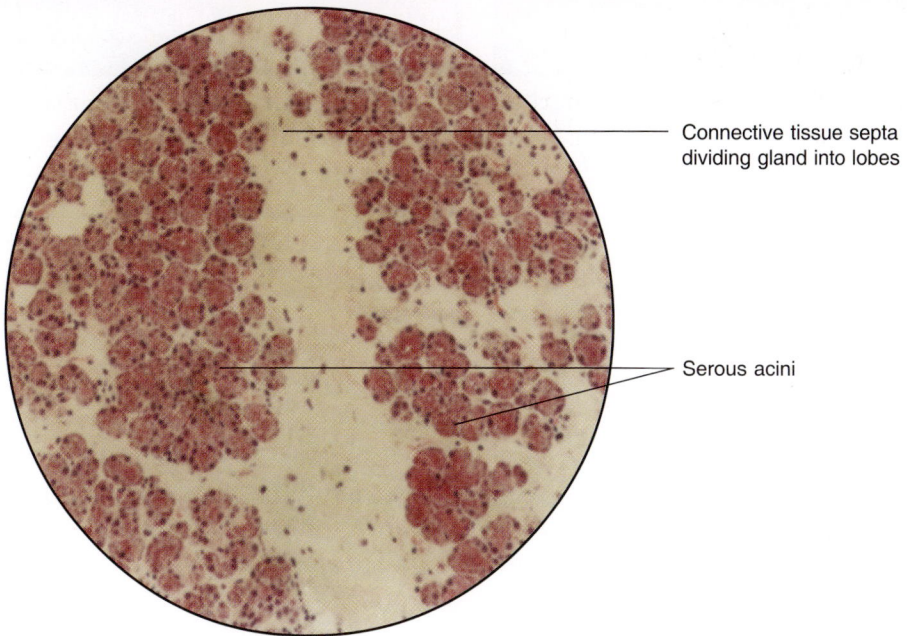

Connective tissue septa
dividing gland into lobes

Serous acini

Serous salivary gland (photomicrograph 10X)

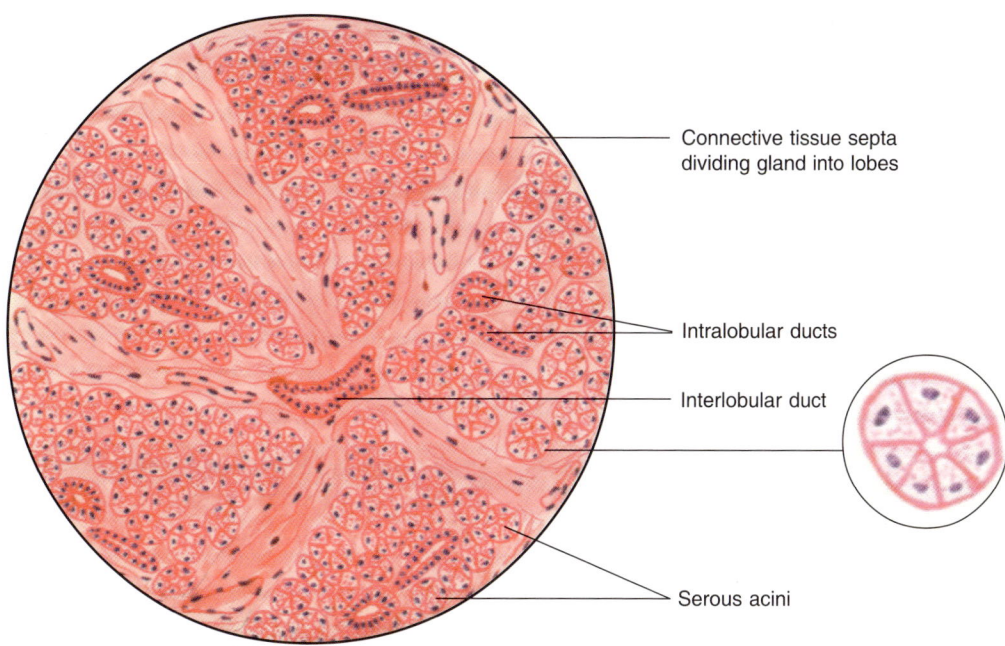

Connective tissue septa
dividing gland into lobes

Intralobular ducts

Interlobular duct

Serous acini

Fig. 11.1: Serous salivary gland

MUCOUS SALIVARY GLAND—SUBLINGUAL GLAND (Fig. 11.2)

Mucous salivary glands have numerous secretory units called mucous acini. These acini are collection of mucous cells. Mucous cells are columnar in shape with nucleus flattened and pressed against the basement membrane. Cytoplasm is restricted to basal region. Apical portion of the cell is filled with mucous secretory droplets and appear empty in H & E stained sections. Mucin can be stained positively using periodic acid–Schiff stain. Mucous cells are arranged to form mucous acini that are ovoid or tubular with large lumen. In a histologic section along with acini intralobular ducts are also seen. Connective tissue septa is present between the acini that shows blood vessels and interlobular ducts.

MIXED SALIVARY GLAND—SUBMANDIBULAR GLAND (Fig. 11.3)

In a mixed salivary gland both serous and mucous acini are seen. The number can vary depending on predominantly serous or mucous. Along with these acini, mixed acini are also seen having both serous and mucous cells. In a mixed acinus the basic secretory unit is a typical mucous acinus in a tubular shape. The blind end of this tubular structure is capped by a group of serous cells that form a crescent-shaped structure. This crescent-shaped structure is called 'demilune of Gianuzzi'. Intralobular and interlobular ducts, connective tissue septa are also seen.

Identification Points (Fig. 11.2)

Mucous Salivary Gland

- Composed of tubular acini with large lumen
- Nucleus of cells is flat and pressed to basal plasma membrane
- Apical cytoplasm appears empty

Identification Points (Fig. 11.3)

Mixed Salivary Gland

- Contains both serous and mucous acini
- The blind end of mucous acini has serous demilunes
- Demilunes are crescent-shaped and named as 'demilune of Gianuzzi'

Table 11.1: Differences between serous and mucous acini

Serous acini	Mucous acini
• Circular or round in shape	• Ovoid or tubular in shape
• Smaller in size	• Larger
• Composed of less number of cells	• More number of cells
• Small lumen	• Wider lumen
• Cells are pyramidal in shape	• Cells are columnar in shape
• Nucleus is round and placed at basal one-third of the cell	• Nucleus is flattened and pressed against basal plasma membrane of the cell
• Apical cytoplasm appears eosinophilic because of zymogen granules	• Apical cytoplasm appears empty in H & E stained sections

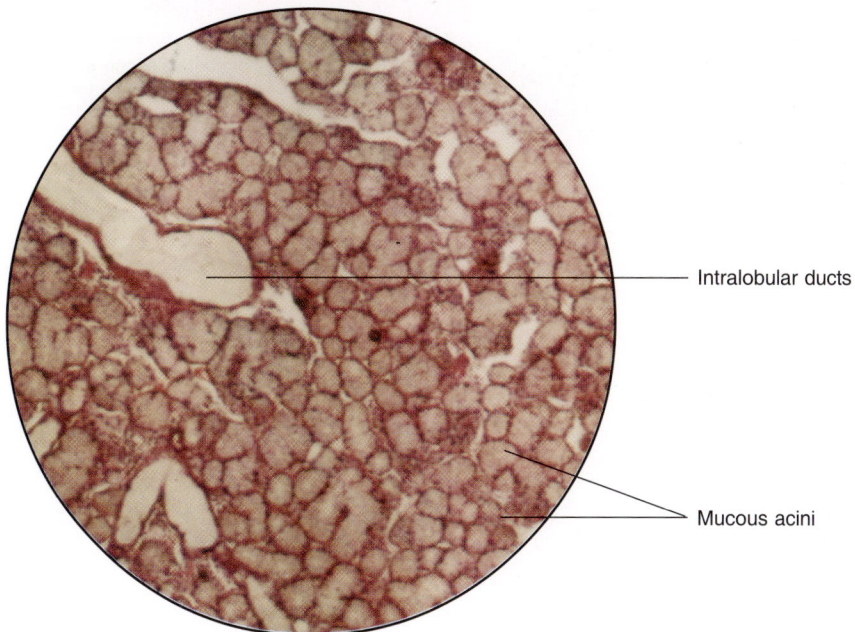

Intralobular ducts

Mucous acini

Mucous salivary gland (photomicrograph 10X)

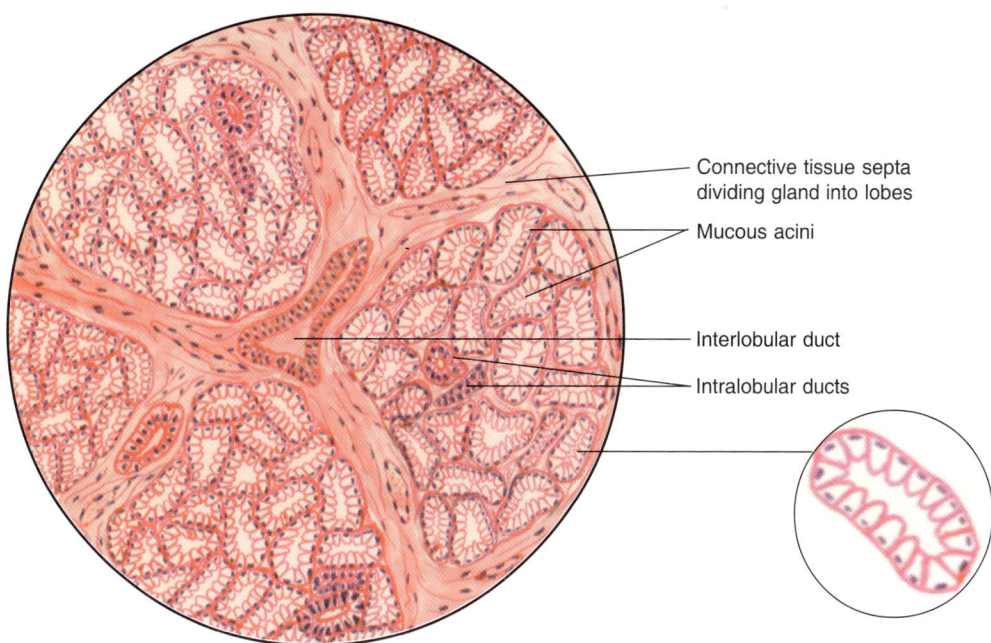

Connective tissue septa
dividing gland into lobes

Mucous acini

Interlobular duct

Intralobular ducts

Fig. 11.2: Mucous salivary gland

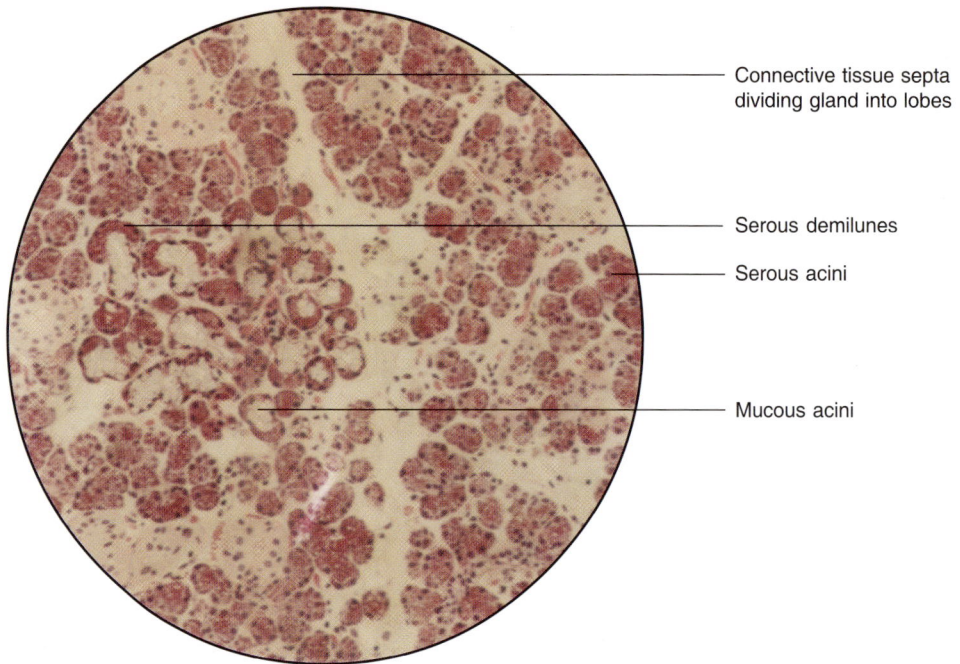

Connective tissue septa
dividing gland into lobes

Serous demilunes

Serous acini

Mucous acini

Mixed salivary gland (photomicrograph 10X)

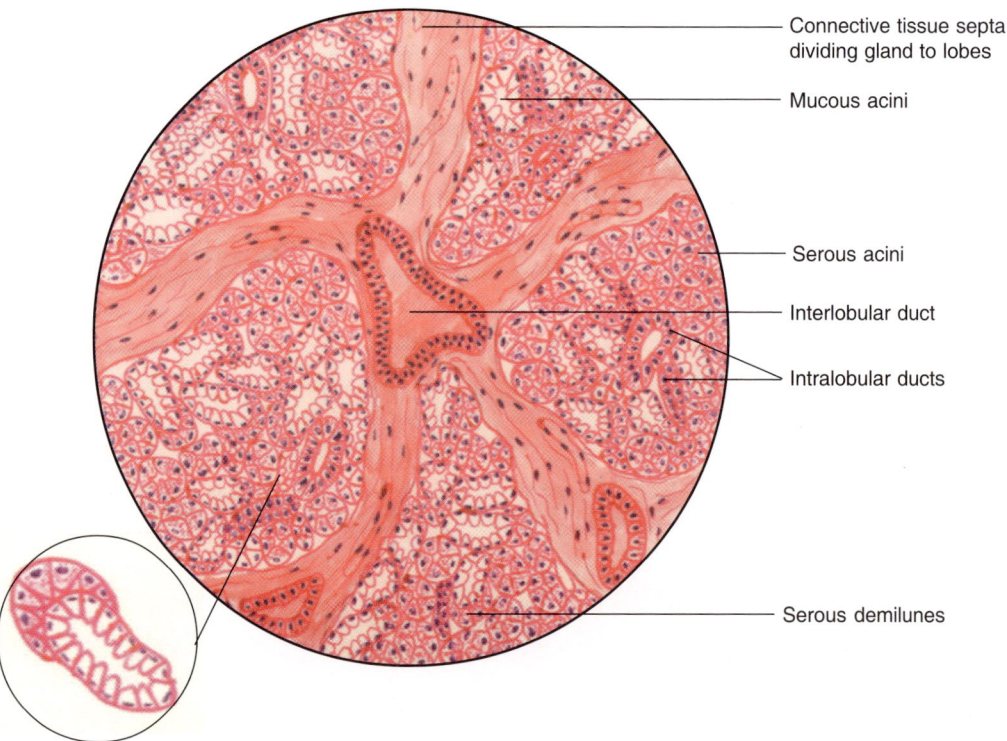

Connective tissue septa
dividing gland to lobes

Mucous acini

Serous acini

Interlobular duct

Intralobular ducts

Serous demilunes

Fig. 11.3: Mixed salivary gland

Oral Pathology

- ❏ **Cysts of Oral Region**

- ❏ **Odontogenic Tumors**

- ❏ **Dental Caries**

- ❏ **Pulp and Periapical Lesions**

- ❏ **Bacterial and Fungal Infections**

- ❏ **Salivary Gland Neoplasms**

- ❏ **Skin Lesions**

- ❏ **Bone Lesions**

- ❏ **Benign and Malignant Tumors of Oral Cavity**

- ❏ **Developmental Disturbances**

12

Cysts of Oral Region

- Odontogenic keratocyst
- Dentigerous cyst
- Eruption cyst
- Calcifying odontogenic cyst
- Lateral periodontal cyst
- Gingival cyst of adults/infants
- Glandular odontogenic cyst
- Radicular cyst/periapical cyst
- Mucocele

Cyst is defined by Kramer as a pathological cavity having fluid, semifluid or gaseous content and which is not formed by accumulation of pus. It is usually but not always lined by epithelium. True cysts have epithelial lining while cysts devoid of epithelial lining are called pseudo cysts. When the epithelium lining the cyst is derived from odontogenic epithelium or its remnants (cell rests of Serres', cell rests of Malassez) the cyst is called as odontogenic cyst.

Cysts have 3 components

1. Cystic cavity or lumen containing fluid or semi fluid materials.
2. Lining epithelium forming a lining of the cystic cavity.
3. Connective tissue capsule that forms the wall of the cyst.

ODONTOGENIC KERATOCYST (OKC)

It is a developmental odontogenic cyst that has characteristic histological features and a high rate of recurrence. Initially these lesions are asymptomatic and do not produce symptoms until it grows to larger size. Symptoms include swelling of jaw, displacement of teeth, pain if secondarily infected and pathologic fracture in later stages.

Histopathology (Fig. 12.1)

Lining epithelium of OKC is characterized by regular parakeratinized stratified squamous epithelium of 5–8 cell layer thickness, without rete ridges formation. Basal cell layer of epithelium is quite distinct with columnar cells having palisading arrangement of nuclei with polarization (nucleus away from basement membrane). This is described as 'tombstone' or 'picket fence' appearance. The superficial parakeratin layer shows characteristic corrugations. Epithelium may show infoldings into the connective tissue capsule and may be separated from capsule in some areas. Connective tissue capsule comprises parallely arranged collagen fibers with a few cells and blood vessels. Satellite cysts or proliferating

Identification Points (Fig. 12.1)

Odontogenic Keratocyst
- Keratinized lining epithelium of 5–8 cell layers thick
- 'Tombstone' appearance of basal cells
- Corrugated parakeratin layer
- Satellite cysts in cystic capsule

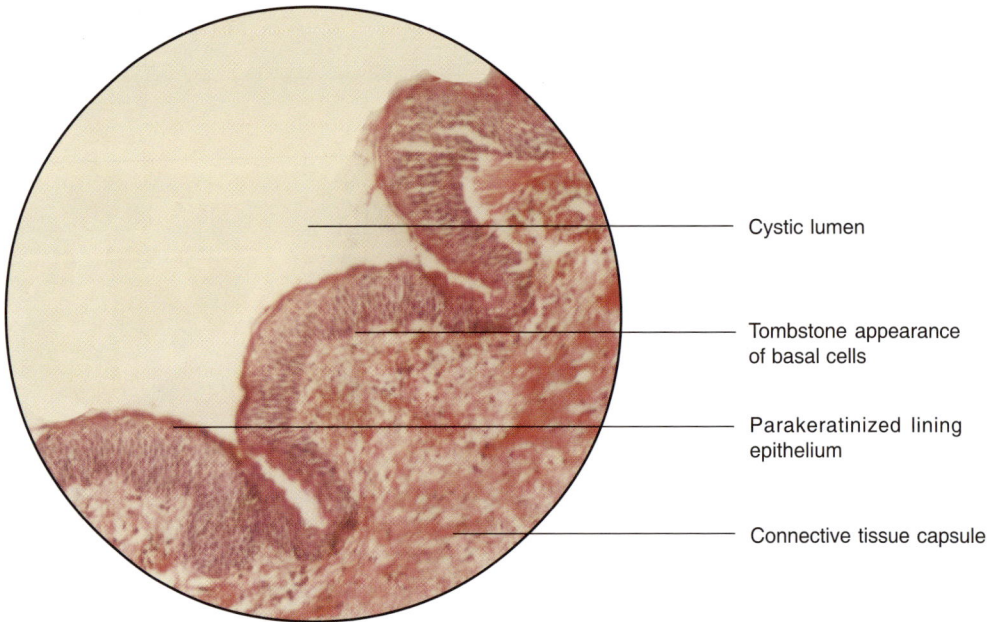

Odontogenic keratocyst (photomicrograph 10X)

Cystic lumen

Tombstone appearance of basal cells

Parakeratinized lining epithelium

Connective tissue capsule

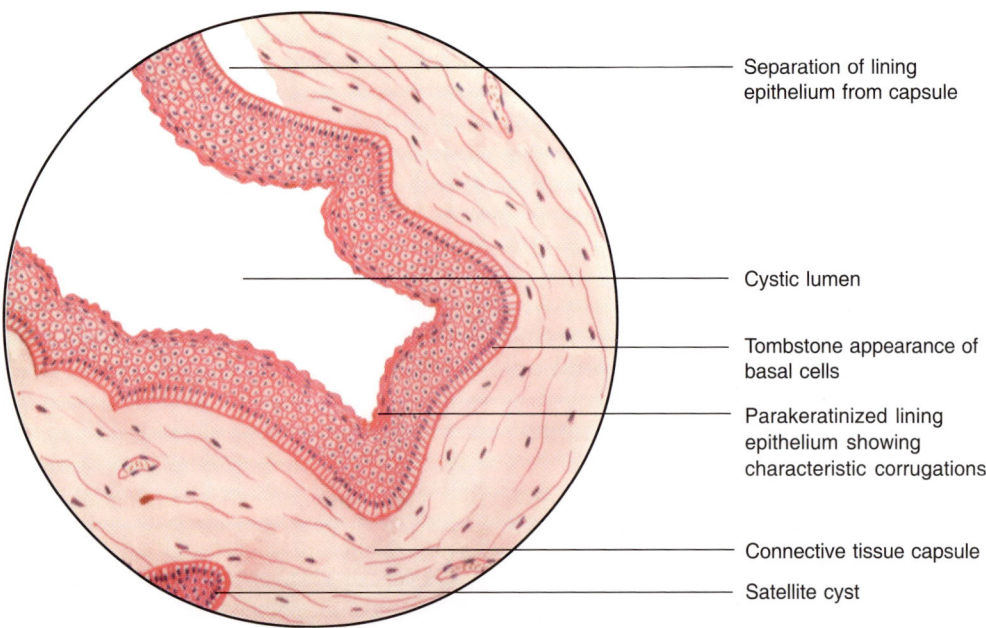

Separation of lining epithelium from capsule

Cystic lumen

Tombstone appearance of basal cells

Parakeratinized lining epithelium showing characteristic corrugations

Connective tissue capsule

Satellite cyst

Fig. 12.1: Odontogenic keratocyst

odontogenic cell rests may be present in the capsule. Cystic lumen contains fluid with low protein level.

DENTIGEROUS CYST (FOLLICULAR CYST)

It is a developmental odontogenic cyst that is formed by expansion of dental follicle and therefore always attached to the neck of an impacted or unerupted tooth. Initially this lesion is asymptomatic, other than a clinically missing tooth. Later stages it causes bony expansion, displacement of teeth and pain if infected.

Histopathology (Fig. 12.2)

The lining epithelium is derived from reduced enamel epithelium and hence appears as uniformly thin nonkeratinized epithelium. The epithelium comprises 2–3 layers of flattened cells and is characteristically devoid of rete ridges. Connective tissue capsule is derived from dental follicle, consists of young fibroblasts widely separated by ground substance rich in mucopolysaccharide. Connective tissue capsule may show odontogenic epithelial remnants. Cystic lumen contains cystic fluid which is thin, watery, or may be blood tinged.

Identification Points (Fig. 12.2)

Dentigerous Cyst
- Non-keratinized epithelium of 2–3 cell layers thick
- Lining epithelium similar to reduced enamel epithelium
- Cyst attached to neck of tooth
- Odontogenic epithelial islands in capsule

ERUPTION CYST

Eruption cyst is a soft tissue counterpart of dentigerous cyst. This occurs, when the eruption process is impeded in soft tissue, probably because of dense fibrous tissue. This results in separation of dental follicle around the crown of erupting tooth. Clinically eruption cyst present as swelling of mucosa in the region of an erupting tooth.

Histopathology (Fig. 12.3)

As in case of dentigerous cyst, lining epithelium of eruption cyst is nonkeratinized

Identification Points (Fig. 12.3)

Eruption Cyst
- Lining epithelium of 2–3 cell layers thick, resembling reduced enamel epithelium
- Cystic capsule resembling dental follicle
- Presence of gingival epithelium and connective tissue

stratified squamous epithelium of 2–3 layers resembling reduced enamel epithelium. Supporting connective tissue capsule is of dental follicular origin and therefore is more basophilic and less collagenous. Overlying compressed gingival epithelium and highly collagenous eosinophilic gingival connective tissue is also observed in the tissue sections

CALCIFYING ODONTOGENIC CYST (GORLIN'S CYST)—SIMPLE CYSTIC TYPE (Type 1-A)

This is a type of developmental odontogenic cyst that has many features of odontogenic tumor. COC can occur as a central (intraosseous) or peripheral (extraosseous) lesion. Extraosseous lesions manifest as gingival swelling. Central lesions are initially asymptomatic, later presents as painless swelling of the jaw.

Histopathology (Fig. 12.4)

Microscopically simple cystic type of COC shows lining epithelium of variable thickness, or may be of regular thickness with 5–10 cell layers thick. Basal cells are columnar with palisading arrangement of hyperchromatic nuclei that are arranged away from basement membrane (resembling ameloblast). Spinous cells are loosely arranged and widely separa-

Identification Points (Fig. 12.4)

Calcifying Odontogenic Cyst
- Lining epithelium of 5–8 cell layers thick
- Basal cells similar to ameloblasts
- Presence of ghost cells
- Dentinoid induction just beneath the lining epithelium

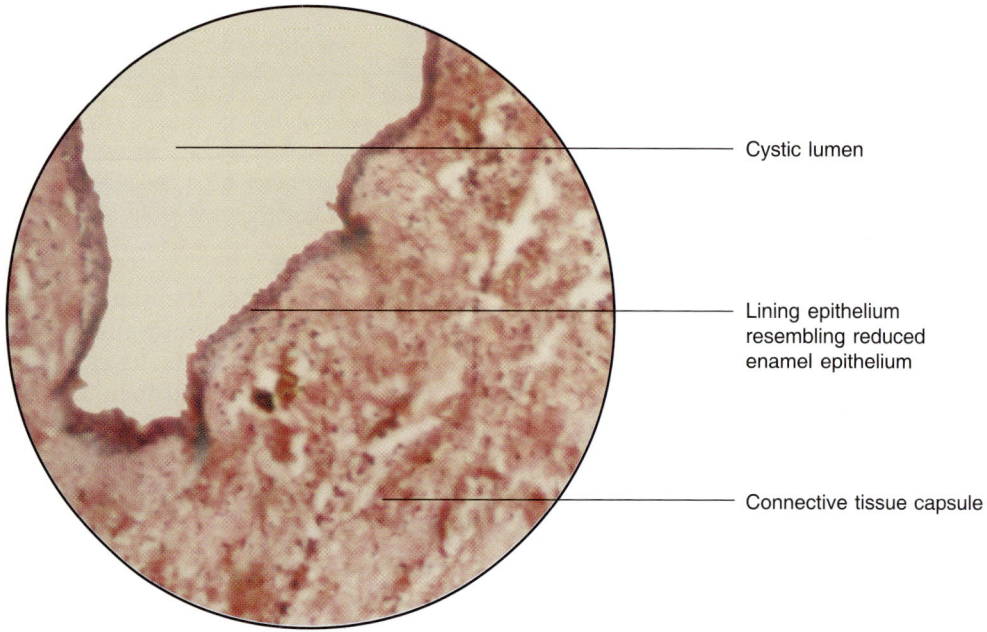

Cystic lumen

Lining epithelium resembling reduced enamel epithelium

Connective tissue capsule

Dentigerous cyst (photomicrograph 10X)

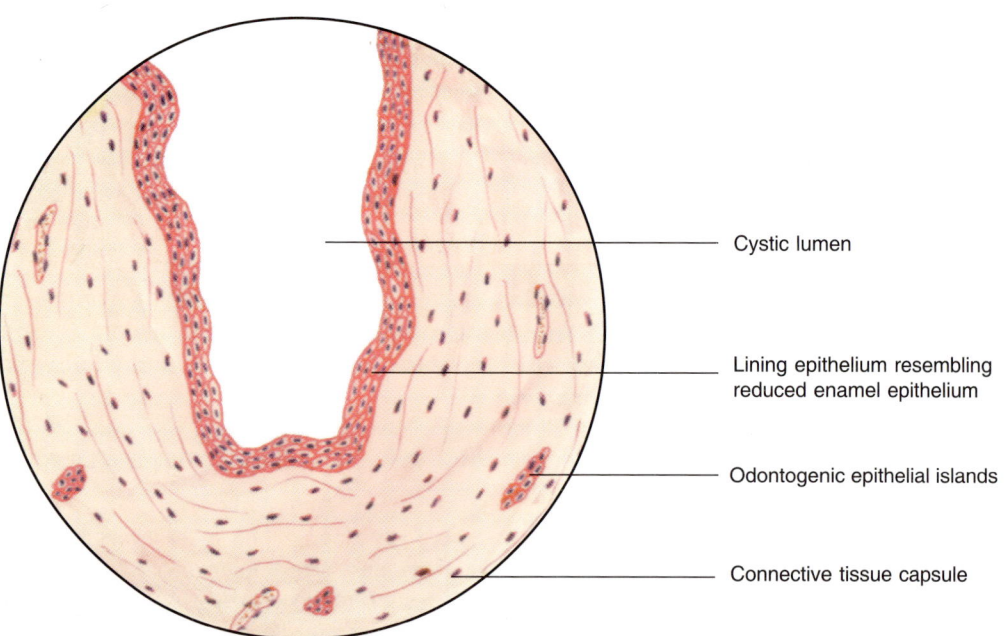

Cystic lumen

Lining epithelium resembling reduced enamel epithelium

Odontogenic epithelial islands

Connective tissue capsule

Fig. 12.2: Dentigerous cyst

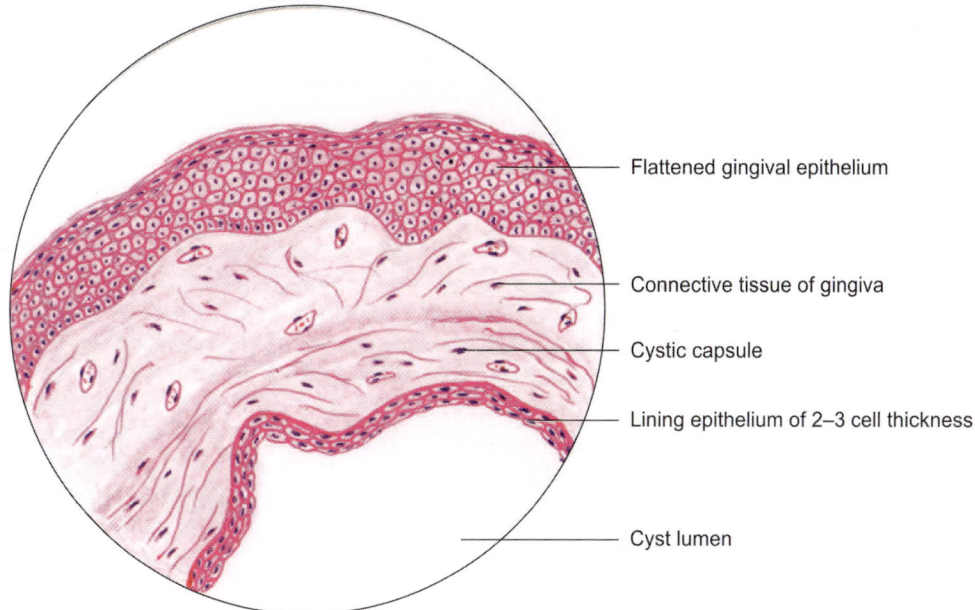

Flattened gingival epithelium

Connective tissue of gingiva

Cystic capsule

Lining epithelium of 2–3 cell thickness

Cyst lumen

Fig. 12.3: Eruption cyst

ted and may appear star-shaped resembling stellate reticulum. One of the remarkable features of COC is presence of **ghost cells**. Ghost cells are degenerating epithelial cells that appear as ovoid, eosinophilic cells with nucleus showing different stages of degeneration. These cells are seen in thickened areas of lining epithelium. Calcifications may be present which are seen as dystrophic deposits in connection with the ghost cells. Another feature of COC is inductive changes in connective tissue adjacent to lining epithelium as areas of eosinophilic matrix material resembling dentinoid. Connective tissue capsule is often scanty and sometimes contain discrete islands of odontogenic cells.

LATERAL PERIODONTAL CYST

Lateral periodontal cyst is a developmental odontogenic cyst which occurs lateral to the roots of a vital teeth. The source of epithelium may be the reduced enamel epithelium of an erupting tooth, rests of the dental lamina or rests of Malassez. The typical radiographic appearance is that of small (up to 1 cm diameter) radiolucency located between the roots of two teeth often in the cuspid-bicuspid region of the mandible. Lateral periodontal cysts must be differentiated from lateral radicular cysts of inflammatory origin, which develop along the lateral canals of non-vital teeth. Multilocular variant of this cyst is Botryoid odontogenic cyst

Histopathology (Fig. 12.5)

Histologically, the lateral periodontal cyst is characterized by a thin, nonkeratinized epithelium usually 1–5 cell layers thick, which resembles the reduced enamel epithelium. The epithelial lining exhibits focal thickenings or plaques (mural plaques), which often show glycogen-containing epithelial cells. The cells in these thickened areas are slightly larger,

Identification Points (Fig. 12.5)

Lateral Periodontal Cyst
- Lining epithelium of 1–5 cell layers thick, resembling reduced enamel epithelium
- Focal thickenings of lining epithelium (mural plaques)
- Glycogen-containing clear epithelial cells in mural plaques

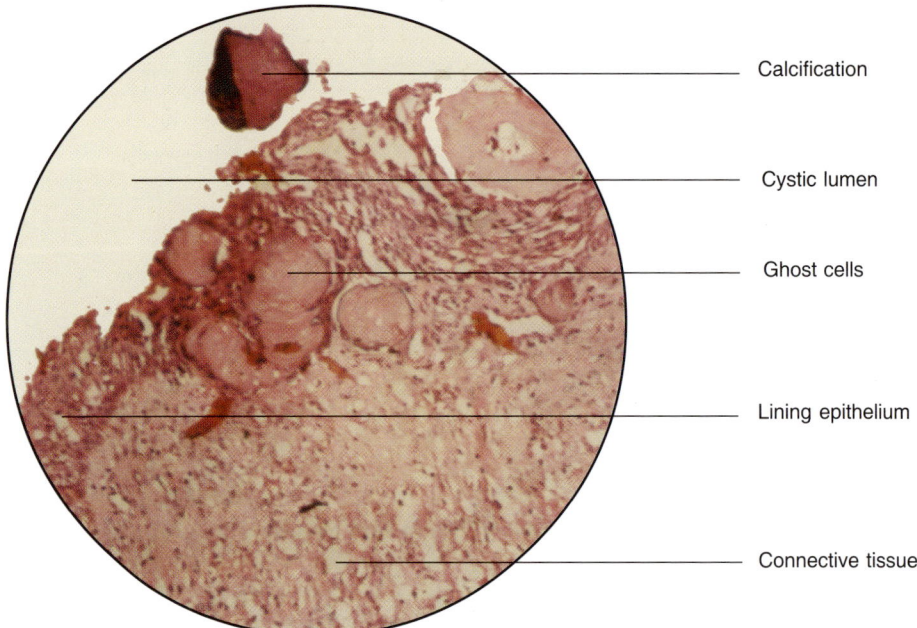

Calcification

Cystic lumen

Ghost cells

Lining epithelium

Connective tissue

Calcifying odontogenic cyst (photomicrograph 10X)

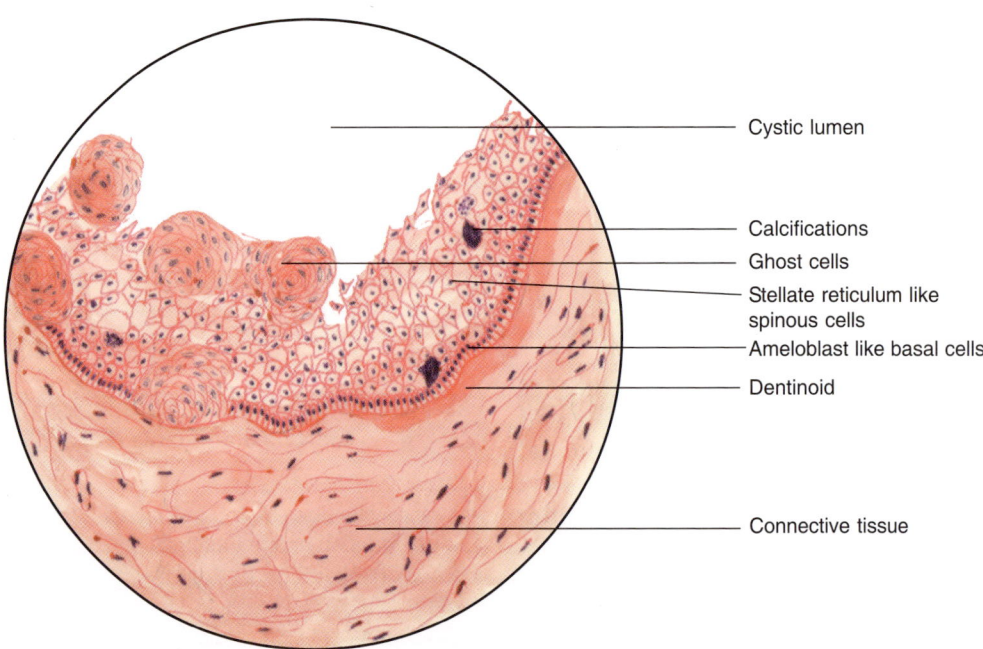

Cystic lumen

Calcifications

Ghost cells

Stellate reticulum like spinous cells

Ameloblast like basal cells

Dentinoid

Connective tissue

Fig. 12.4: Calcifying odontogenic cyst

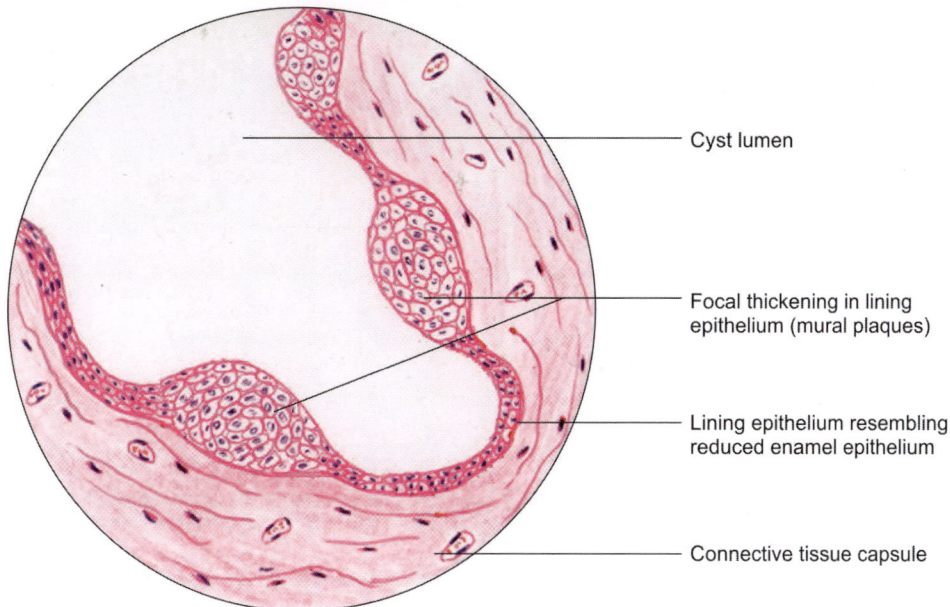

Cyst lumen

Focal thickening in lining epithelium (mural plaques)

Lining epithelium resembling reduced enamel epithelium

Connective tissue capsule

Fig. 12.5: Lateral periodontal cyst

more round with clear or empty (clear cells) cytoplasm. The connective tissue capsule is fibrous in nature.

GINGIVAL CYSTS OF ADULTS/INFANTS

Gingival cysts are developmental odontogenic cyst arise from epithelial rests of dental lamina (cell rests of Serres) located in connective tissue of gingiva. Clinically, gingival cysts of adults present as solitary, well circumscribed swelling involving facial gingiva of mandibular/maxillary canines and premolars, usually less than 0.5 cm size. This may cause superficial pressure resorption of underlying alveolar bone causing a superficial "cupping out" effect. Gingival cysts of infants occur as multiple small swelling in alveolar mucosa of newborn.

Histopathology (Fig. 12.6)

Gingival cyst presents as unicystic structure lined with non-keratinized low cuboidal or stratified squamous epithelium of 1–3 layer thickness with a flat interface with connective

Identification Points (Fig. 12.6)

Gingival Cysts of Adult
- Lining epithelium of 1–3 cell layers thick
- Focal thickenings of lining epithelium
- Overlying gingival epithelium

tissue capsule. Cyst lining epithelium may show focal thickened areas, which may have clear cells. Connective tissue capsule is relatively uninflamed, fibrovascular tissue. Compressed overlying gingival tissue may be observed if it is included in biopsy.

GLANDULAR ODONTOGENIC CYST

Glandular odontogenic cyst (GOC) is a rare developmental cyst of the jaws mostly occurring in middle-aged men, especially in the anterior mandible, clinically present as asymptomatic slow-growing swelling. Radiographically, GOC presents as well-defined uni- or multilocular radiolucency.

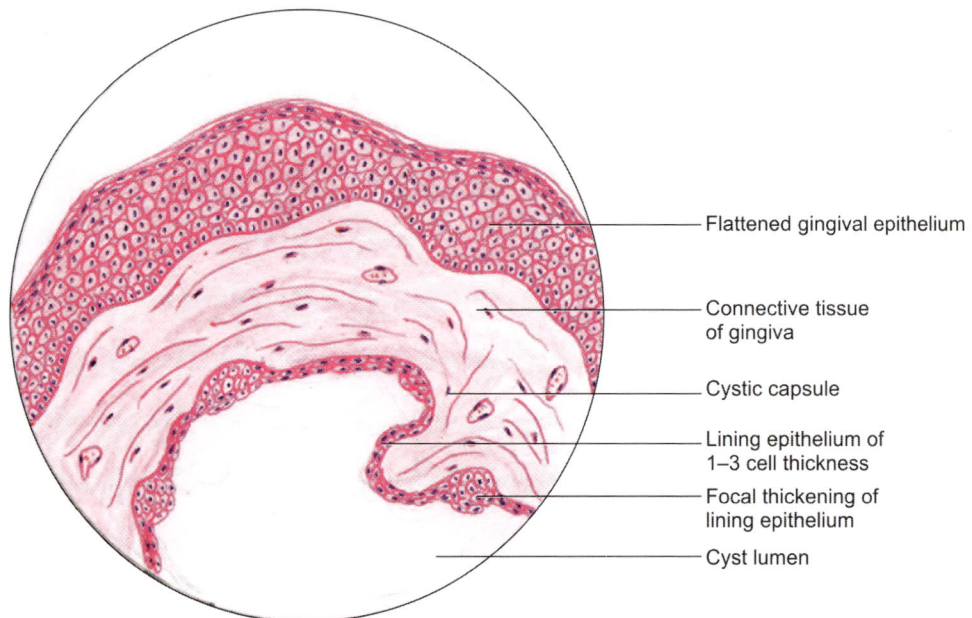

Flattened gingival epithelium

Connective tissue of gingiva

Cystic capsule

Lining epithelium of 1–3 cell thickness

Focal thickening of lining epithelium

Cyst lumen

Fig. 12.6: Gingival cysts of adult

Histopathology (Fig. 12.7)

In GOC cystic cavity is lined by nonkeratinized, stratified, squamous epithelium, of variable thickness with a flat epithelial—connective tissue interface. Presence of localized plaque-like thickenings or epithelial whorls or spheres within the lining, variable numbers of PAS-positive mucus secreting cells with microcystic areas lined by single layer of cuboidal or columnar cells are characteristic features of GOC. The superficial layer of the epithelium consists of eosinophilic cuboidal cells or columnar cells with cilia (hobnail cells). The subepithelial connective tissue is usually free of inflammation.

RADICULAR CYST/PERIAPICAL CYST

Radicular cyst or apical periodontal cyst is an inflammatory odontogenic cyst that develop in the periapical region of a non-vital tooth. The source of epithelium is cell rests of Malassez and proliferation is stimulated by inflammation. Radiographic picture shows a well defined radiolucency at the root apex.

Histopathology (Fig. 12.8)

Cystic lumen is filled with fluid containing cholesterol crystals. Lining epithelium is non-keratinized stratified squamous epithelium of variable thickness. Epithelium shows spongiosis and inflammatory cell infiltration. Proliferating epithelium exhibits characteristic arcading

Identification Points (Fig. 12.7)

Glandular Odontogenic Cyst
- Nonkeratinized lining epithelium of variable thickness
- Focal thickenings of lining epithelium
- Mucous cells and mucin containing microcyst in lining epithelium
- Superficial cuboidal/columnar (hobnail) cells

Identification Points (Fig. 12.8)

Radicular Cyst
- Nonkeratinized lining epithelium of variable thickness
- Arcading patterns of epithelium
- Dense inflammation of cystic capsule
- Cholesterol clefts in capsules

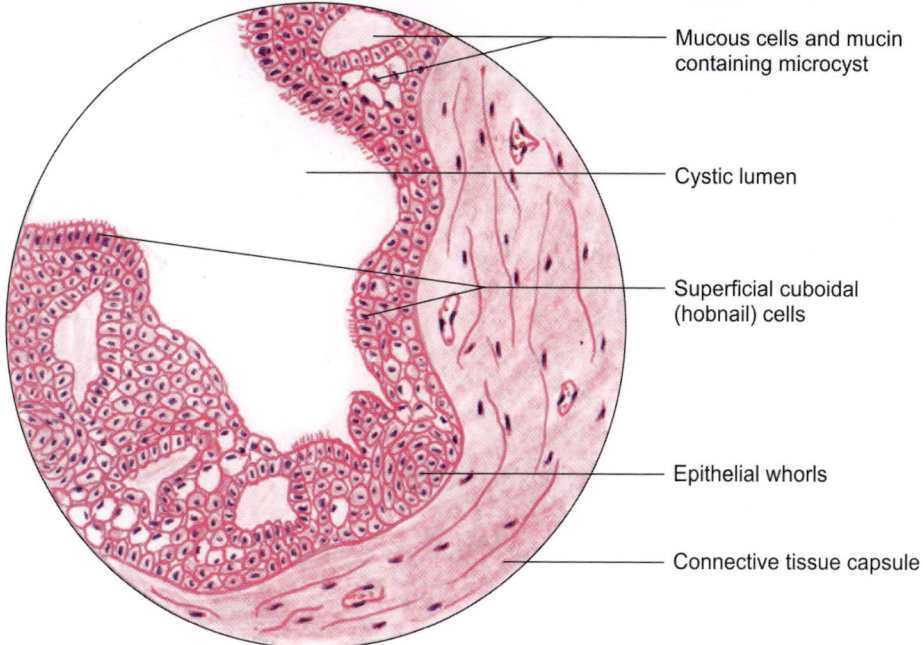

Mucous cells and mucin containing microcyst

Cystic lumen

Superficial cuboidal (hobnail) cells

Epithelial whorls

Connective tissue capsule

Fig. 12.7: Glandular odontogenic cyst

pattern where arcades of epithelium enclosing a densely inflamed connective tissue. Epithelium may also show arc-shaped hyaline structures called Rushton bodies. Connective tissue capsule adjacent to lining epithelium is delicate with dense inflammatory cell infiltration. Deeper portion of connective tissue capsule is more fibrous with relatively less inflammation.

Connective tissue capsule may also show cleft-like spaces (Fig. 12.9) filled with cholesterol that are seen as spindle-shaped spaces. The presence of these cholesterol crystals evoke a granulomatous reaction in the connective tissue.

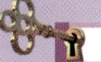 **Identification Points (Fig. 12.9)**

Cholesterol Clefts in Radicular Cyst
- Seen as spindle-shaped clear spaces in the connective tissue capsule
- Surrounding connective tissue shows granulation tissue reaction

MUCOCELE (MUCOUS EXTRAVASATION CYST)

This is a common soft tissue cyst, occurring in the oral mucosa due to trauma to the minor salivary duct. Trauma leads to rupture of duct followed by spillage of mucin to the surrounding tissue evoking an inflammatory reaction. Mucocele is seen as a fluctuant dome-shaped swelling ranging from 1 to 8 mm size. This lesion is common on lower lip and patient may give a definite history of trauma.

Histopathology (Fig. 12.10)

Basic feature of mucocele is a pseudocyst with granulation tissue wall. There is no lining epithelium. The lesion shows a central irregular mucin spilled area surrounded by granulation tissue wall. Granulation tissue comprises delicate collagen bundles, plump fibroblasts, proliferating endothelial cells,

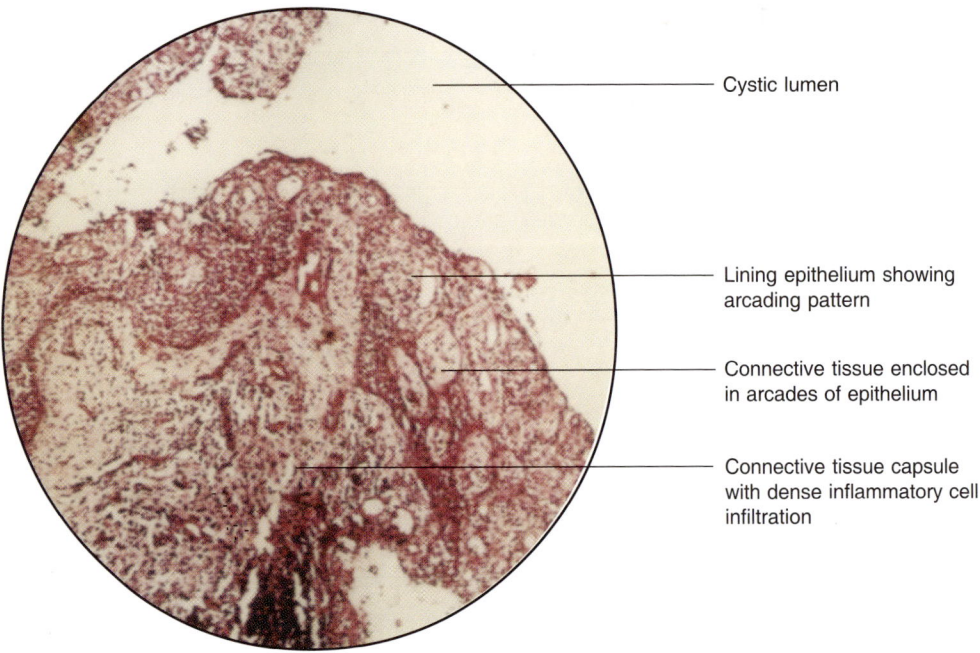

Cystic lumen

Lining epithelium showing
arcading pattern

Connective tissue enclosed
in arcades of epithelium

Connective tissue capsule
with dense inflammatory cell
infiltration

Radicular cyst (photomicrograph 10X)

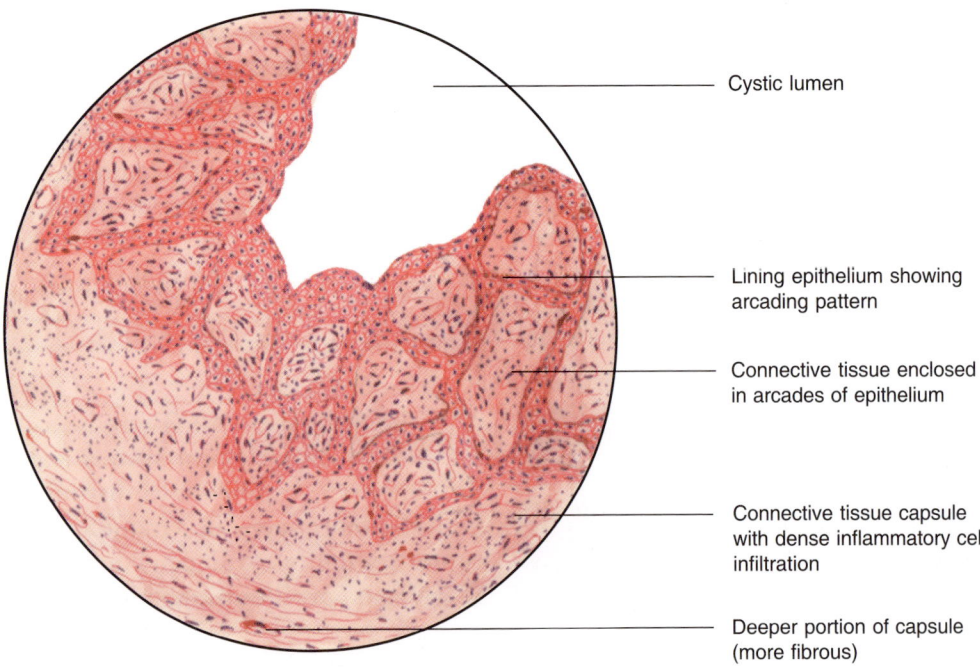

Cystic lumen

Lining epithelium showing
arcading pattern

Connective tissue enclosed
in arcades of epithelium

Connective tissue capsule
with dense inflammatory cell
infiltration

Deeper portion of capsule
(more fibrous)

Fig. 12.8: Radicular cyst

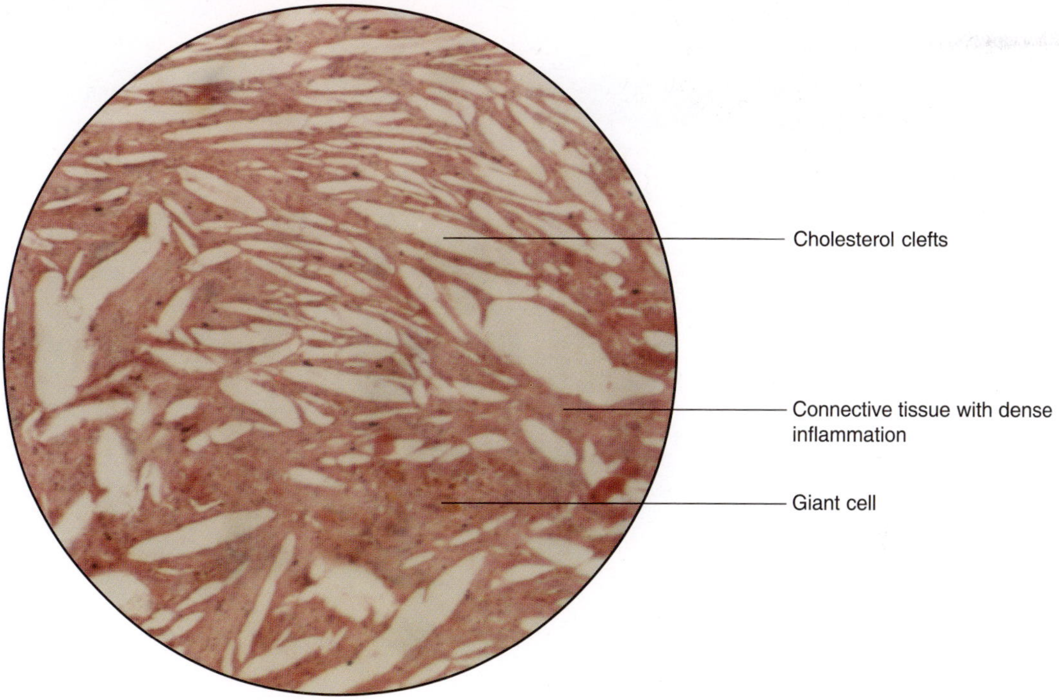

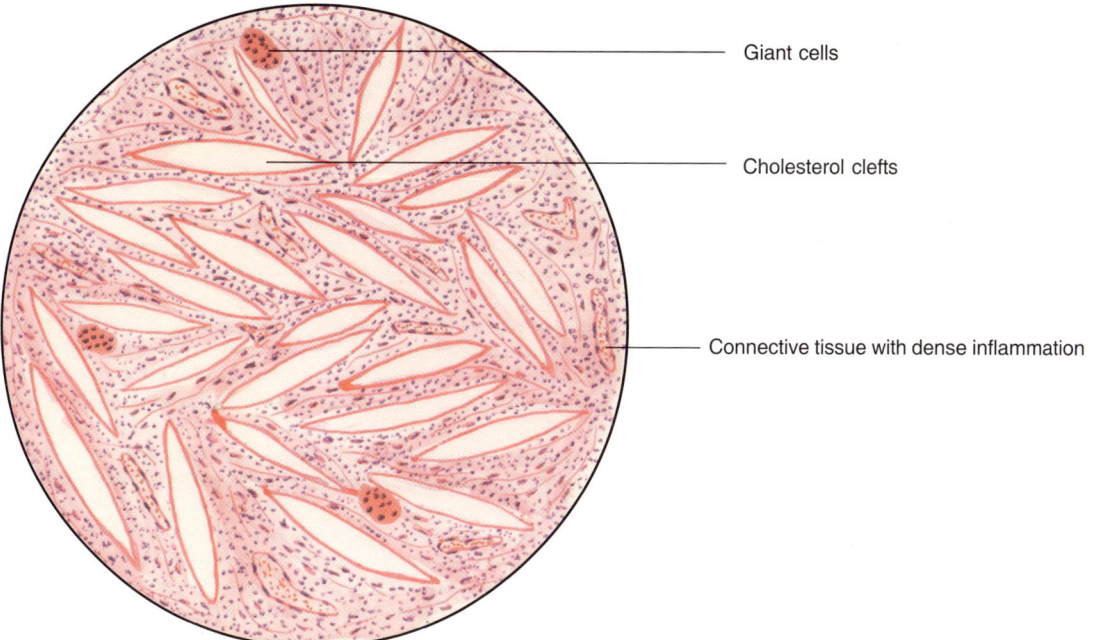

Cholesterol clefts in radicular cyst (photomicrograph 10X)

Fig. 12.9: Cholesterol clefts in radicular cyst

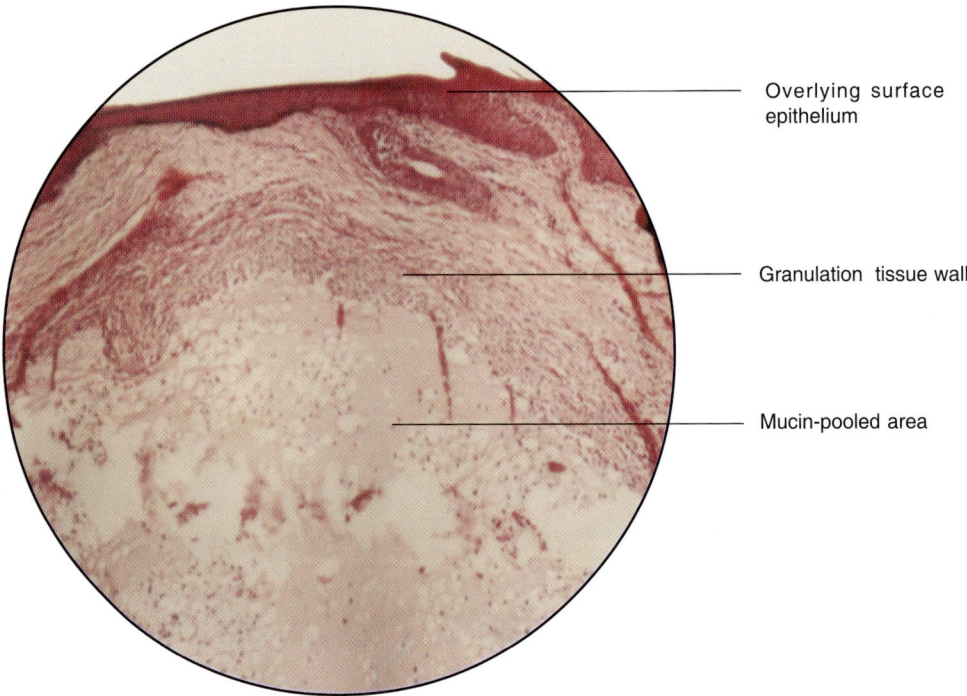

Overlying surface epithelium

Granulation tissue wall

Mucin-pooled area

Mucocele (photomicrograph 10X)

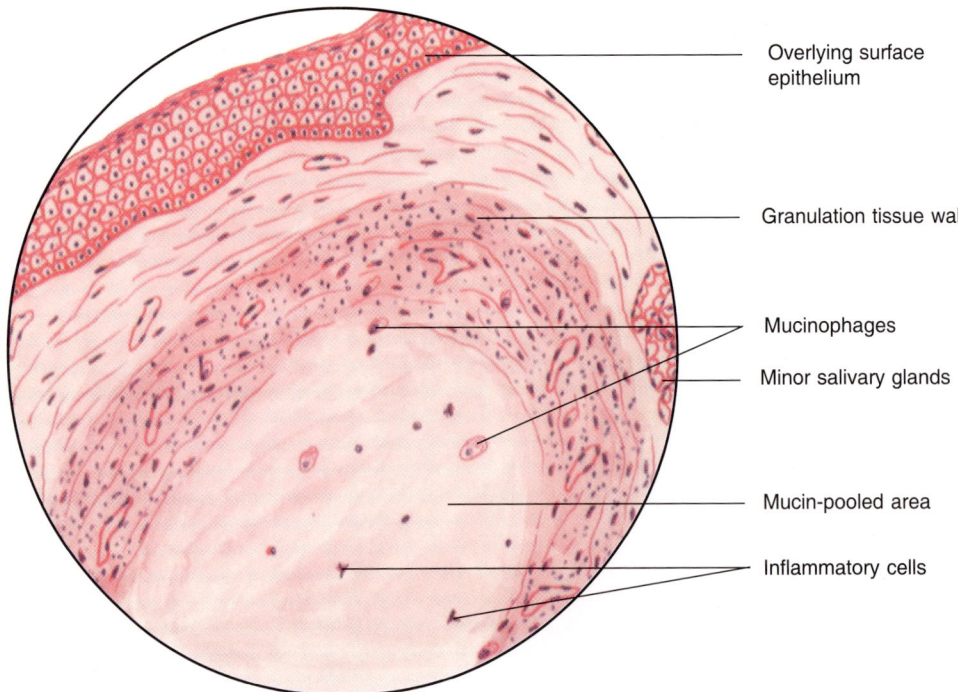

Overlying surface epithelium

Granulation tissue wall

Mucinophages

Minor salivary glands

Mucin-pooled area

Inflammatory cells

Fig. 12.10: Mucocele

budding capillaries and chronic inflammatory cells. Muciphages or mucin-engulfed macrophages are seen in the mucin-pooled area and in lining. Adjacent minor salivary gland and a ruptured salivary duct (feeder duct) may be seen.

Identification Points (Fig. 12.10)

Mucocele
- Mucin pooled area
- Granulation tissue wall surrounding mucin
- Presence of mucinophages and inflammatory cells

13

Odontogenic Tumors

- Ameloblastoma
- Calcifying epithelial odontogenic tumor
- Adenomatoid odontogenic tumor
- Ameloblastic fibroma
- Central cementifying fibroma

Tumors developing from the odontogenic tissue (any component of tooth germ or its remnants) are called odontogenic tumors. These tumors may develop from epithelial component or ectomesenchymal component, or both (mixed tumors). Based on biological behavior odontogenic tumors can be benign and malignant.

AMELOBLASTOMA

Ameloblastoma is a locally aggressive benign neoplasm of odontogenic epithelial origin. According to the World Health Organization, ameloblastomas are classified into the following types: Conventional (solid/multicystic type), unicystic, peripheral and desmoplastic. Conventional ameloblastoma mainly affect the posterior region of mandible. This lesion is initially asymptomatic, slowly progressing to cause bony expansion. Ameloblastoma can grow to massive size and typically present in a radiograph as a multilocular radiolucency described as "honeycomb" or "soap bubble" appearance.

Histopathology

Histological variants of **conventional solid/multicystic type** ameloblastoma are:

1. *Follicular ameloblastoma (Fig. 13.1):* In this variant, tumor cells are arranged in the form of a few follicles distributed in connective tissue stroma. Follicles have a peripheral layer of ameloblast like cells, i.e. columnar cells that have nucleus arranged away from the base of the cells. Central portion of the follicle has loosely arranged cells resembling stellate reticulum. In this variant, cyst formation can take place within the follicle by the cystic degeneration of stellate reticulum like cells (intrafollicular cysts).

Identification Points (Fig. 13.1)

Follicular Ameloblastoma
- Odontogenic epithelial cells arranged to form follicles
- Peripheral ameloblast like cells
- Central stellate reticulum like cells
- Intrafollicular cyst formation

2. *Acanthomatous type (Fig. 13.2):* In this histological variant, tumor cells are arranged in the form of follicles with peripheral ameloblast like cells and central

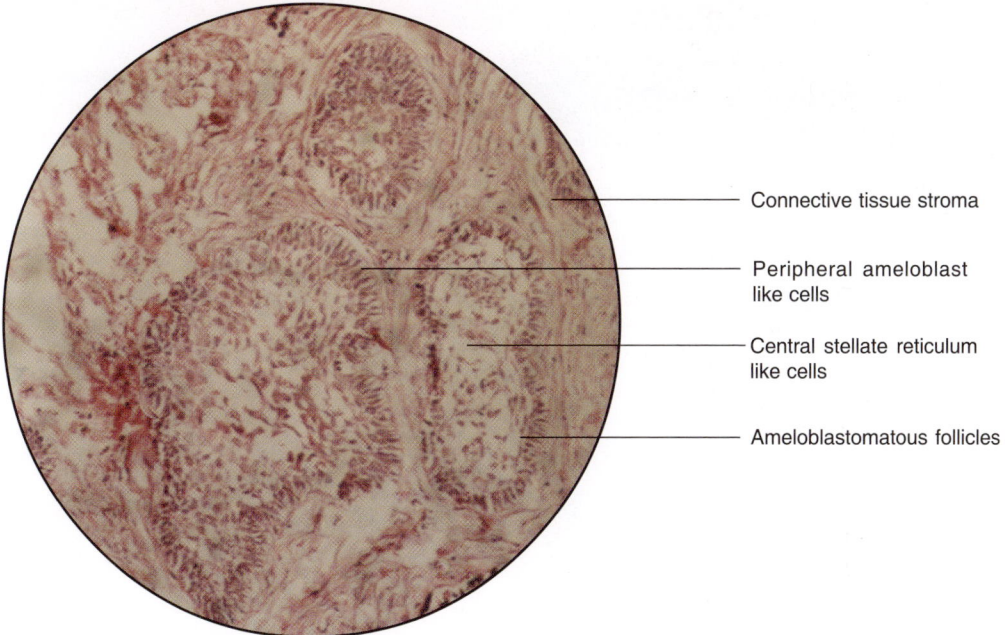

Connective tissue stroma

Peripheral ameloblast like cells

Central stellate reticulum like cells

Ameloblastomatous follicles

Ameloblastoma—follicular type (photomicrograph 10X)

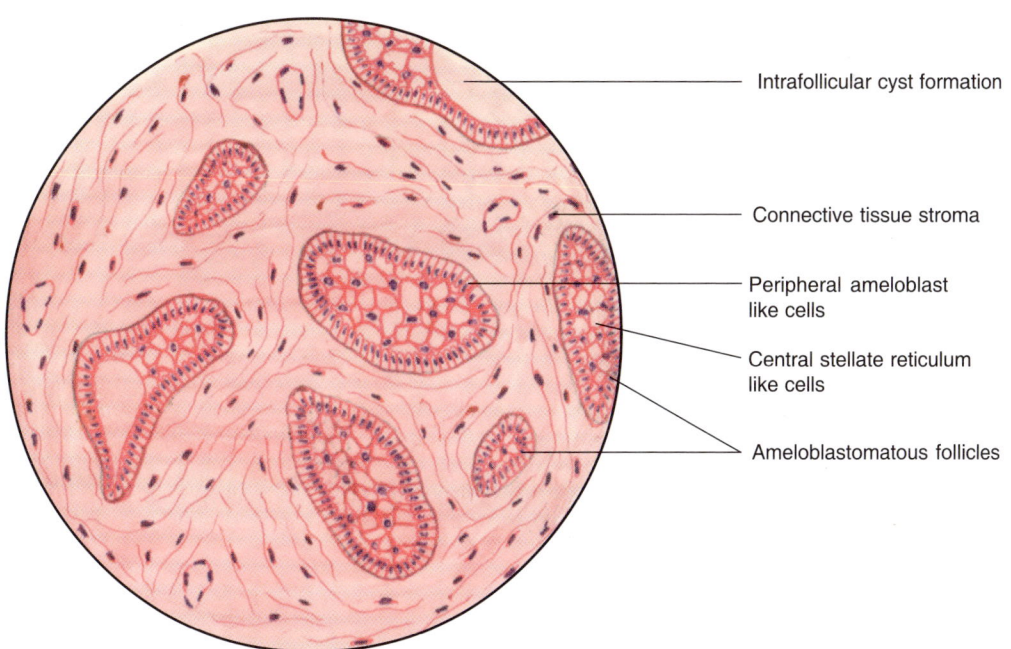

Intrafollicular cyst formation

Connective tissue stroma

Peripheral ameloblast like cells

Central stellate reticulum like cells

Ameloblastomatous follicles

Fig. 13.1: Ameloblastoma—follicular type

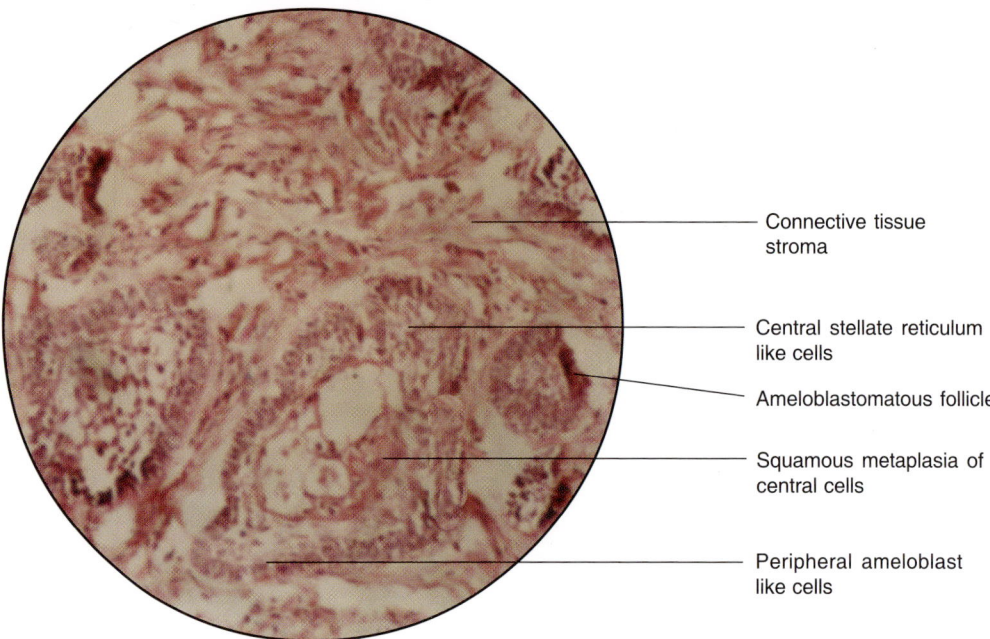

Connective tissue stroma

Central stellate reticulum like cells

Ameloblastomatous follicle

Squamous metaplasia of central cells

Peripheral ameloblast like cells

Ameloblastoma—acanthomatous type (photomicrograph 10X)

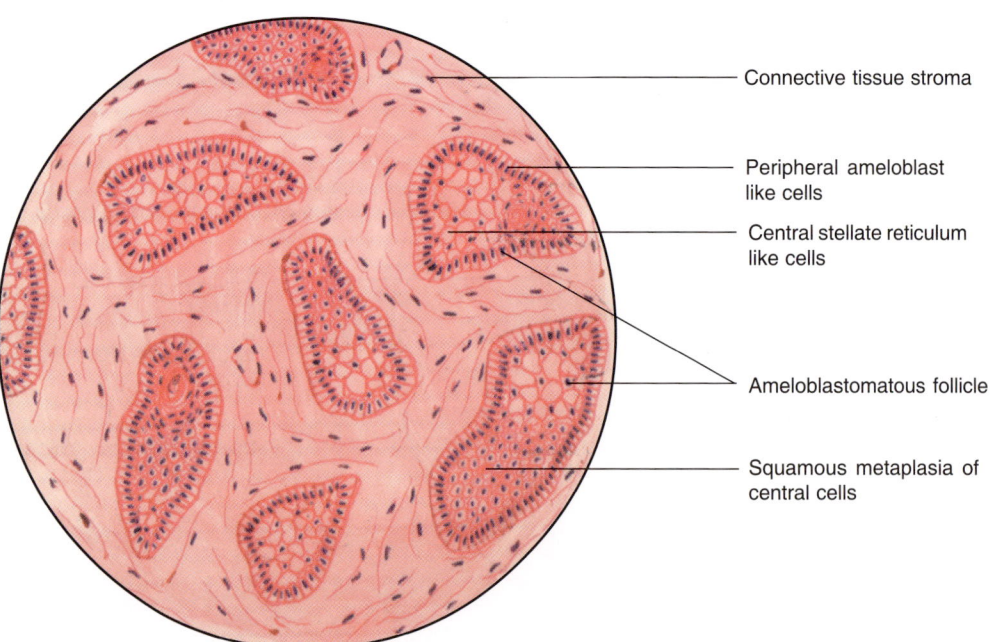

Connective tissue stroma

Peripheral ameloblast like cells

Central stellate reticulum like cells

Ameloblastomatous follicle

Squamous metaplasia of central cells

Fig. 13.2: Ameloblastoma—acanthomatous type

stellate reticulum like cells. In some of the follicles the central cells are transformed in to squamous cells and may show the evidence of keratinization.

3. *Basal cell ameloblastoma (Fig. 13.3)*: This is a rare histologic variant of ameloblastoma. In this type arrangement of proliferating odontogenic epithelial cells are in follicular pattern with peripheral cuboidal or low columnar with a little evidence of palisading. The central cells of the follicle are typical basaloid cells having hyperchromatic nucleus almost filling the cells and scanty cytoplasm. However, some follicles may show classic features of conventional ameloblastomatous follicle.

4. *Granular cell ameloblastoma (Fig. 13.4)*: This is also a rare histological variant of ameloblastoma where the central stellate reticulum cells of ameloblastomatous follicles show extensive granular cell transformation. These granular cells are large cells with abundant granular eosinophilic cytoplasm and piknotic nucleus. The granules are identified as numerous lysosomes accumulated in the cytoplasm

attributed to degenerative changes. Sometimes this change, may be so extensive that the peripheral columnar cells may also be replaced by granular cells.

5. *Plexiform ameloblastoma (Fig. 13.5)*: In this pattern, ameloblast like cells are arranged in the form of long anastomosing cords or as irregular strands. These strands are bounded by ameloblast like cells on either side having back to back arrangement with stellate reticulum like cells in between. Stellate reticulum cells are less prominent than in follicular pattern. Connective tissue stroma is seen enclosed between the networks of odontogenic epithelial cells. Cystic degeneration may be observed within the stroma (stromal cysts).

DESMOPLASTIC AMELOBLASTOMA
(Fig. 13.6)

This is a distinct variant of ameloblastoma which is characterized by extensive stromal collagenization or desmoplasia surrounding irregular islands of odontogenic epithelium. Proliferating odontogenic tumor islands will be compressed in highly collagenized stroma

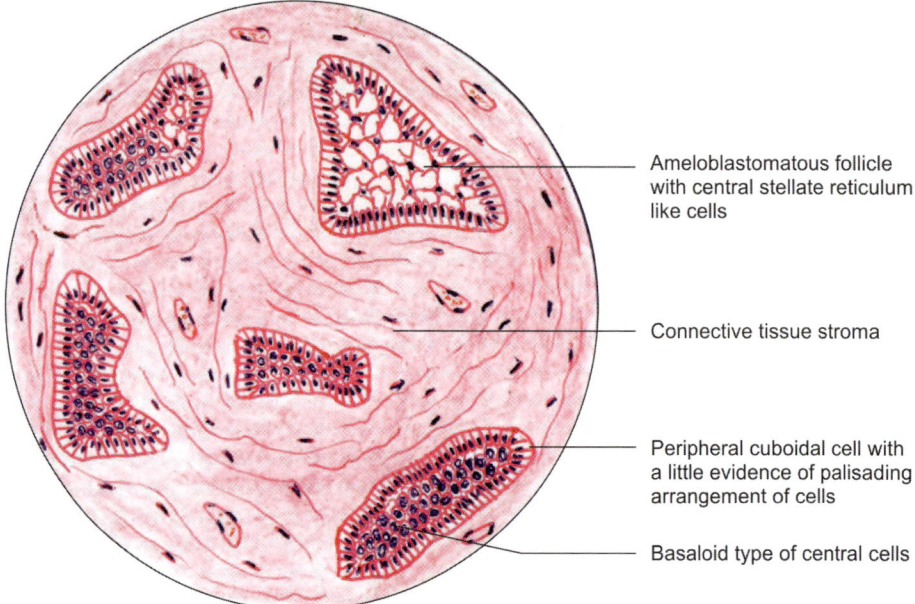

Ameloblastomatous follicle
with central stellate reticulum
like cells

Connective tissue stroma

Peripheral cuboidal cell with
a little evidence of palisading
arrangement of cells

Basaloid type of central cells

Fig. 13.3: Ameloblastoma—basal cell type

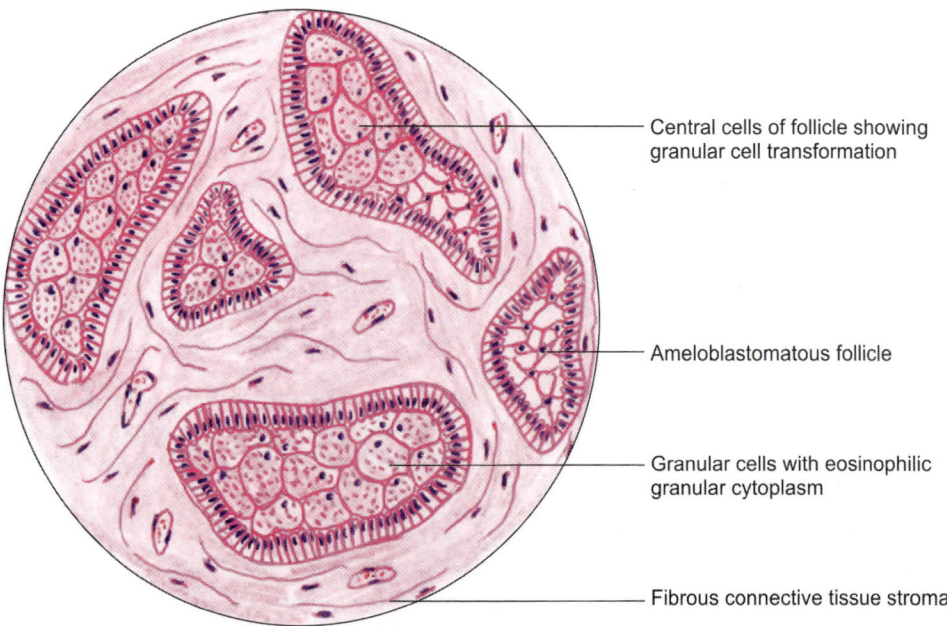

Central cells of follicle showing
granular cell transformation

Ameloblastomatous follicle

Granular cells with eosinophilic
granular cytoplasm

Fibrous connective tissue stroma

Fig. 13.4: Granular cell ameloblastoma

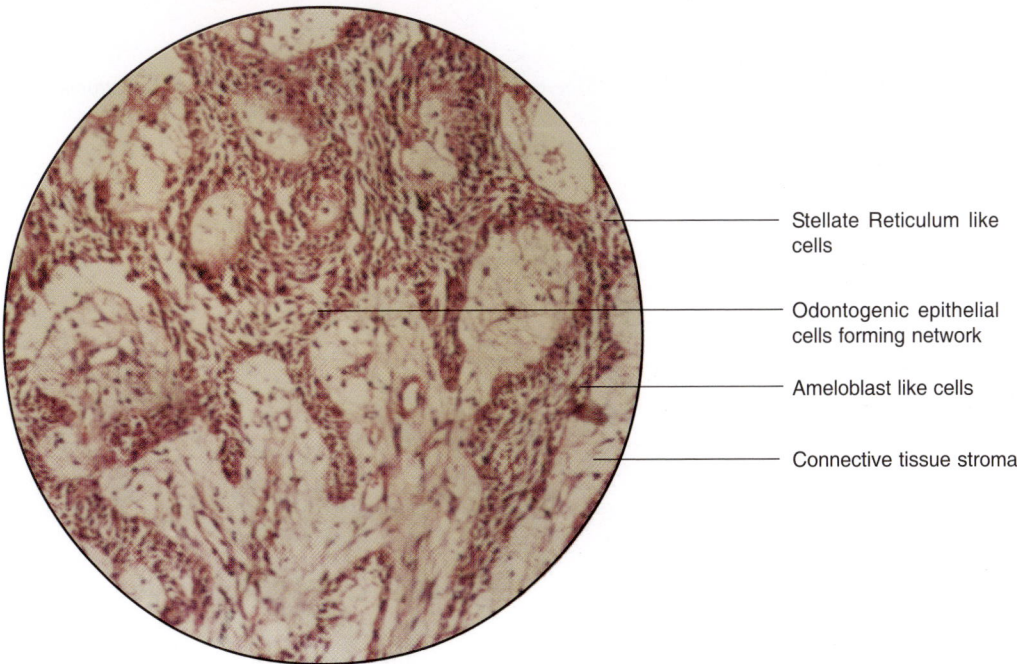

Stellate Reticulum like cells

Odontogenic epithelial cells forming network

Ameloblast like cells

Connective tissue stroma

Ameloblastoma—plexiform type (photomicrograph 10X)

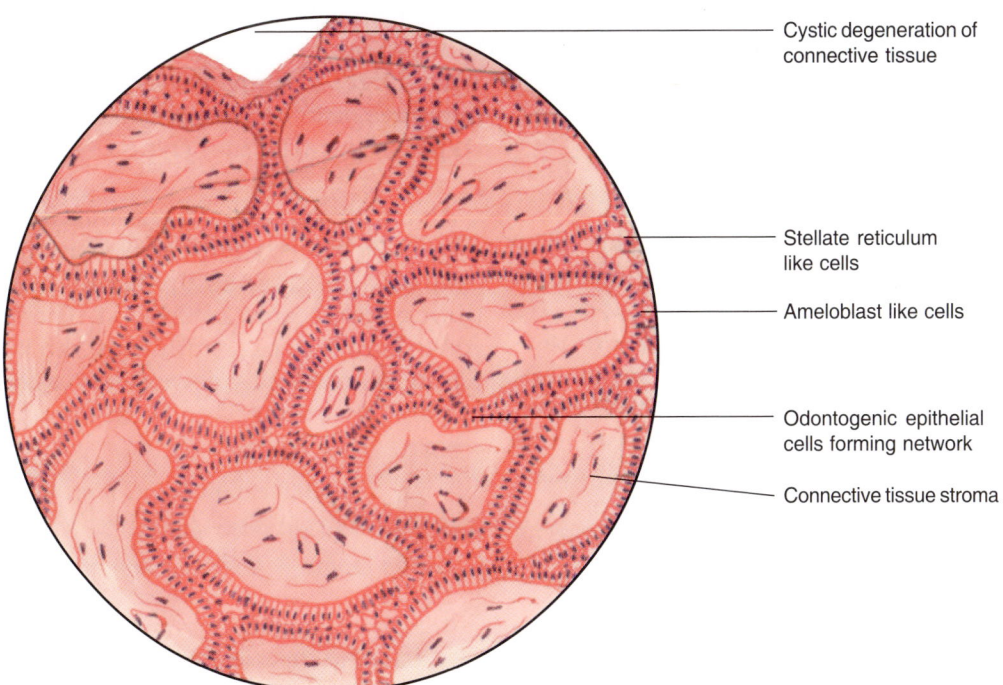

Cystic degeneration of connective tissue

Stellate reticulum like cells

Ameloblast like cells

Odontogenic epithelial cells forming network

Connective tissue stroma

Fig. 13.5: Ameloblastoma—plexiform type

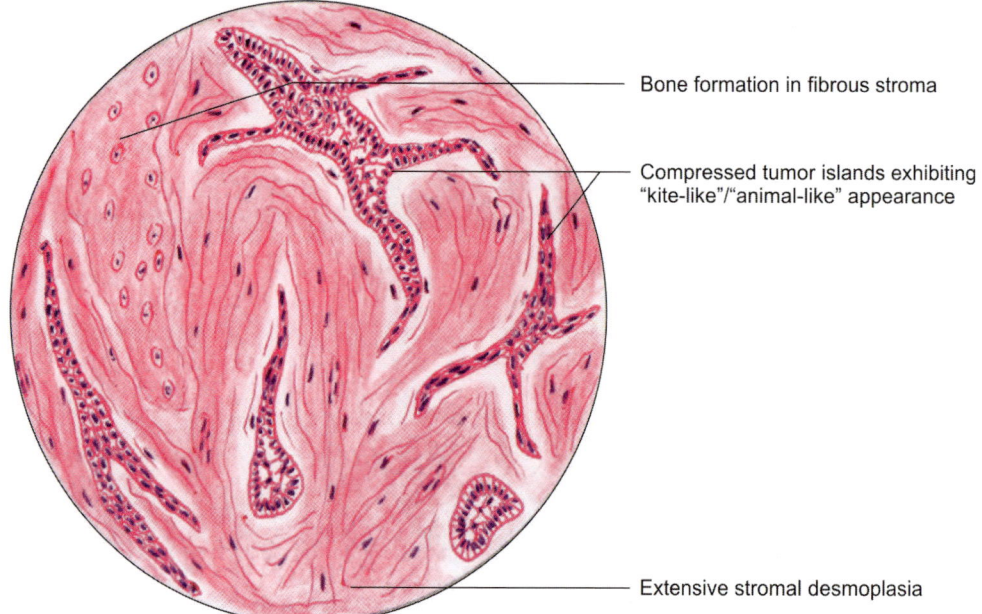

Bone formation in fibrous stroma

Compressed tumor islands exhibiting "kite-like"/"animal-like" appearance

Extensive stromal desmoplasia

Fig. 13.6: Desmoplastic ameloblastoma

Identification Points (Fig. 13.6)

Desmoplastic Ameloblastoma
- Odontogenic epithelial cells in highly collagenized stroma
- Compressed tumor islands showing "kite-like" or "animal-like" appearance
- Central spindle or squamoid cells
- Calcifications in fibrous stroma

and may show a pointed, stellate or "kite-like" or "animal-like" appearance. The epithelial cells at the periphery of the islands are cuboidal and occasionally show hyperchromatic nuclei and typical ameloblast-like peripheral cells demonstrating reversed nuclear polarity are rarely observed. The center of the islands may contain spindle-shaped or squamoid epithelial cells. Calcifications, at times even bone formation may be noted in fibrous stroma.

UNICYSTIC AMELOBLASTOMA

Unicystic ameloblastoma refers to a variant of ameloblastoma that shows features of a cystic

lesion on clinical, radiographic, or gross presentation, but on histologic examination shows a typical ameloblastomatous epithelium lining the cyst cavity, with or without luminal and/or mural tumor growth. Accordingly Ackermann classified this entity into three histologic groups, namely luminal (type 1), intraluminal (type 2) and mural patterns (type 3).

Unicystic ameloblastoma—luminal type (Fig. 13.7): In this type the ameloblastomatous change is confined to the luminal surface (lining epithelium) of the cyst. The lesion consists of a dense, uniformly thickened, fibrous connective tissue capsule, that consists of parallely arranged collagen fibers; lined

Identification Points (Fig. 13.7)

Unicystic Ameloblastoma—Luminal Type
- Cystic cavity lined by stratified squamous epithelium of variable thickness
- The ameloblastomatous change is confined to the lining epithelium of the cyst
- Tall columnar basal cells with hyperchromatic palisading nuclei

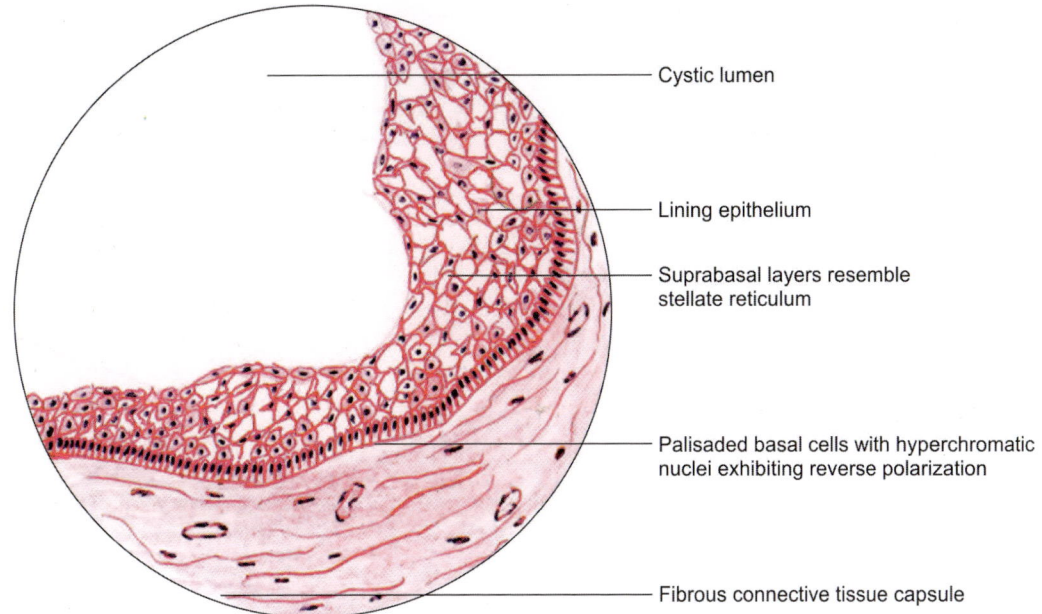

Cystic lumen

Lining epithelium

Suprabasal layers resemble stellate reticulum

Palisaded basal cells with hyperchromatic nuclei exhibiting reverse polarization

Fibrous connective tissue capsule

Fig. 13.7: Unicystic ameloblastoma—luminal type

totally or partially by ameloblastic epithelium, lining the cystic lumen. The epithelial lining has hyperchromatic basal cells exhibiting palisading arrangement and reverse polarization of the nucleus. The remaining layers resemble stellate reticulum.

Unicystic ameloblastoma—intraluminal type (Fig. 13.8): The cystic lining epithelium is thickened with projections extending into the lumen exhibiting ameloblastomatous proliferation that resembles the plexiform pattern seen in conventional ameloblastomas.

Unicystic ameloblastoma—mural type (Fig. 13.9): When the thickened lining exhibiting ameloblastomatous change penetrates

Identification Points (Fig. 13.8)

Unicystic Ameloblastoma—Intraluminal Type
- Cystic cavity lined by stratified squamous epithelium of variable thickness
- Projections of thickened epithelium extending into the lumen
- Epithelial projection showing ameloblastomatous proliferation

the adjacent capsular tissue, it is termed a mural type. The extent and depth of the ameloblastic infiltration may vary considerably.

Identification Points (Fig. 13.9)

Unicystic Ameloblastoma—Mural type
- Cystic cavity lined by stratified squamous epithelium of variable thickness
- Thickened lining epithelium exhibiting ameloblastomatous change penetrating the adjacent capsular tissue

CALCIFYING EPITHELIAL ODONTOGENIC TUMOR (PINDBORG'S TUMOR)

This benign epithelial odontogenic tumor is first described by Pindborg, so it is also called Pindborg's tumor. Clinically Pindborg's tumor may occur as extraosseous lesions manifesting as gingival swelling, or as intraosseous lesions. In intraosseous lesions present as asymptomatic slowly growing tumor of jaw bone, causing facial asymmetry. Radiographically this tumor shows 'driven snow' appearance.

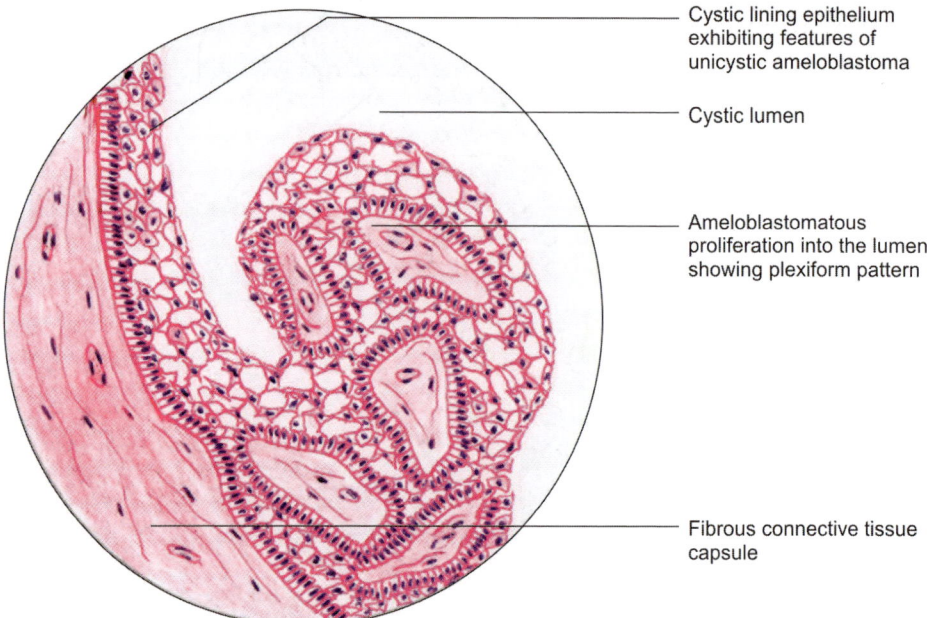

Fig. 13.8: Unicystic ameloblastoma—intraluminal type

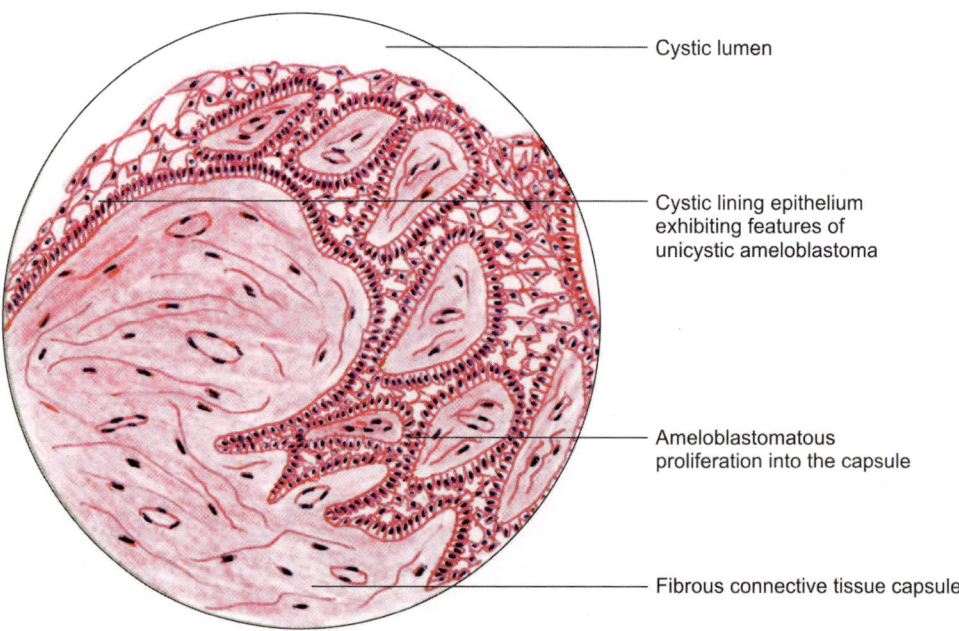

Fig. 13.9: Unicystic ameloblastoma—mural type

Histopathology (Fig. 13.10)

Calcifying epithelial odontogenic tumor is composed of sheets or islands of polyhedral odontogenic epithelial cells. These cells have distinct cellular outline and prominent inter-cellular bridges. The nuclei of these cells may show variation in size and shape, although mitotic figures are rare. The epithelial component encloses a homogeneous, eosinophilic amyloid like material. Another characteristic feature of Pindborg's tumor is calcifications that may be in the form of concentric rings called 'Liesegang ring' of calcification.

Connective tissue is bland and fibrous in nature.

Identification Points (Fig. 13.10)

Pindborg's Tumor
- Sheets of polyhedral cells with prominent inter-cellular bridges
- Nucleus shows pleomorphism
- Eosinophilic, amyloid like material among the cells
- Calcifications in the form of 'Liesegang ring'

ADENOMATOID ODONTOGENIC TUMOR

This is a benign epithelial odontogenic tumor which occurs commonly in the anterior region of maxilla, and present as asymptomatic lesion which may gradually produce facial asymmetry.

Histopathology (Fig. 13.11)

AOT is composed of epithelial cells, poly-hedral or spindle-shaped or ameloblast like cells arranged to form different patterns like island, sheets, strands, whorled mass, rosettes, duct-like pattern or convoluted pattern. One of the characteristic features of this tumor is duct-like or tubular arrangement of ameloblast like cells (therefore the name adenomatoid odontogenic tumor). The ameloblast like cells have nucleus arranged at the periphery away from the central space. The central space may

Identification Points (Fig. 13.11)

Adenomatoid Odontogenic Tumor
- Cells arranged in various patterns like strands, sheets, island etc.
- Ameloblast-like cells arranged to form duct-like pattern
- Amyloid-like material in the midst of cells
- Presence of scattered calcifications

contain eosinophilic material. Amorphous eosinophilic material also may be found in the midst of cells arranged as nests. Foci of calcification also may be scattered throughout the tumor. Connective tissue is scanty.

AMELOBLASTIC FIBROMA

Ameloblastic fibroma is a benign neoplasm of odontogenic epithelium and mesenchymal tissues, and therefore categorized as mixed odontogenic tumors. The lesion may occur in either jaw, more predominantly in the mandible, usually in the premolar-molar area. The tumor enlarges by gradual expansion to cause facial asymmetry and often follows an asymptomatic clinical course.

Histopathology (Fig. 13.12)

Microscopically, ameloblastic fibroma is characterized by the proliferation of odonto-genic epithelium supported by connective tissue stroma that resembles primitive

Identification Points (Fig. 13.12)

Ameloblastic Fibroma
- Proliferation of odontogenic epithelium and ectomesenchyme
- Connective tissue stroma resembles primitive ectomesenchyme/dental papilla of the developing tooth germ
- Odontogenic epithelial component as nests, buds, or cords
- No calcifications in connective tissue stroma

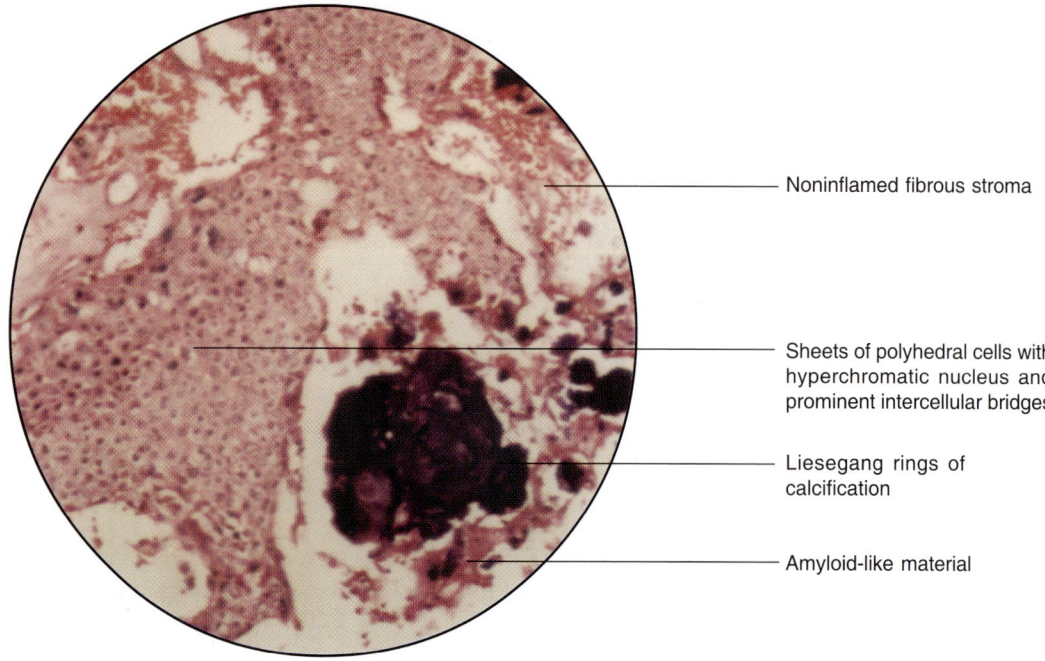

Noninflamed fibrous stroma

Sheets of polyhedral cells with hyperchromatic nucleus and prominent intercellular bridges

Liesegang rings of calcification

Amyloid-like material

Calcifying epithelial odontogenic tumor (photomicrograph 10X)

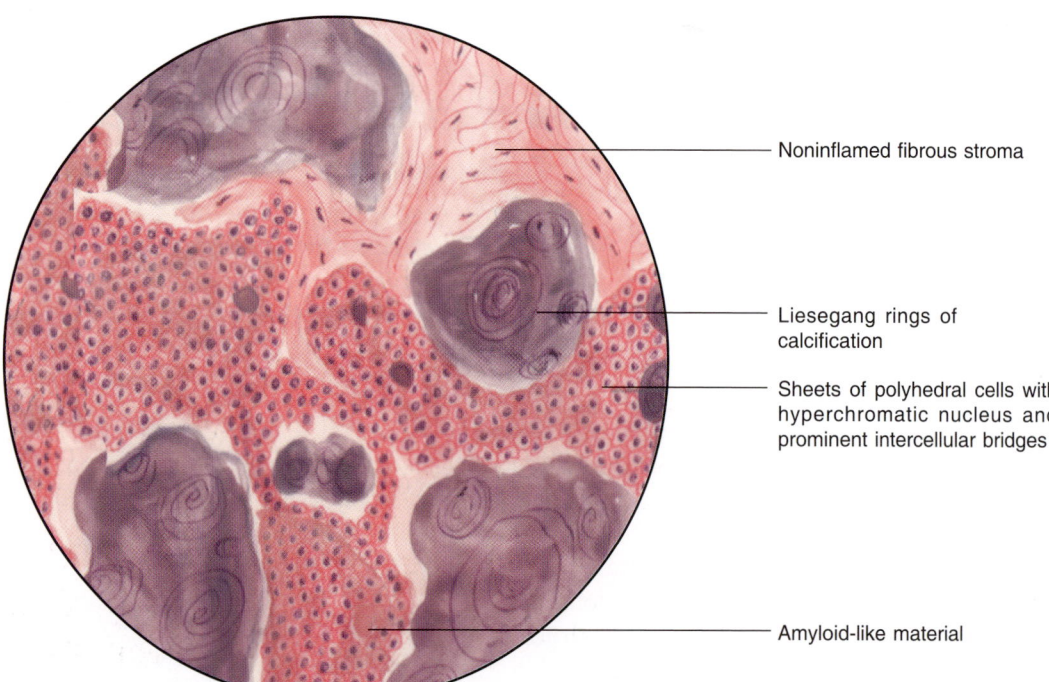

Noninflamed fibrous stroma

Liesegang rings of calcification

Sheets of polyhedral cells with hyperchromatic nucleus and prominent intercellular bridges

Amyloid-like material

Fig. 13.10: Calcifying epithelial odontogenic tumor

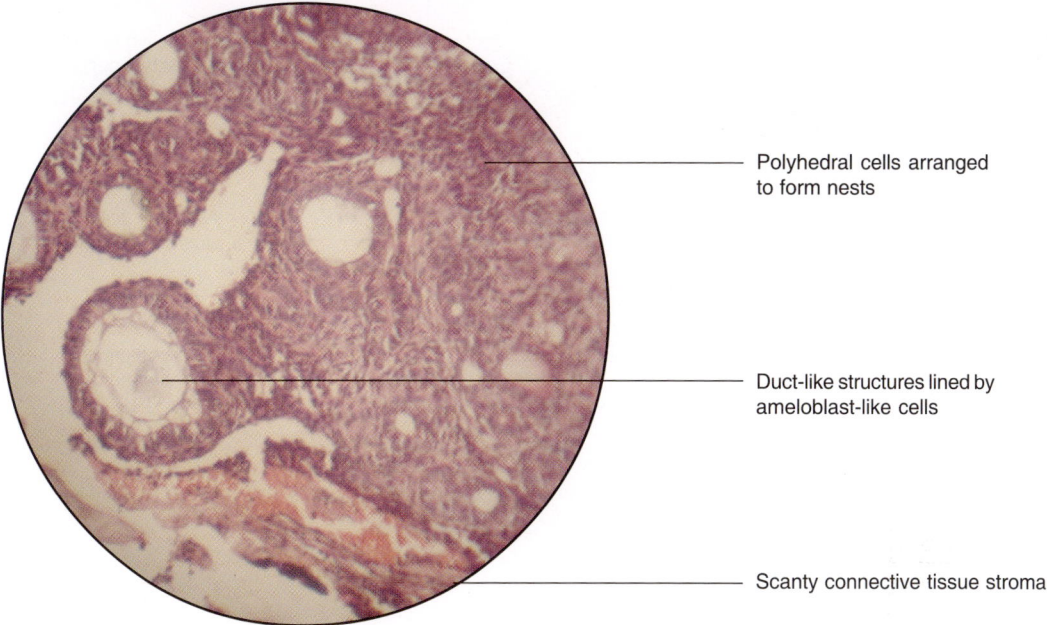

Polyhedral cells arranged to form nests

Duct-like structures lined by ameloblast-like cells

Scanty connective tissue stroma

Adenomatoid odontogenic tumor (photomicrograph 10X)

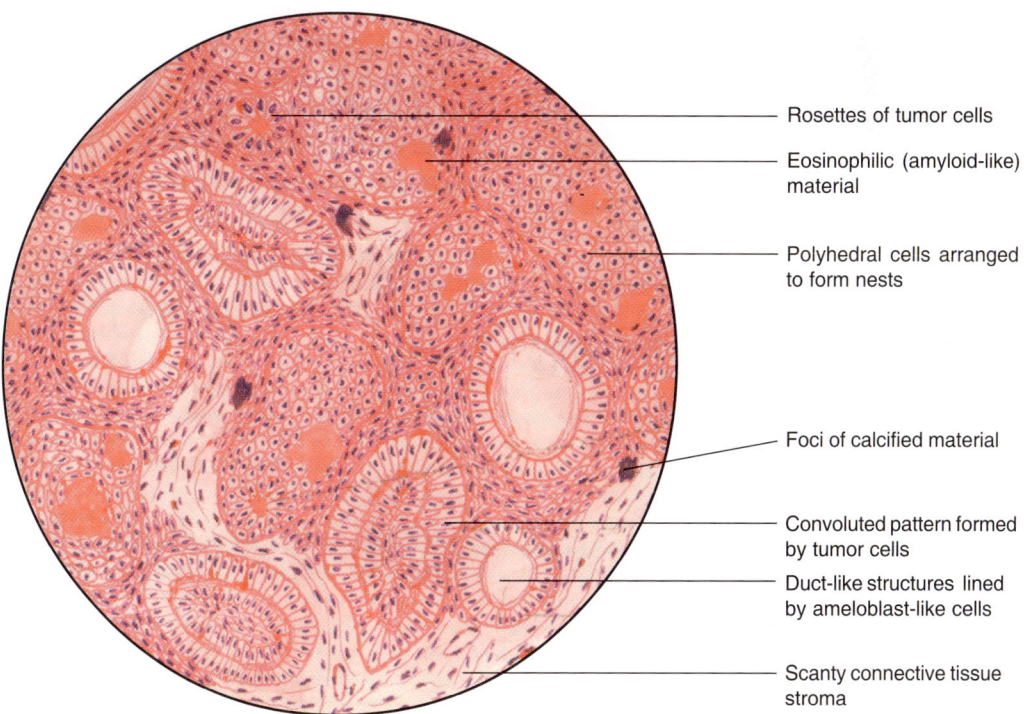

Rosettes of tumor cells

Eosinophilic (amyloid-like) material

Polyhedral cells arranged to form nests

Foci of calcified material

Convoluted pattern formed by tumor cells

Duct-like structures lined by ameloblast-like cells

Scanty connective tissue stroma

Fig. 13.11: Adenomatoid odontogenic tumor

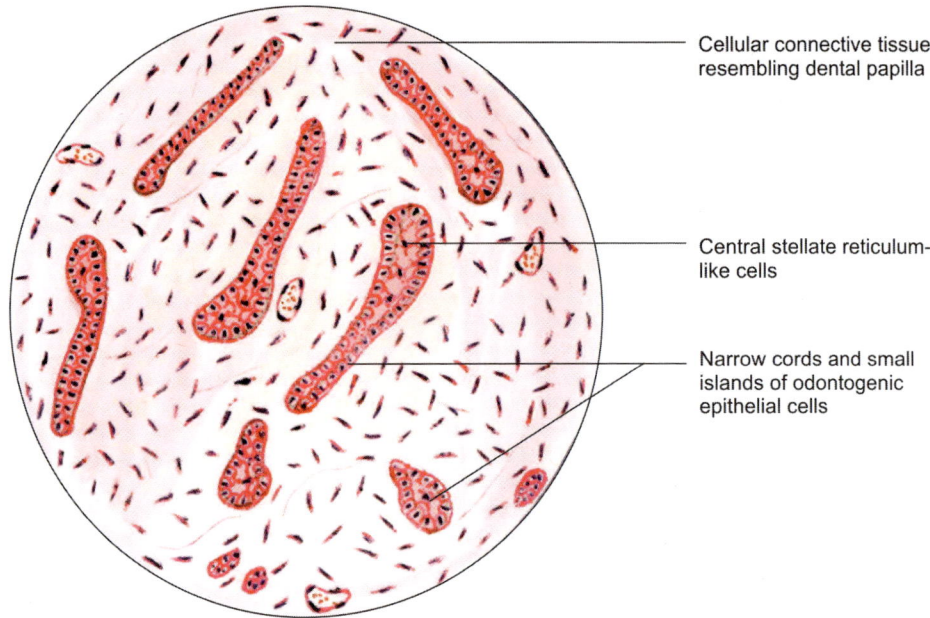

Cellular connective tissue resembling dental papilla

Central stellate reticulum-like cells

Narrow cords and small islands of odontogenic epithelial cells

Fig. 13.12: Ameloblastic fibroma

ectomesenchyme/dental papilla of the developing tooth germ. The mesenchymal component is highly cellular, composed of spindle-shaped cells with a little collagen, imparting a myxomatous appearance. The odontogenic epithelial component is made up of nests, buds, or cords of cuboidal/columnar hyperchromatic cells of two cell layers thick. Larger nests may show a central area of stellate reticulum. The ameloblastic fibroma contains no calcified tissue elements.

CENTRAL CEMENTIFYING FIBROMA

Central cementifying fibroma is a benign tumor of odontogenic mesenchymal origin. This lesion is considered as a fibro-osseous lesion. Clinically this tumor present as a central lesion of the bone that enlarges to cause facial asymmetry and displacement of the teeth.

Histopathology (Fig. 13.13)

Central cementifying fibroma is composed of highly cellular connective tissue that has large number of plump fibroblasts and cementoblasts. Foci of basophilic calcification (cementum like material) is scattered in this stroma. Calcifications may be round, ovoid or slightly irregular in shape. In mature lesions these cementum like materials fuse to form large mass. Some lesions may also show a few bony trabeculae along with cementum like material. Such lesions are called cemento-ossifying fibromas.

Identification Points (Fig. 13.13)

Central Cementifying Fibroma
- Highly cellular connective tissue
- Scattered cementum-like material in the stroma

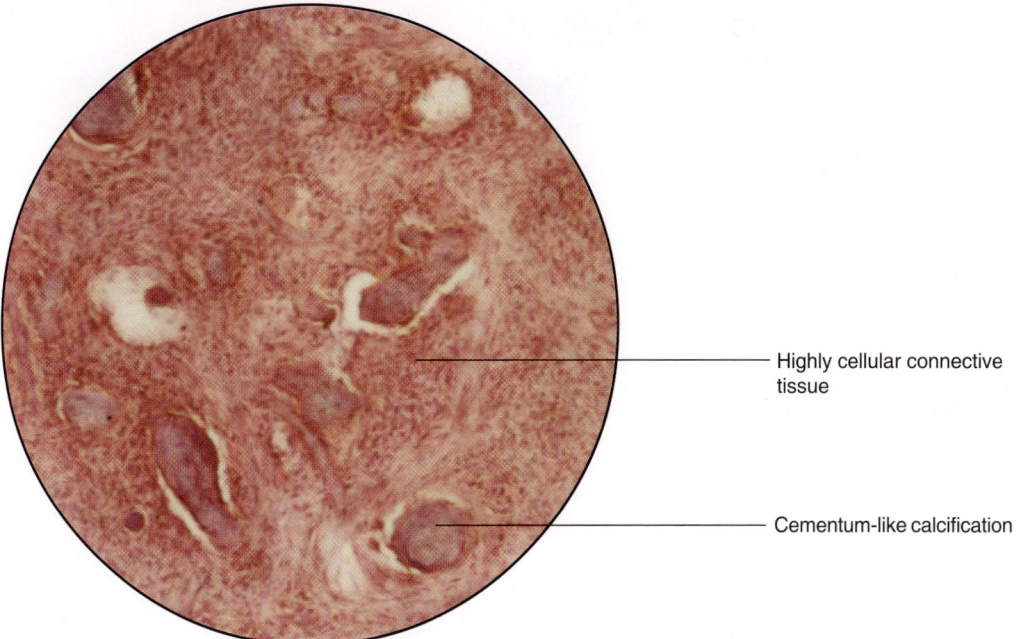

Highly cellular connective tissue

Cementum-like calcification

Central cementifying fibroma (photomicrograph 10X)

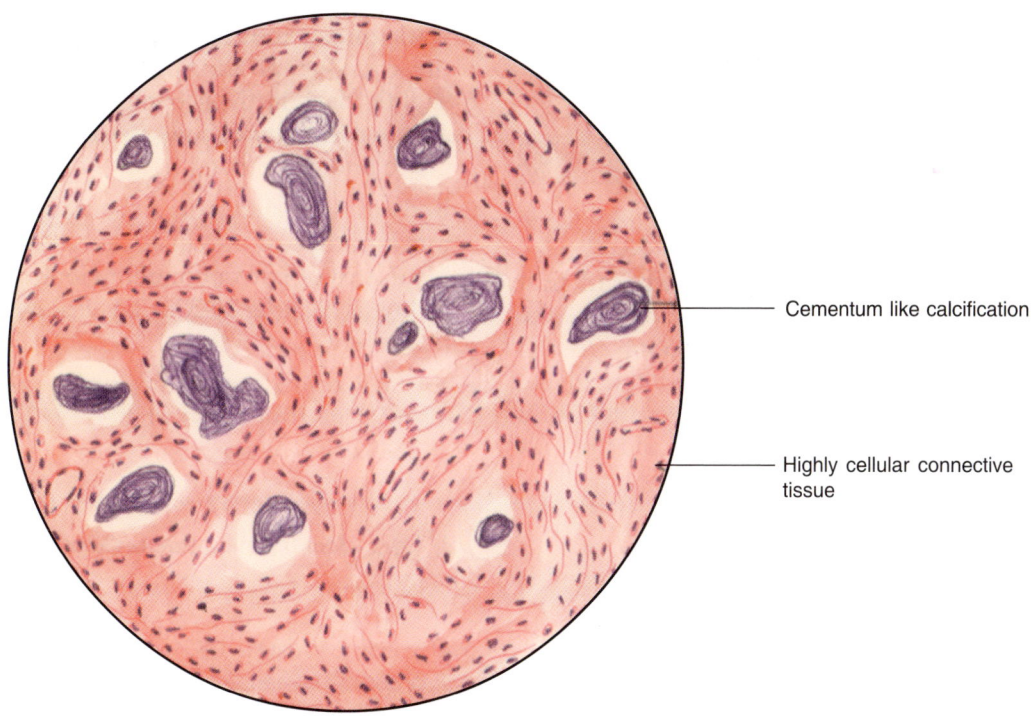

Cementum like calcification

Highly cellular connective tissue

Fig. 13.13: Central cementifying fibroma

14

Dental Caries

- Enamel caries
  - Pit and fissure
  - Smooth surface
- Dentinal caries

Dental caries is an irreversible, infectious, microbial disease affecting the hard tissue portion of the tooth exposed to the oral cavity, characterized by demineralization of inorganic components and destruction of organic components, resulting in cavitation.

ENAMEL CARIES

In enamel, caries process may start in the pits and fissures or in the smooth surface.

Caries in pit and fissures spread in a triangular pattern with the base towards the dentinoenamel junction and apex towards the surface. In smooth surface caries although the spread follows a triangular pattern the base is towards the surface of the enamel and the apex towards the dentinoenamel junction.

Histopathology

Microscopically both pit and fissure (Fig. 14.1) and smooth surface enamel caries (Fig. 14.2) shows four zones.

1. **Translucent zone:** This zone is the innermost zone at the advancing end of the caries. This zone is not always present.

Identification Points (Fig. 14.1)

Enamel Caries (Pit and Fissure)
- Triangular in shape with base towards the DEJ and apex towards the surface
- *Four zones are seen*: Translucent zone, dark zone, body of the lesion and surface zone
- Striae of Retzius is prominent in the body of lesion

2. **Dark zone** is the zone immediately above the translucent zone and this appears slightly dark in the section. Dark zone is always present and shows positive birefringence under polarized light.

3. **Body of the lesion:** This zone occupies the major portion of the caries lesion and this is the area of maximum demineralization. In this zone striae of Retzius appear more prominent.

4. **Surface zone:** This is the intact zone of 40 microns thickness at the surface of enamel caries lesion.

Identification Points (Fig. 14.2)

Enamel Caries (Smooth Surface)
- Triangular shape with base towards the surface and apex towards the DEJ
- *Four zones are seen*: Translucent zone, dark zone, body of the lesion and surface zone
- Striae of Retzius is prominent in the body of lesion

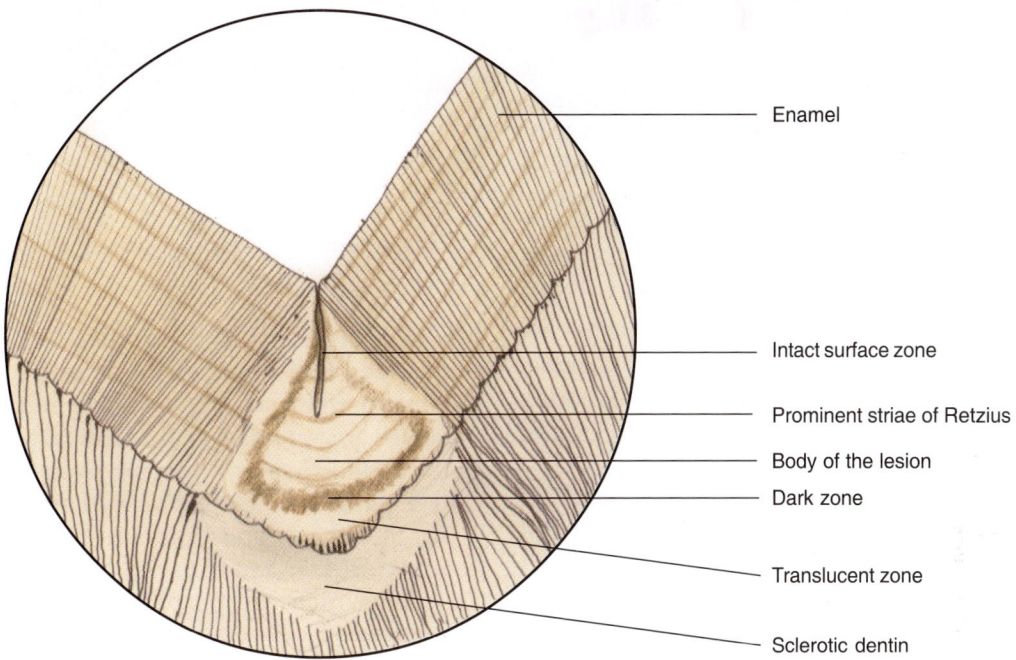

Fig. 14.1: Enamel caries (pit and fissure—ground section)

Enamel

Intact surface zone

Prominent striae of Retzius

Body of the lesion

Dark zone

Translucent zone

Sclerotic dentin

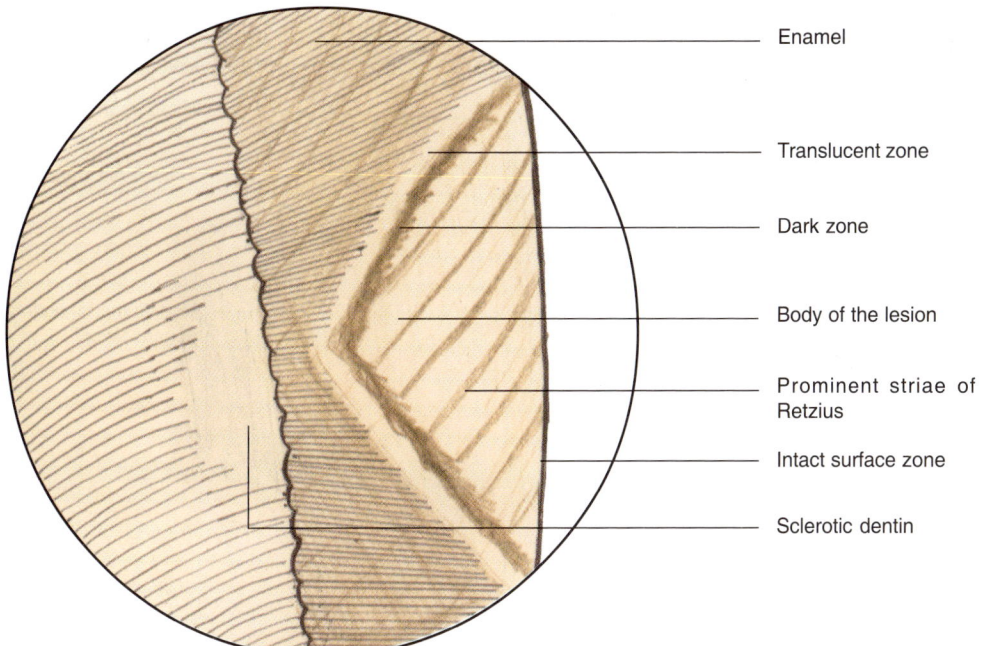

Enamel

Translucent zone

Dark zone

Body of the lesion

Prominent striae of Retzius

Intact surface zone

Sclerotic dentin

Fig. 14. 2: Enamel caries (smooth surface—ground section)

DENTINAL CARIES

Once the caries process spreads to dentin, the microorganisms invade the dentinal tubules and release acids. The spread of caries follows a triangular pattern with the base towards the dentino-enamel junction and apex towards the pulp. Apex will be located more apical to the base.

Histopathology (Fig. 14.3)

Microscopically five different zones are seen:
1. Zone of fatty degeneration of Tomes' dentinal fibers is the initial change seen at the advancing front of dentinal caries near the pulpal surface. In this zone deposition of fat globules are seen in the odontoblast process.
2. Translucent zone where the dentinal tubules are sclerosed.
3. Zone of demineralization in which the dentin shows decalcification without evidence of bacterial invasion.
4. *Zone of bacterial invasion*: In this zone dentin is intact but shows dense bacterial invasion of dentinal tubules. The walls of dentinal

Identification Points (Fig. 14.3)

Dentinal Caries
Five zones are seen:
- Zone of fatty degeneration
- Zone of dentinal sclerosis
- Zone of demineralization
- Zone of bacterial invasion
- Zone of decomposed dentin

tubules are softened due to demineralization and get distorted by the dense packing of microorganisms. The resulting elliptical-shaped areas parallel to the dentinal tubules are called 'Miller's foci of liquefaction degeneration. Lateral spread of organisms through the lateral branches of dentinal tubules results in formation of 'transverse clefts' which are perpendicular to the tubules.
5. *Zone of decomposed dentin*: This is the most superficial layer of dentinal caries where the architecture of dentin is lost due to bacterial destruction.

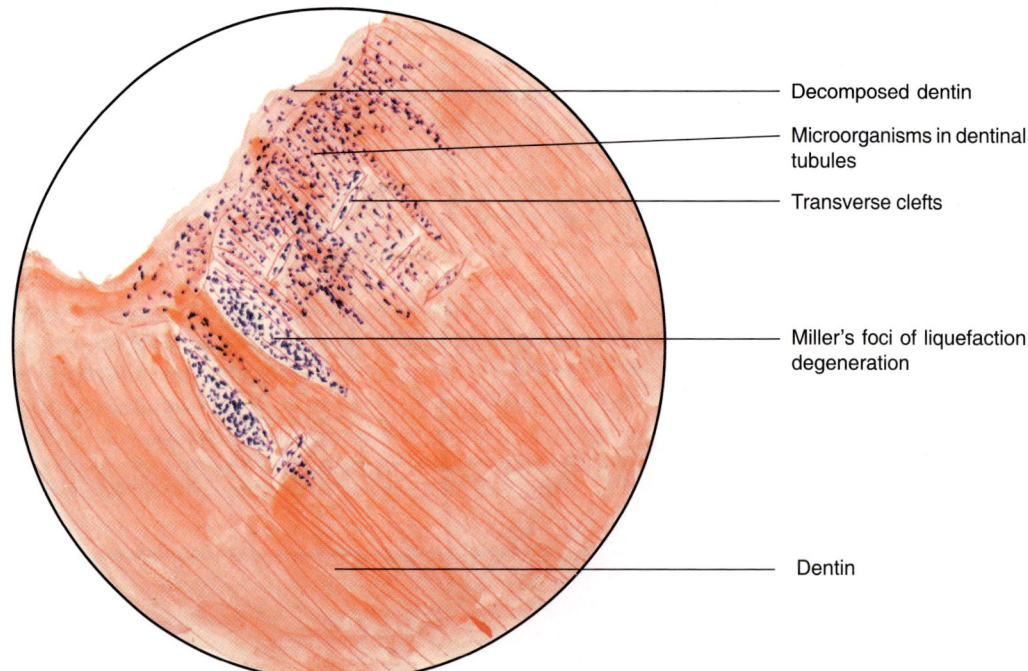

Fig. 14.3: Dentinal caries (decalcified section)

Labels: Decomposed dentin; Microorganisms in dentinal tubules; Transverse clefts; Miller's foci of liquefaction degeneration; Dentin

15

Pulp and Periapical Lesions

- Pulpal hyperemia
- Pulp abscess
- Pulp polyp
- Periapical granuloma

Pulp is vital tissue and it responds to bacterial infection or any other stimulus by an inflammatory reaction. Inflammation of pulp is called pulpitis and this can be acute or chronic, may involve focal area (partial or focal pulpitis) or most of the pulp tissue (total or generalized pulpitis).

PULP HYPEREMIA (FOCAL REVERSIBLE PULPITIS)

This is the earliest form of pulpitis. This condition is also called reversible pulpitis because the changes are reversible if irritants are removed before the pulp is severely damaged. The affected tooth is sensitive to thermal stimulus which disappears after the removal of the stimulus.

Histopathology (Fig. 15.1)

Characteristic microscopic feature is multiple dilated blood vessels filled with RBCs. Pulp

may also show edematous changes, extravasation of RBCs and a few inflammatory cells.

ACUTE PULPITIS (PULP ABSCESS)

Acute pulpitis may be a sequel to focal reversible pulpitis or due to acute exacerbation of chronic pulpitis. This condition is associated with severe lancinating pain. Tooth is sensitive to thermal changes which persists even after the removal of the stimulus.

Histopathology (Fig. 15.2)

Microscopically acute pulpitis is characterized by infiltration of polymorphs in the pulpal tissue. There may be localized destruction of pulpal tissue and formation of pulp abscess. Pulp abscess contain pus arising from break down of leukocytes, bacteria and tissue. Pulp abscess is seen as a small void surrounded by dense band of leukocytic infiltration. The odontoblasts near the region of the abscess undergo degeneration. Adjacent pulpal tissue may show hyperemic changes.

Identification Points (Fig. 15.1)

Pulp Hyperemia
- Multiple dilated capillaries filled with RBCs
- Edematous changes in the pulp tissue
- Presence of inflammatory cells

Identification Points (Fig. 15.2)

Pulp Abscess
- Abscess is seen as small void
- Dense inflammatory cell infiltration around the abscess
- Hyperemic changes in the surrounding areas

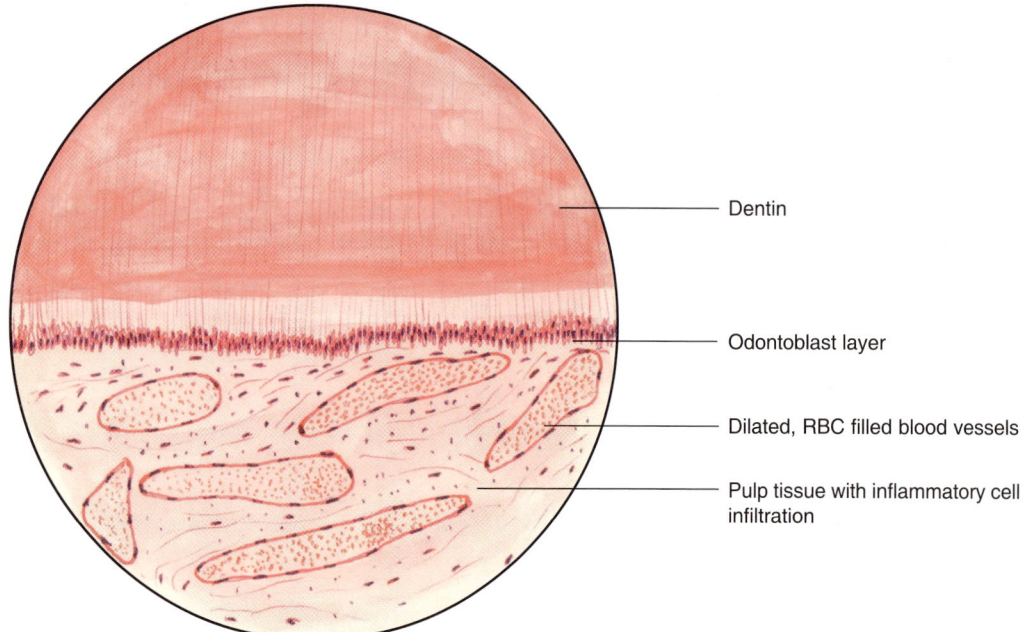

Fig. 15.1: Pulp hyperemia

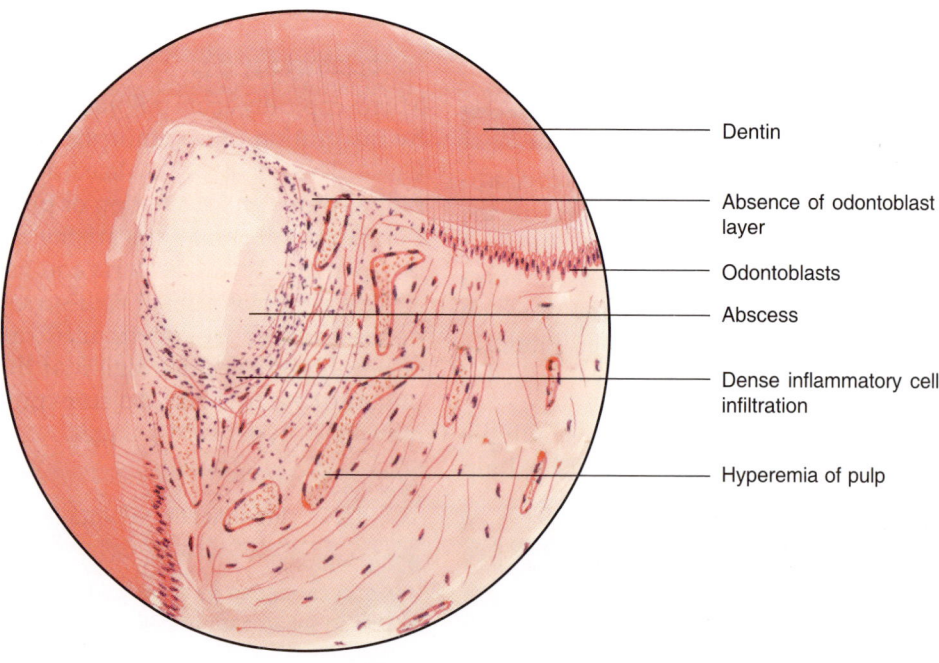

Fig. 15.2: Pulp abscess

CHRONIC HYPERPLASTIC PULPITIS (PULP POLYP)

This is a specific type of pulpitis in which pulp respond with an exuberant proliferation, to an irritation or stimulus. Most commonly involved teeth are deciduous molars and first permanent molars. These teeth have excellent blood supply due to large apical foramen. This, along with high tissue resistance in young individuals lead to proliferation of pulp. Clinically pulp polyp presents as a pink soft tissue mass filling the large carious lesion.

Histopathology (Fig. 15.3)

Microscopically pulp polyp present as granulation tissue covered by stratified squamous epithelium. Granulation tissue comprises delicate connective tissue exhibiting proliferating endothelial cells, budding capillaries and chronic inflammatory cells. Continuity to the pulpal tissue is evident which also shows inflammatory cell infiltration.

Identification Points (Fig. 15.3)

Pulp Polyp
- Chronic proliferative reaction of pulp
- Granulation tissue covered by epithelium
- Connection to pulp is seen

PERIAPICAL GRANULOMA

Periapical granuloma is a sequel to pulpitis that occur as a collection of granulation tissue at the root apex (periapical—around the apex). The affected tooth is nonvital but relatively asymptomatic and this condition is identified in radiograph as a well-defined radiolucency, often less than 2 cm size.

Histopathology (Fig. 15.4)

Histopathologically periapical granuloma comprises granulation tissue attached to the root apex. Granulation tissue exhibits mixed inflammatory cell infiltrate consisting of lymphocytes, plasma cells, histiocytes and a few polymorphonuclear leukocytes. A few giant cells, cholesterol clefts, Russel bodies (collection of gamma globulins produced by plasma cells) and a few epithelial cell rests of Malassez are also seen in granulation tissue.

Identification Points (Fig. 15.4)

Periapical Granuloma
- Granulation tissue attached to the root apex
- Mixed inflammatory cells, cholesterol clefts and Russel bodies may be seen
- Epithelial cell rests of Malassez may be present

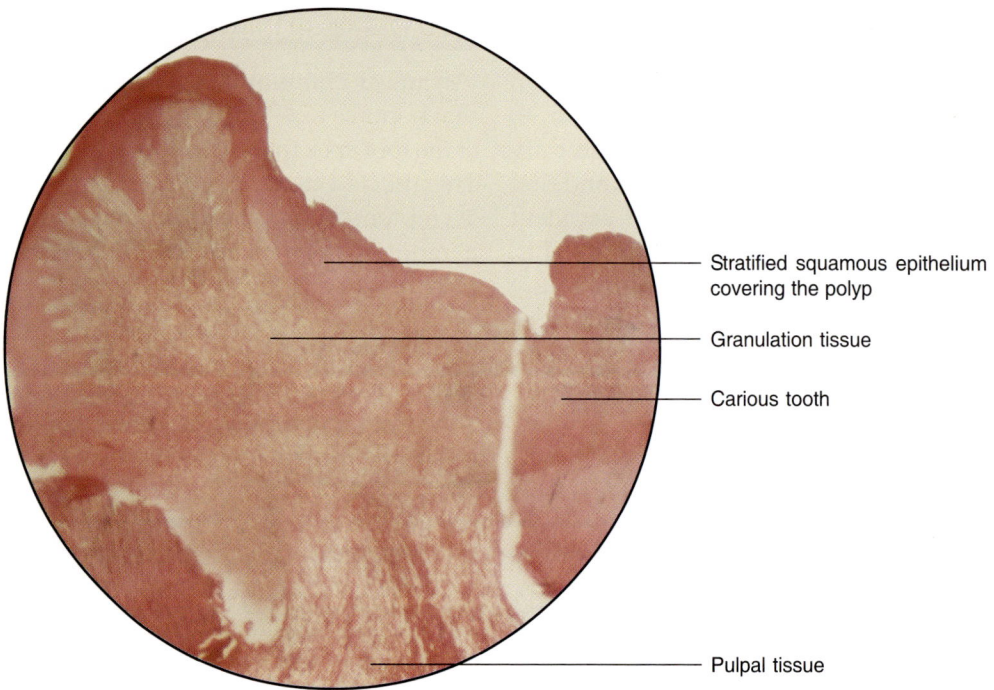

Stratified squamous epithelium covering the polyp

Granulation tissue

Carious tooth

Pulpal tissue

Pulp polyp (photomicrograph 4X)

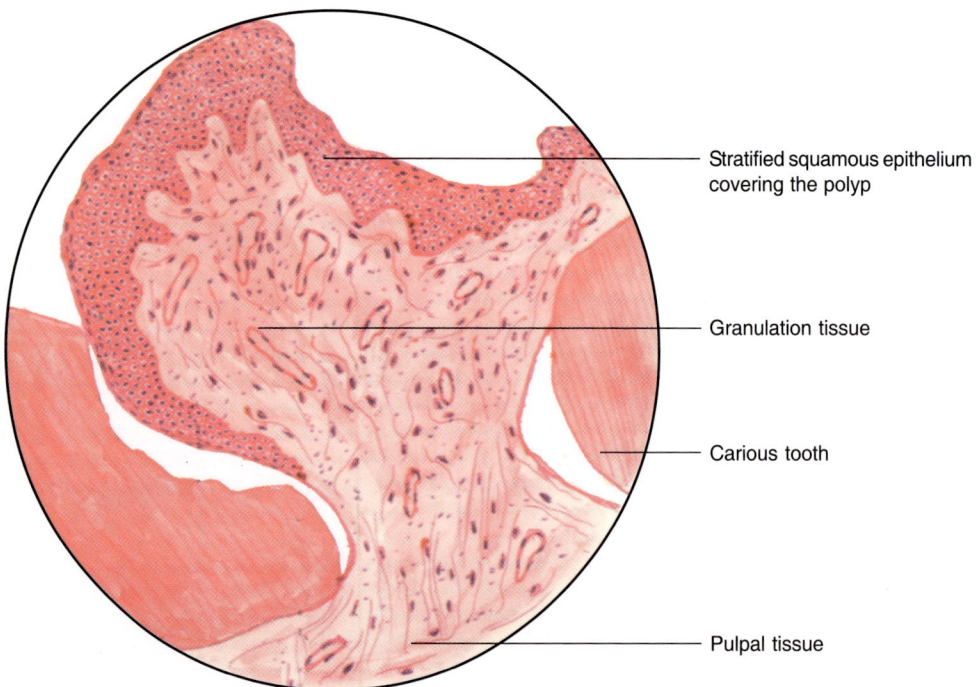

Stratified squamous epithelium covering the polyp

Granulation tissue

Carious tooth

Pulpal tissue

Fig. 15.3: Pulp polyp

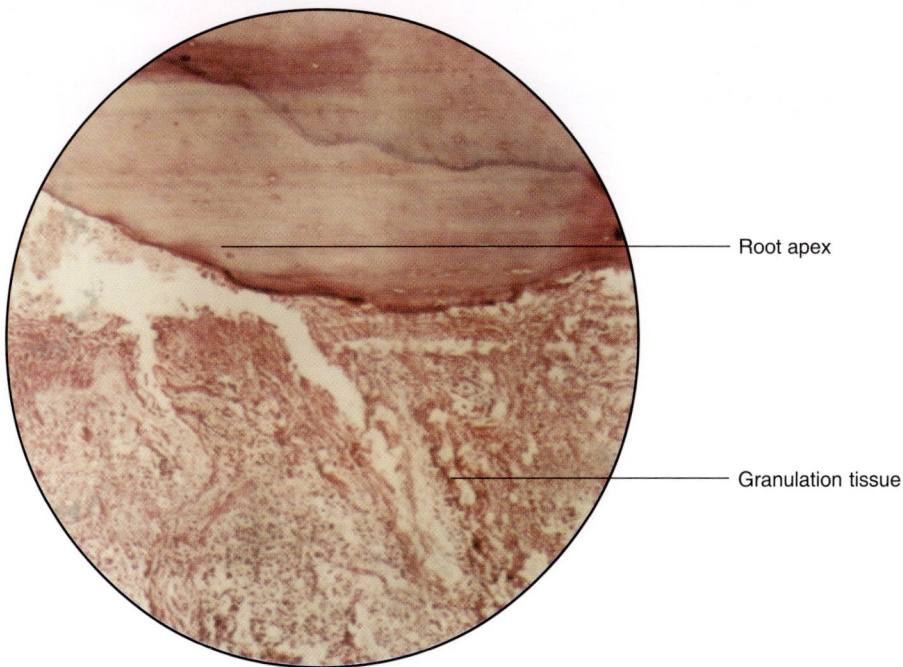

Root apex

Granulation tissue

Periapical granuloma (photomicrograph 4X)

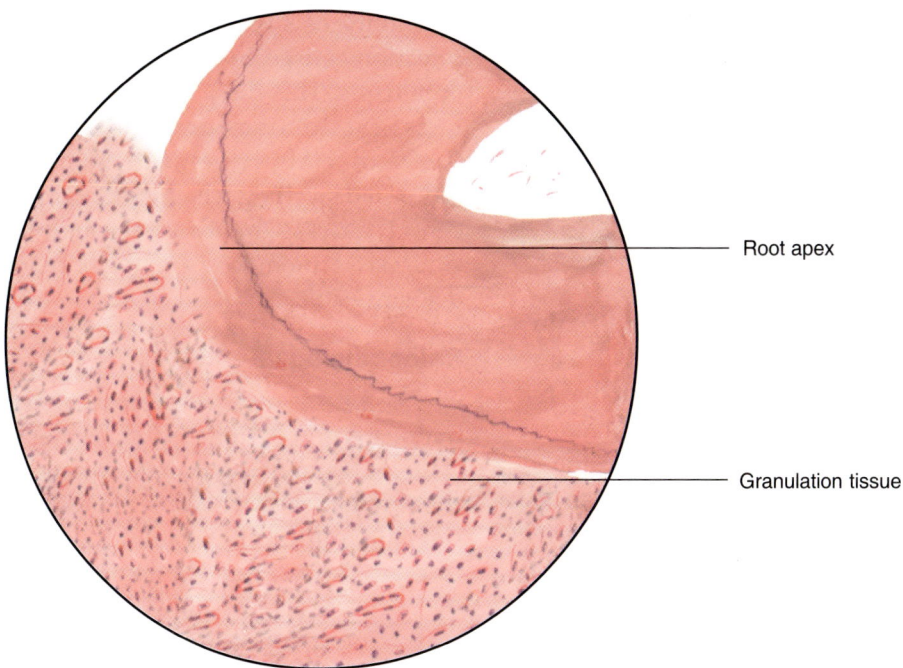

Root apex

Granulation tissue

Fig. 15.4: Periapical granuloma

16

Bacterial and Fungal Infections

- Tuberculosis
- Actinomycosis
- Candidiasis

TUBERCULOSIS

Tuberculosis is a specific bacterial infection caused by *Mycobacterium tuberculosis*. Oral tuberculosis usually represents secondary infection from pulmonary lesions. Common oral manifestation is in the form of oral ulceration, mainly involving the tongue. Tuberculosis also manifest in the oral cavity as tubercular gingivitis, tubercular granuloma and osteomyelitis. Cervical lymph node involvement is referred to as scrofula.

Histopathology (Fig. 16.1)

Microscopic presentation of tuberculosis is in the form of granulomas, which are circumscribed lesions. These granulomas have a central area of caseous necrosis surrounded by multinucleated giant cells and epithelioid cells. The nuclei of multinucleated giant cells are seen at the periphery, having a horse shoe shaped arrangement and these cells are called Langhans' giant cells. This is surrounded by a zone of lymphocytic infiltration and fibrosis. Tubercular organisms may be demonstrated by Ziehl-Neelsen or other acid-fast stains.

Identification Points (Fig. 16.1)

Tuberculosis
- Granuloma with central caseation necrosis
- Presence of Langhans' giant cells and epithelioid cells
- Peripheral zone of lymphocytes

ACTINOMYCOSIS

Actinomycosis is a chronic granulomatous infection caused by Actinomyces species of organisms. This disease manifest as cervico-facial, abdominal or pulmonary forms. Cervicofacial actinomycosis manifest as indurated swelling which eventually develop central abscess that drain through multiple sinuses. Actinomycosis may also manifest as osteomyelitis.

Histopathology (Fig. 16.2)

Classic lesions of actinomycosis are granulomatous with central abscess formation. The central area may show characteristic colonies that appear to be floating in a collection of polymorphonuclear leukocytes. These colonies appear round or lobulated and made up of meshwork of filamentous organisms that stain hematoxylin and show eosinophilia of peripheral clubs. Since the colonies have peripheral radiating filaments forming a

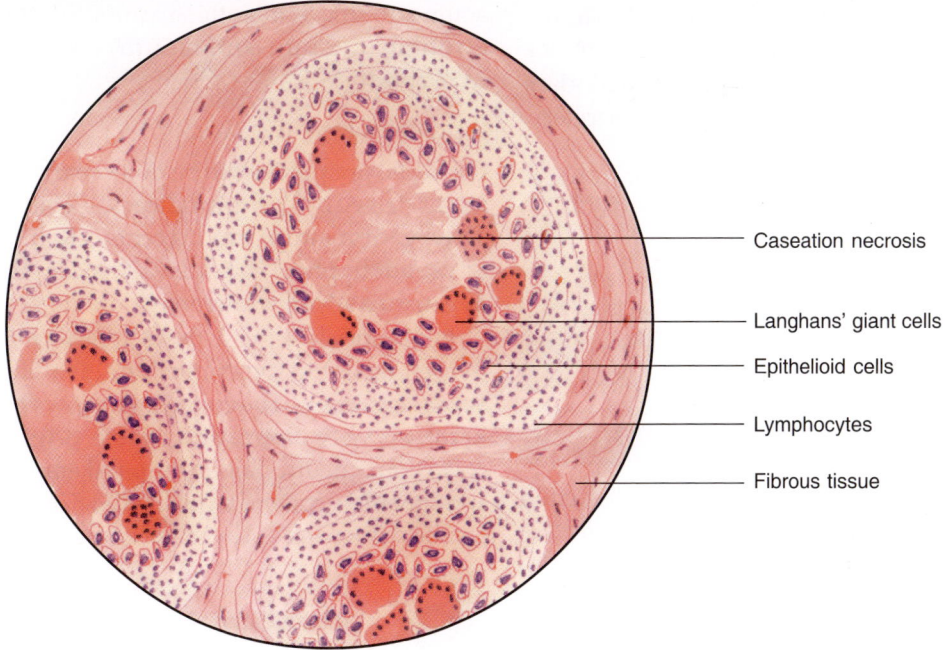

Caseation necrosis

Langhans' giant cells

Epithelioid cells

Lymphocytes

Fibrous tissue

Fig. 16.1: Tubercular granuloma

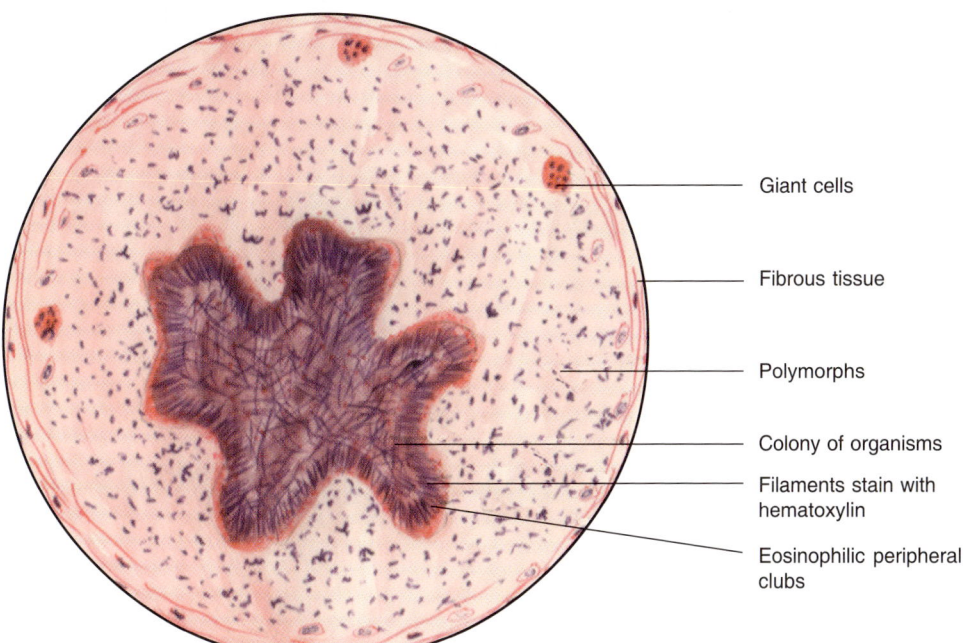

Giant cells

Fibrous tissue

Polymorphs

Colony of organisms

Filaments stain with hematoxylin

Eosinophilic peripheral clubs

Fig. 16. 2: Actinomycosis

rosette pattern, these are referred to as 'ray fungus'. Around the polymorphs there is a zone of histiocytes and multinucleated giant cells. A zone of fibrosis is seen at the periphery.

Identification Points (Fig. 16.2)

Actinomycosis
- Colony of organisms described as 'ray fungus'
- Organisms surrounded by polymorphs
- Presence of a few multinucleated giant cells and histiocytes

CANDIDIASIS

Candidiasis is the commonest fungal infection affecting oral cavity caused by *Candida albicans* and other related organisms. *Candida albicans* are the commensal organisms of the oral cavity. Invasion of the oral mucosa by these organisms occur in certain conditions, producing candidiasis. Although there are various predisposing factors, the most important one is immunosuppression.

Oral candidiasis may manifest in different forms—acute pseudomembranous (thrush), acute atrophic (antibiotic sore mouth), chronic atrophic (denture sore mouth) and chronic hyperplastic.

Histopathology (Fig. 16.3)

Candidal organisms can be demonstrated in a smear stained by PAS (periodic acid–Schiff) stain. The organisms appear as magenta color hyphae or pseudohyphae. Hyphae vary in length and approximately of 2 microns in diameter.

In a biopsy specimen, these hyphae are seen perpendicular to the epithelium invading the superficial layers. The epithelium shows hyperkeratosis with elongation of rete ridges and collection of neutrophils in the parakeratin layer and superficial spinous layer. Candidal organisms can be demonstrated by silver stains also.

Identification Points (Fig. 16.3)

Candidiasis
- PAS positive candidal hyphae invading the epithelium
- Epithelium may show hyperkeratosis and elongated rete ridges
- Collection of neutrophils in the epithelium

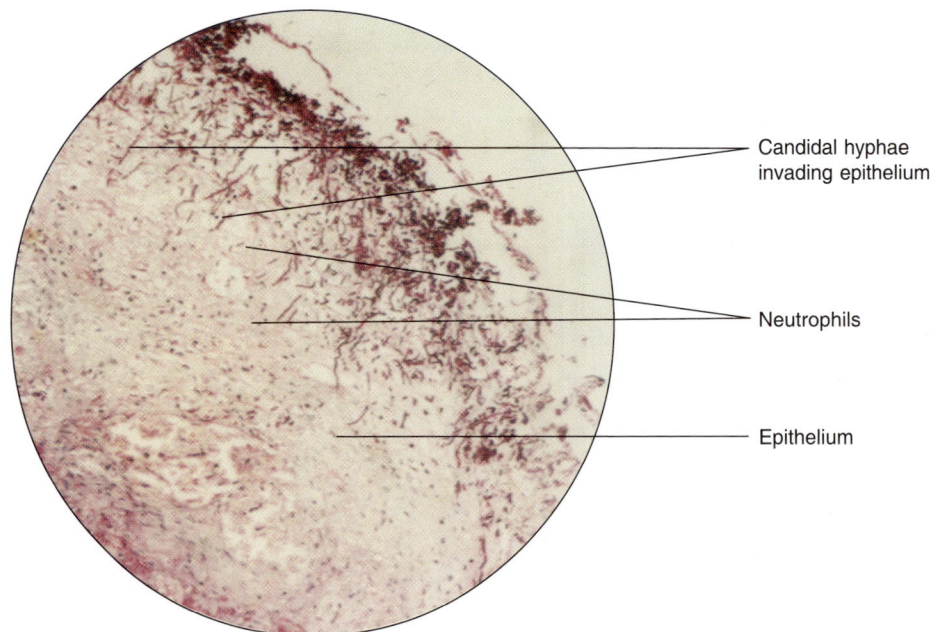

Candidal hyphae invading epithelium

Neutrophils

Epithelium

Candidiasis (PAS stain) (photomicrograph 10X)

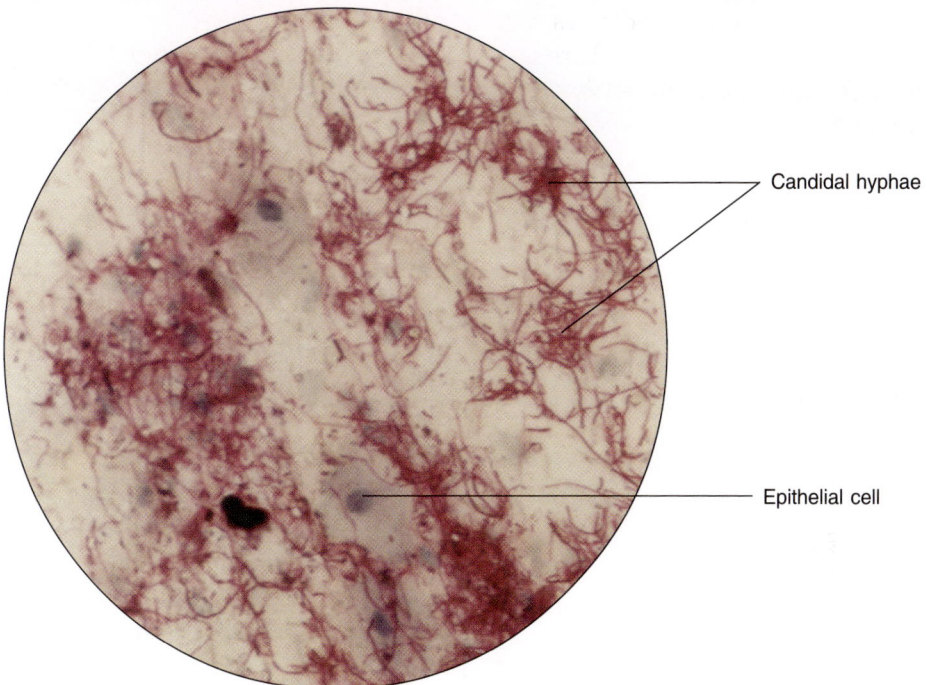

Candidal hyphae

Epithelial cell

Candidal hyphae in PAS stained smear preparation (photomicrograph 10X)

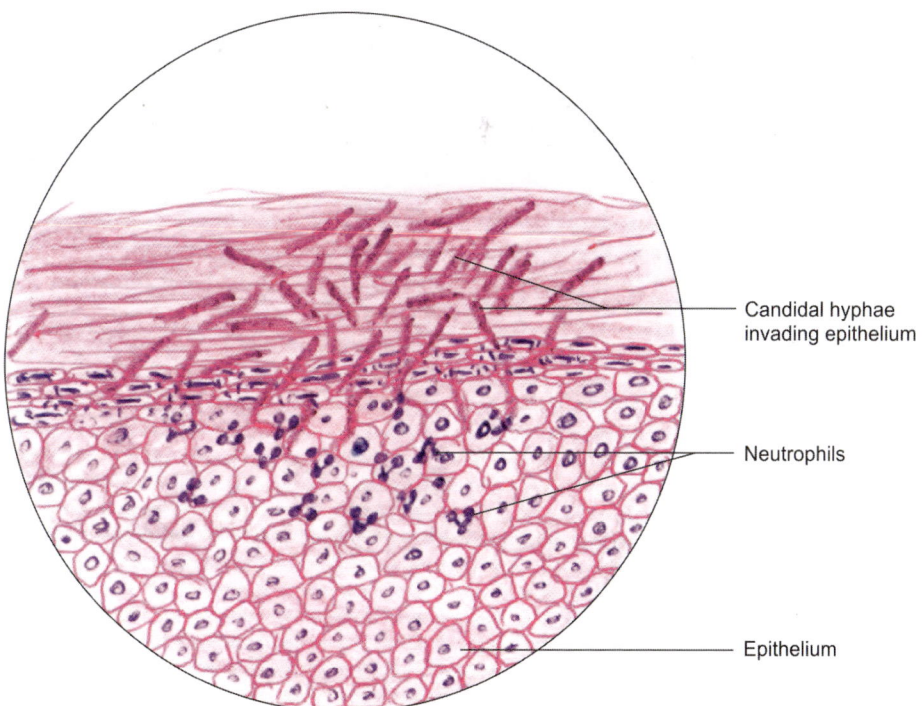

Candidal hyphae
invading epithelium

Neutrophils

Epithelium

Fig. 16.3: Candidiasis (PAS stain)

17

Salivary Gland Neoplasms

- Pleomorphic adenoma
- Warthin's tumor
- Adenoid cystic carcinoma
- Mucoepidermoid carcinoma

Salivary gland tumors constitute major group of neoplasms of oral cavity. These may be broadly classified into benign or malignant neoplasms based on the biological behavior.

PLEOMORPHIC ADENOMA

Pleomorphic adenoma is the commonest benign salivary gland neoplasm mainly affecting parotid gland. It is also called mixed tumor of salivary gland because of presence of different types of tissues observed in a microscopic section. Clinically this lesion presents as slow growing painless firm mass without fixation to the surrounding structures.

Histopathology (Fig. 17.1)

Pleomorphic adenoma is a well circumscribed tumor with complete or partial encapsulation with dense fibrous tissue. Tumor has epithelial and mesenchymal components. Epithelial components include proliferating ductal and myoepithelial cells, forming ductal structures containing eosinophilic material. These cells

also may form sheets, strands or islands. Ductal cells are cuboidal in shape with scanty cytoplasm. Myoepithelial cells have varying morphology, angular, spindle-shaped or plasmacytoid appearance. Metaplastic changes of epithelial component may lead to formation of squamous cells, sometimes even with keratin pearl formation. This lesion also shows mesenchymal components in the form of loose myxoid tissue or mucoid, chondroid or osseous areas and foci of hyalinized connective tissue.

Identification Points (Fig. 17.1)

Pleomorphic Adenoma
- Mixture of different types of tissues
- Cells arranged in cords, sheets or duct-like pattern containing eosinophilic material
- Myxoid, chondroid, osseous, mucoid or hyalinized areas of connective tissue

WARTHIN'S TUMOR (PAPILLARY CYSTADENOMA LYMPHOMATOSUM)

This is a benign tumor of salivary gland, mainly involving the parotid gland. Warthin's tumor usually present as a slow growing, painless, nodular mass of the parotid gland, firm or fluctuant, affecting elderly individuals.

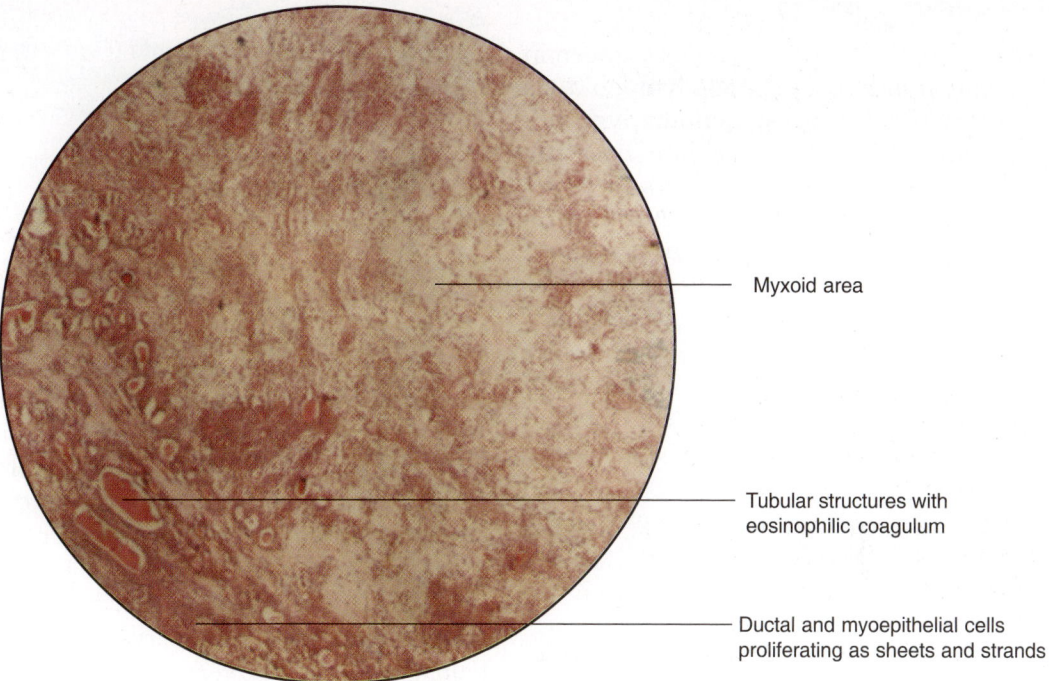

— Myxoid area

— Tubular structures with eosinophilic coagulum

— Ductal and myoepithelial cells proliferating as sheets and strands

Pleomorphic adenoma (photomicrograph 10X)

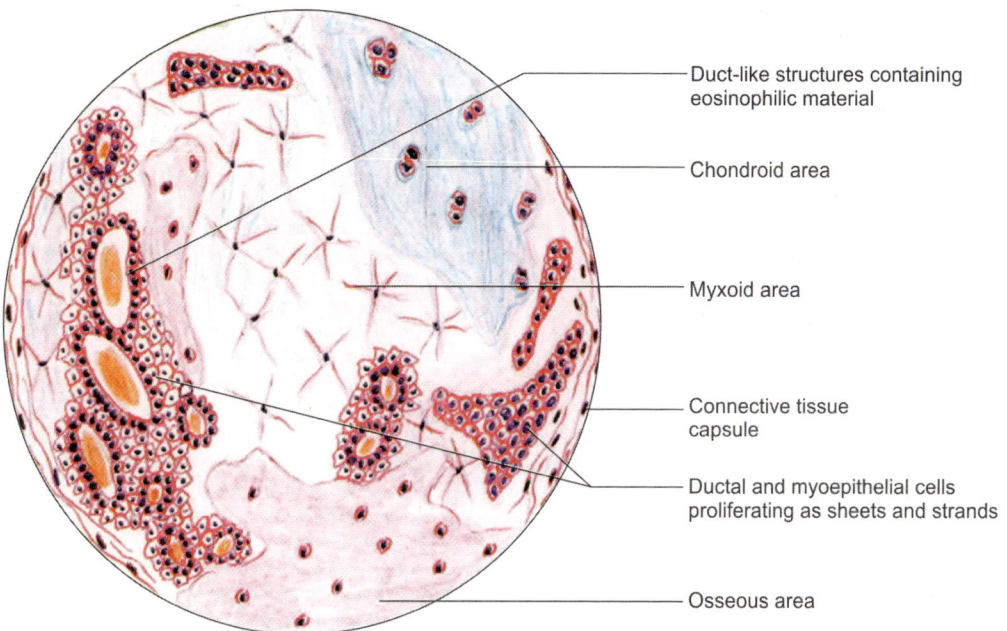

— Duct-like structures containing eosinophilic material

— Chondroid area

— Myxoid area

— Connective tissue capsule

— Ductal and myoepithelial cells proliferating as sheets and strands

— Osseous area

Fig. 17.1: Pleomorphic adenoma

Histopathology (Fig. 17.2)

Microscopically two components are seen in Warthin's tumor, epithelial and lymphoid. As the name papillary cystadenoma lymphomatosum indicates, this lesion is basically cystic, with papillary processes lined by epithelium, projecting in to the cystic space. Connective tissue has abundant lymphoid component exhibiting germinal center.

Epithelium lining the papillary projections is bilayered with inner cuboidal cells and outer columnar cells. Columnar cells are regularly arranged having palisading arrangement of nuclei. Cystic space may contain eosinophilic material.

Identification Points (Fig. 17.2)

Warthin's Tumor
- Papillary projections into cystic spaces
- Bilayered epithelium lining the projections with inner cuboidal and outer columnar cells
- Lymphoid component exhibiting germinal centers

ADENOID CYSTIC CARCINOMA (CYLINDROMA)

Adenoid cystic carcinoma is a malignant salivary gland tumor. Clinically this tumor present with slow growing swelling which may show typical features of malignancy like, local pain fixation to surrounding structures, surface ulceration, facial nerve paralysis, etc.

Histopathology (Fig. 17.3)

The tumor is composed of uniform cells, resembling basal cells arranged in anastomosing cords or duct-like pattern. Some of these duct-like areas contain a mucoid material. The above mentioned feature gives rise to the characteristic appearance described as cribriform, 'honeycomb' or 'Swiss cheese' pattern. There may be areas where the cells show a tubular or more solid pattern. The connective tissue component is often hyalinized, and surrounding the tumor cells, forming a structural pattern of cylinders. The term cylindroma is given because of this cylindrical pattern.

Identification Points (Fig. 17.3)

Adenoid Cystic Carcinoma
- 'Cribriform' or 'Swiss cheese' pattern
- Uniform tumor cells resembling basal cells
- Hyalinized connective tissue

MUCOEPIDERMOID CARCINOMA

Mucoepidermoid carcinoma is a malignant salivary gland neoplasm arising from epithelium of large ducts of salivary glands. Although parotid is commonly affected, minor salivary glands also may be involved. Clinical features can vary depending on grades of malignancy. Low grade lesions are slow growing and painless. High grade lesions on the other hand show rapid growth, fixation to adjacent structures, facial nerve paralysis and pain as an early symptom.

Histopathology (Fig. 17.4)

Microscopically 3 types of cells are seen, dispersed in connective tissue stroma. One type is the epidermoid cells which are squamous with distinct intercellular bridges, rarely with evidence of keratin formation. Another type is mucus secreting cells which are ovoid, filled with mucin and peripherally placed nucleus. These cells appear as clear cells in H & E stained sections and positively stain with PAS and mucicarmine stain. Intermediate cells are another type of cells, ovoid with small darkly staining nucleus and scanty eosinophilic cytoplasm.

Identification Points (Fig. 17.4)

Mucoepidermoid Carcinoma
- Three types of cells, mucous secreting cells, epidermoid cells, intermediate cells
- Cystic spaces containing PAS positive mucin material
- Histologically lesions can be graded into low, intermediate or high grade

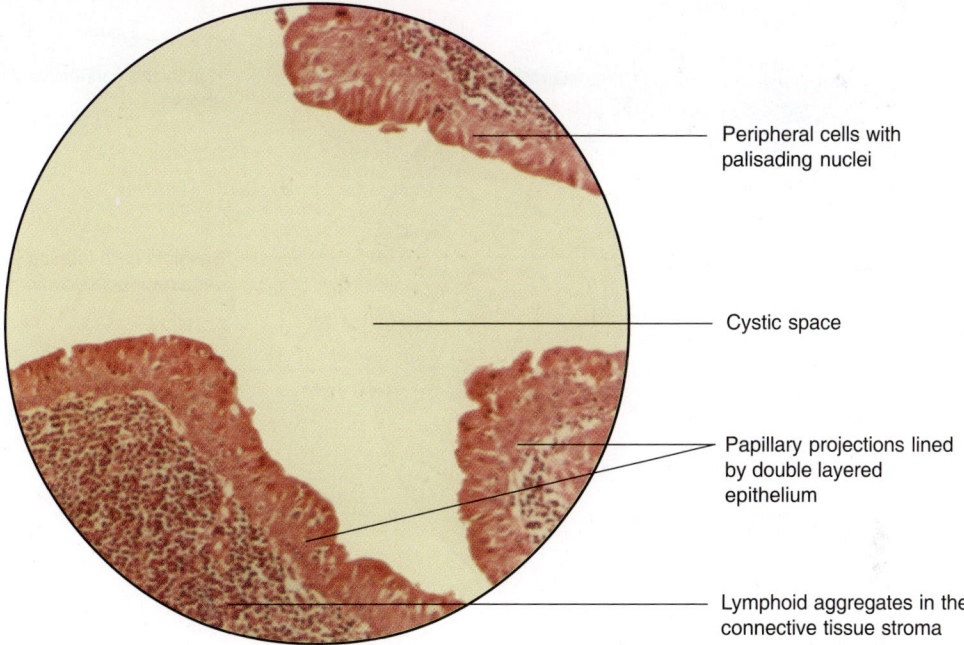

Peripheral cells with
palisading nuclei

Cystic space

Papillary projections lined
by double layered
epithelium

Lymphoid aggregates in the
connective tissue stroma

Warthin's tumor (photomicrograph 10X)

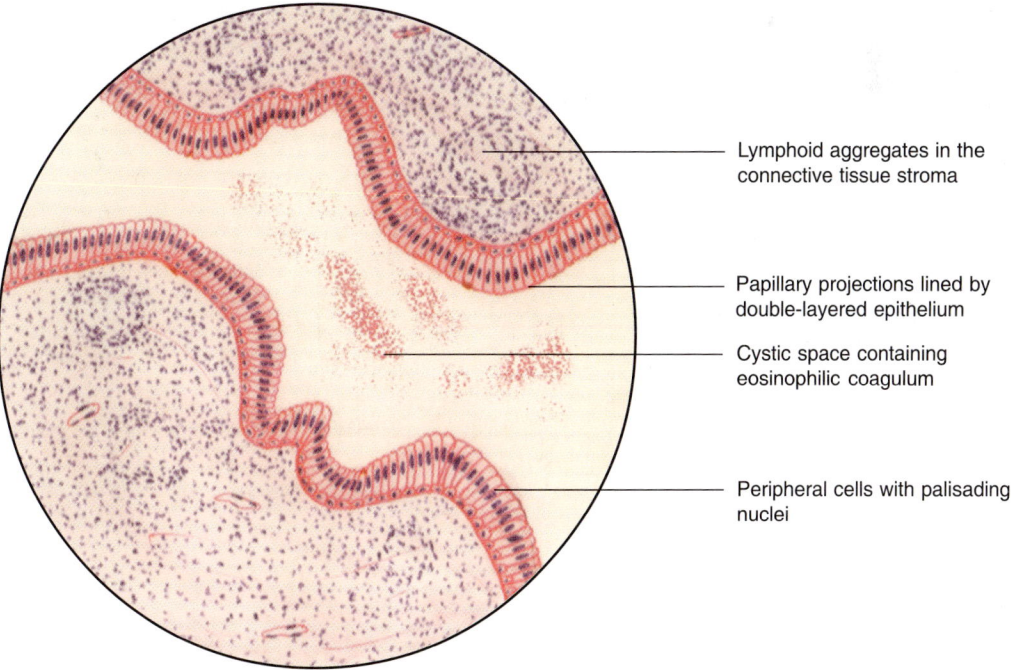

Lymphoid aggregates in the
connective tissue stroma

Papillary projections lined by
double-layered epithelium

Cystic space containing
eosinophilic coagulum

Peripheral cells with palisading
nuclei

Fig. 17.2: Warthin's tumor

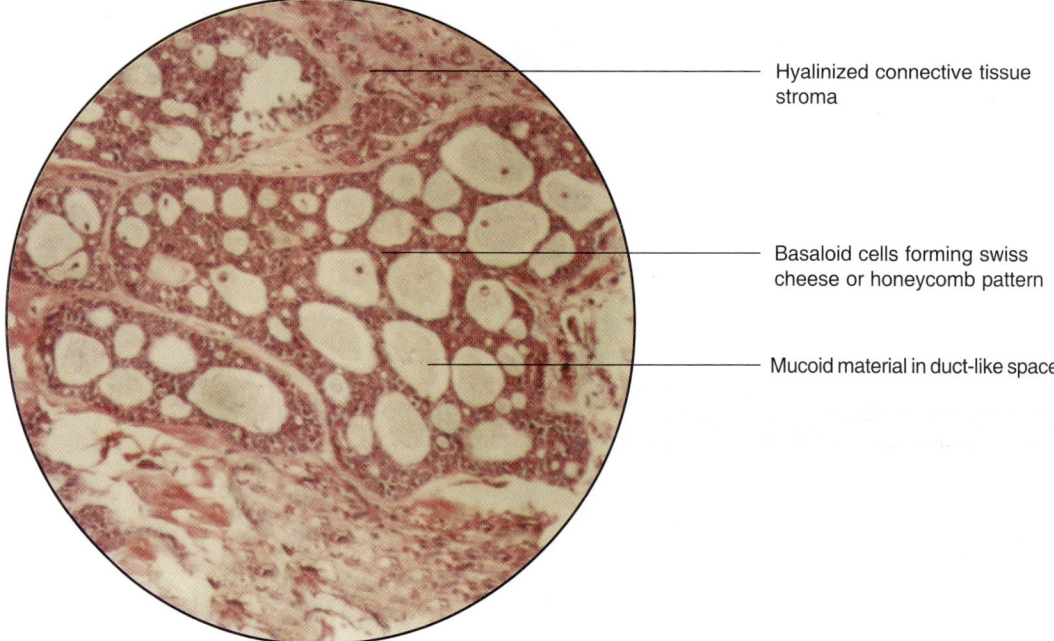

Hyalinized connective tissue stroma

Basaloid cells forming swiss cheese or honeycomb pattern

Mucoid material in duct-like space

Adenoid cystic carcinoma (photomicrograph 10X)

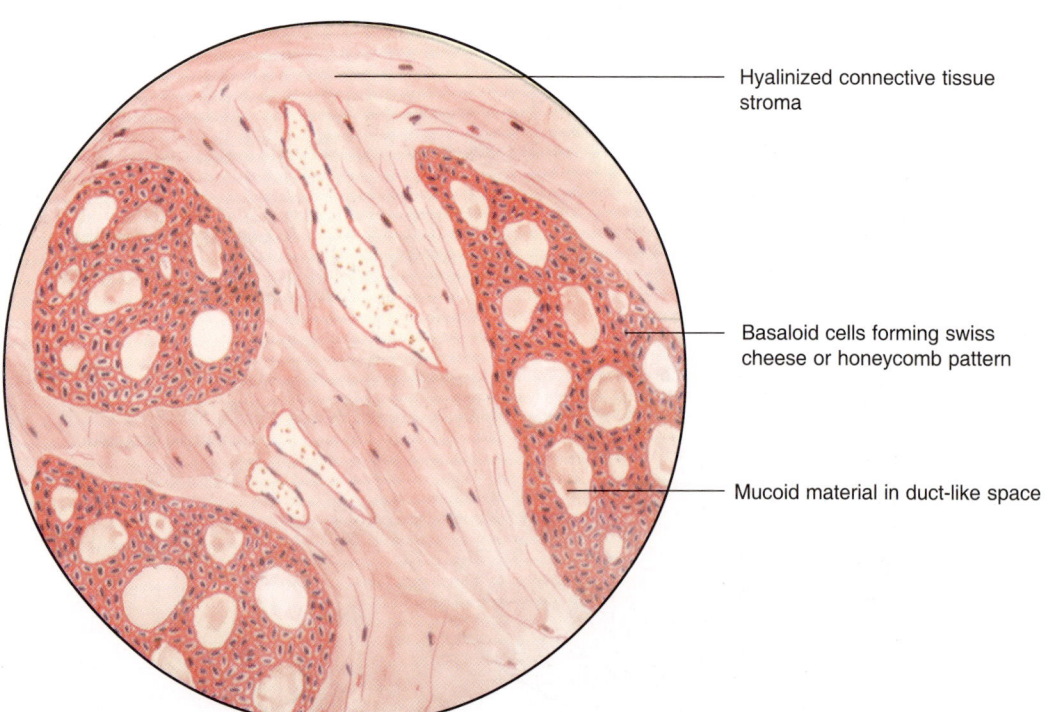

Hyalinized connective tissue stroma

Basaloid cells forming swiss cheese or honeycomb pattern

Mucoid material in duct-like space

Fig. 17.3: Adenoid cystic carcinoma

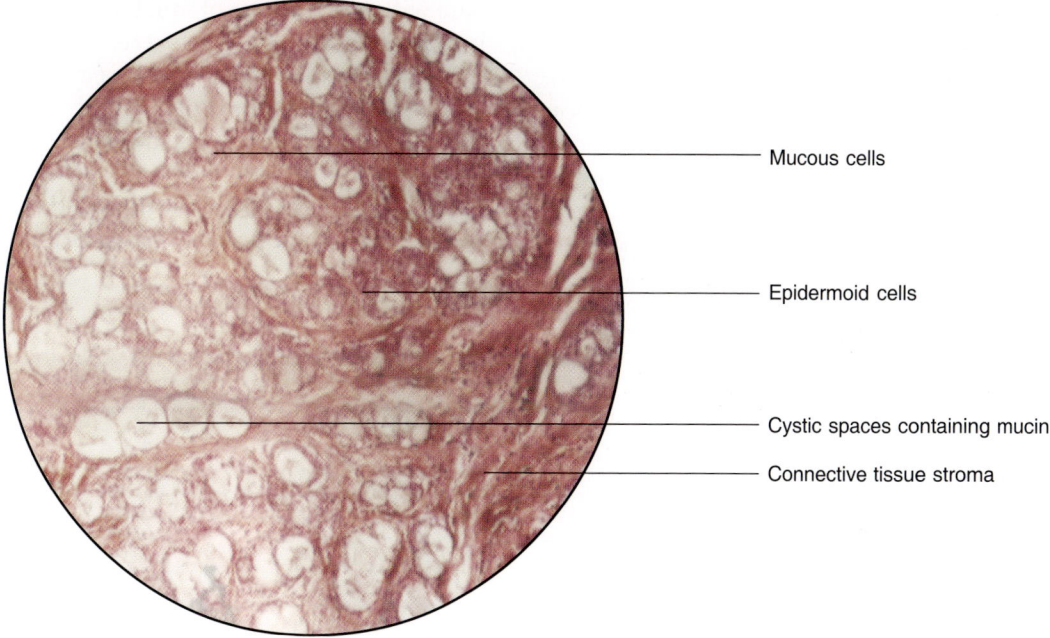

Mucous cells

Epidermoid cells

Cystic spaces containing mucin

Connective tissue stroma

Mucoepidermoid carcinoma (photomicrograph 4X)

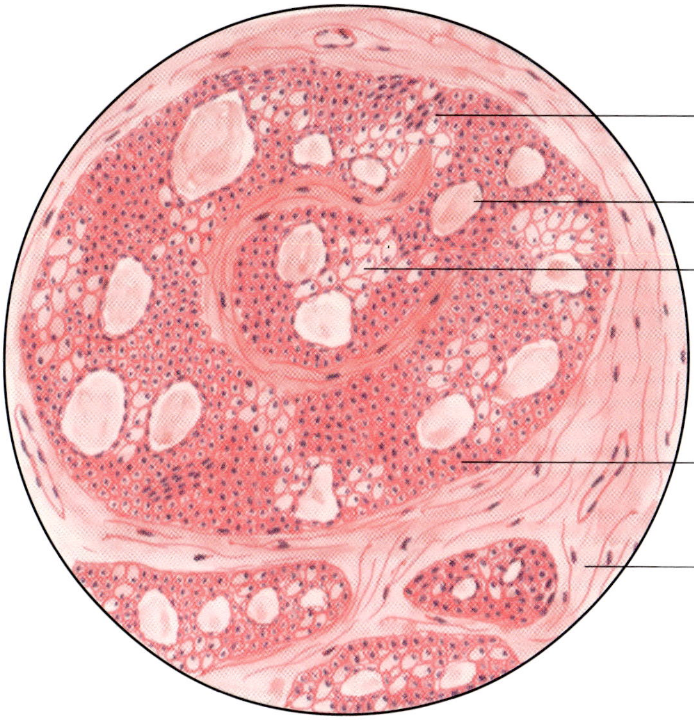

Intermediate cells

Cystic spaces containing mucin

Mucous cells

Epidermoid cells

Connective tissue stroma

Fig. 17.4: Mucoepidermoid carcinoma

Based on histopathological findings muco-epidermoid carcinoma is graded as low, intermediate or high grade malignancy.

Low grade malignancy shows predominantly mucous cells with many microcystic spaces containing mucin. Epidermoid and intermediate cells are less in number. In high grade malignancy, epidermoid cells predominate with less number of mucus secreting and intermediate cells. Cells are arranged in clusters with more solid and less cystic areas. Neoplastic cells show atypical changes. Intermediate grade lesions show intermediate histological features between low and high grades showing both epidermoid and mucous cells. Intermediate cells seldom predominate.

18

Skin Lesions

- Lichen planus
- Pemphigus
- Pemphigoid

LICHEN PLANUS

Lichen planus is a chronic mucocutaneous disorder manifested in various forms in the oral cavity. The most characteristic pattern is reticular type with interlacing white striae called Wickham's striae.

Histopathology (Fig. 18.1)

Microscopically lichen planus shows changes in all layers of epithelium and connective tissue. The epithelium is hyper, ortho- or parakeratotic, with prominent stratum granulosum. Spinous layer shows acanthosis or atrophy. One of the characteristic feature is liquefaction degeneration of basal cells and eosinophilic material is seen replacing the basal cell layer. Rete ridges may be showing a

---

Identification Points (Fig. 18.1)

Lichen Planus
- Hyper-, ortho- or parakeratosis
- Basal cell degeneration
- Saw tooth rete ridges
- Subepithelial band of lymphocytic infiltration

'Saw tooth' appearance. Another significant finding in lichen planus is subepithelial band of lymphocytic infiltration. Deeper part of the connective tissue is free from inflammation. Civatte bodies (eosinophilic apoptotic bodies) may be present in subepithelial connective tissue and in deeper spinous layer of epithelium.

PEMPHIGUS

Pemphigus is a tissue specific autoimmune disease affecting the skin and mucosa. Clinical manifestation is in the form of vesiculobullous lesions that rupture to form ulcers and erosions. Vesiculobullous lesions develop due to immune-mediated acantholysis causing intraepithelial vesicle formation.

Histopathology (Fig. 18.2)

Characteristic microscopic picture of pemphigus is intraepithelial vesicle formation that occurs in the suprabasal layer. Basal layer is intact and is attached to the connective tissue. Spinous cell layer shows acantholysis or destruction of intercellular junctions resulting in separation of cells. Loose cells are found in the vesicle which appear as round cells with degenerative changes like enlarged nuclei and hyperchromatic staining. These cells are called acantholytic cells or 'Tzanck cells'. A

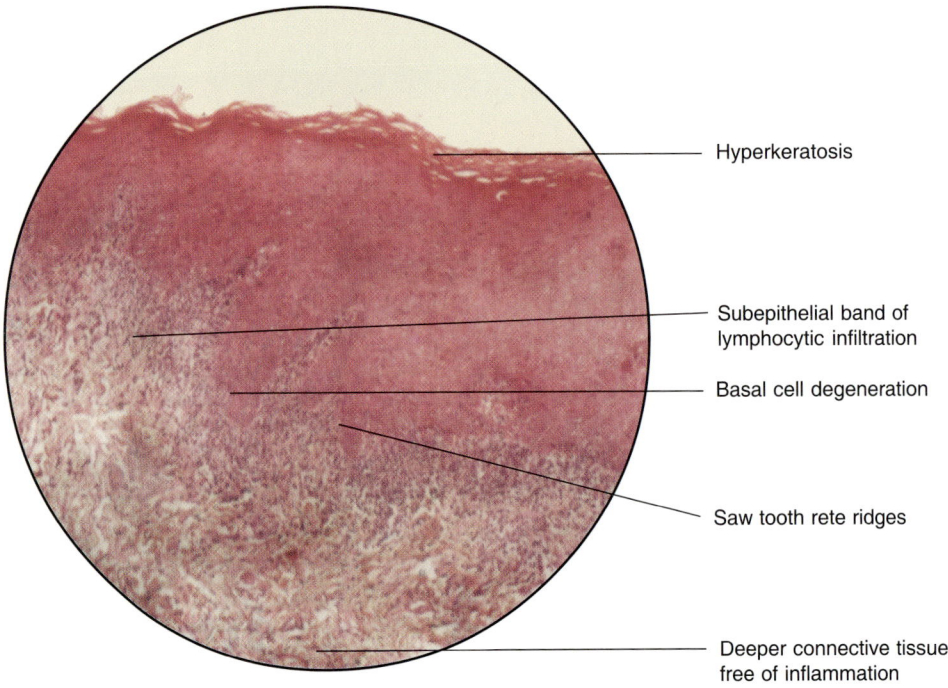

Lichen planus (photomicrograph 10X)

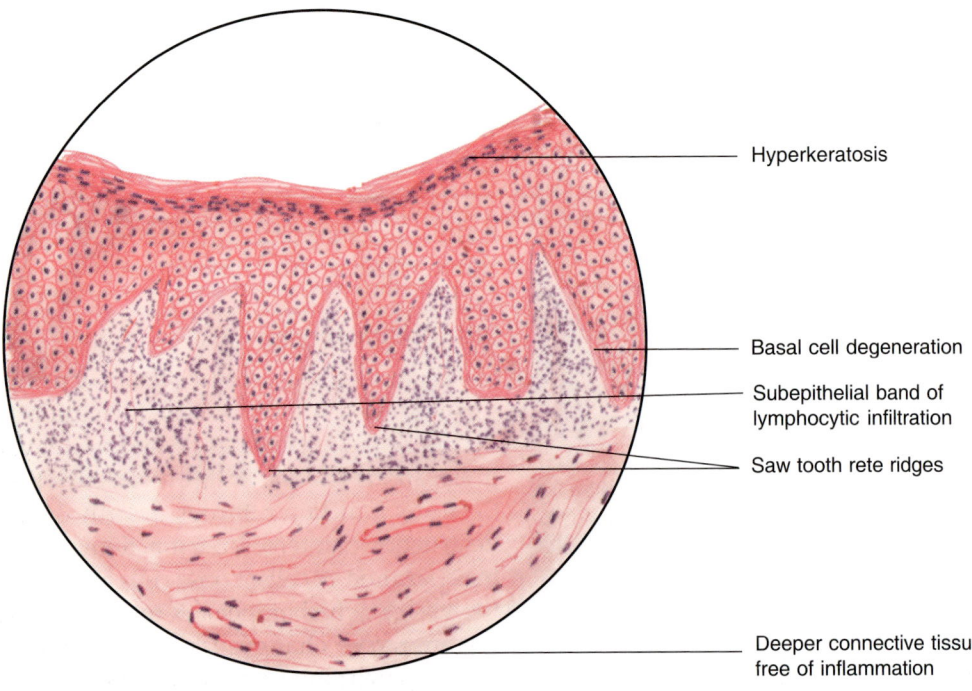

Fig. 18.1: Lichen planus

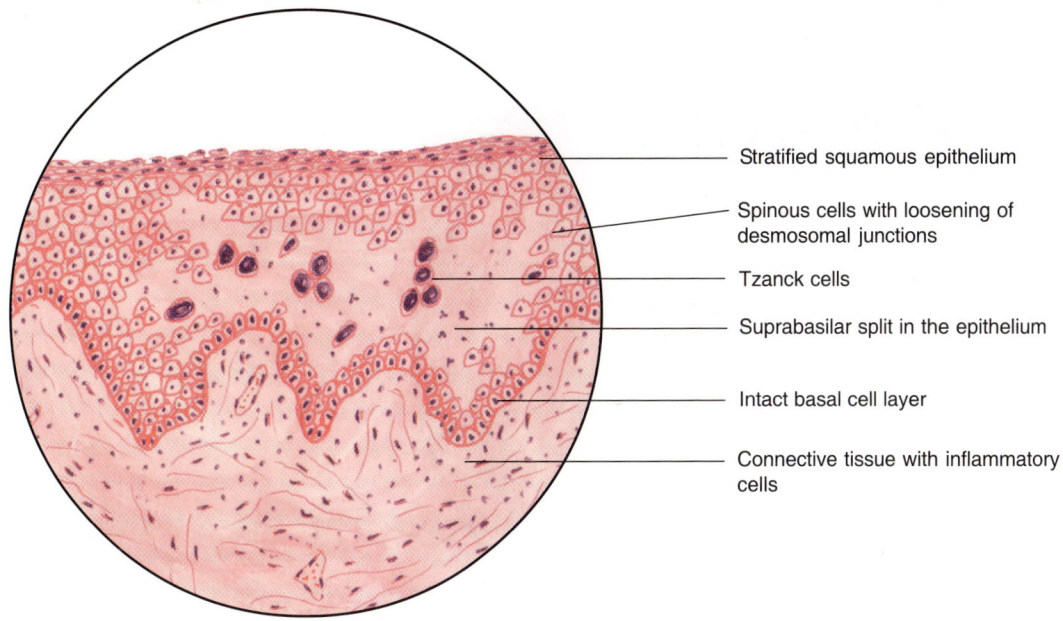

Fig. 18.2: Pemphigus

Identification Points (Fig. 18.2)

Pemphigus
- Suprabasal vesicle formation
- Intact basal layer attached to connective tissue
- Presence of Tzanck cells in the vesicle

sparse inflammatory infiltrate may be occasionally associated with vesicle and sub-epithelial connective tissue.

PEMPHIGOID

Pemphigoid is a vesiculobullous lesion that develops due to an autoimmune reaction directed against some components of base-ment membrane. This results in separation of epithelium from the connective tissue with subepithelial vesicle formation. Bullous pemphigoid and cicatricial pemphigoid are two different types of pemphigoid lesions.

Histopathology (Fig. 18.3)

Characteristic feature of pemphigoid is sub-epithelial vesicle formation. A split or a separation of epithelium from connective tissue is seen at the basement membrane zone. Epithelium is intact without any evidence of acantholysis. Connective tissue shows inflammatory cell infiltration.

Identification Points (Fig. 18.3)

Pemphigoid
- Subepithelial vesicle formation
- Intact epithelium without acantholysis
- Inflammatory cells in the connective tissue

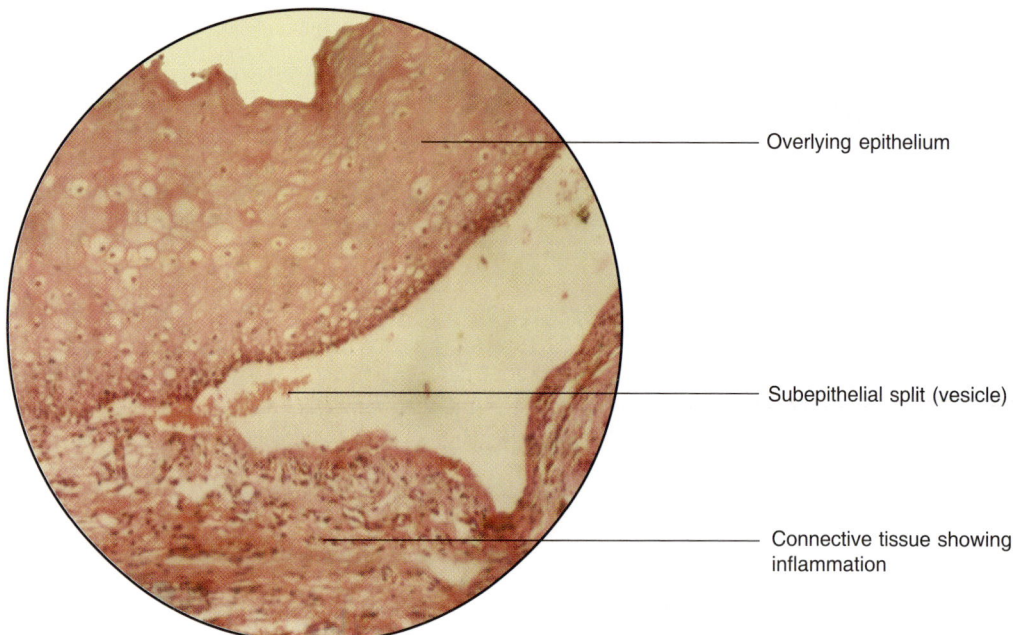

Overlying epithelium

Subepithelial split (vesicle)

Connective tissue showing inflammation

Pemphigoid (photomicrograph 10X)

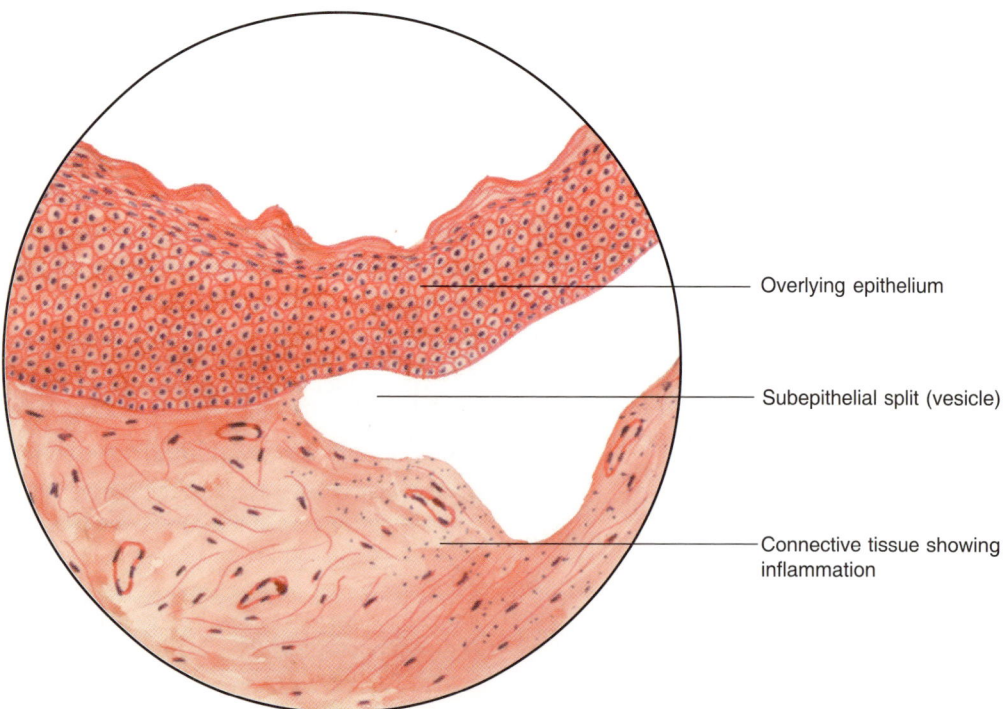

Overlying epithelium

Subepithelial split (vesicle)

Connective tissue showing inflammation

Fig. 18.3: Pemphigoid

19

Bone Lesions

- Fibrous dysplasia
- Paget's disease

FIBROUS DYSPLASIA

Fibrous dysplasia is a fibro-osseous lesion characterized by replacement of bone by fibrous tissue in which metaplastic bone formation takes place.

Fibrous dysplasia may involve single bone (monostotic) or multiple bone (polyostotic). Maxilla is affected more frequently than mandible and clinically present as painless swelling of the affected bone causing facial asymmetry. Characteristic radiographic feature is the 'ground glass' appearance of affected bone.

Histopathology (Fig. 19.1)

The lesional tissue of fibrous dysplasia shows cellular, loosely arranged fibrous connective tissue stroma. Irregular trabeculae of woven bone, which may be C-shaped or 'Chinese character'-shaped (Chinese letter pattern) are

distributed in the stroma. Bony trabeculae lack osteoblastic rimming. Lesional tissue merges with adjacent normal bone.

PAGET'S DISEASE

Paget's disease is a bone disorder that occur due to abnormal bone remodeling resulting in deformed functionally inefficient bone. Involvement of jaw bone results in progressive enlargement causing facial asymmetry. The characteristic radiographic presentation of Paget's disease is 'cotton wool' appearance.

Histopathology (Fig. 19.2)

The lesions of Paget's disease show irregular trabeculae of mature lamellated bone with basophilic resting and reversal lines resulting in a 'jigsaw-puzzle' or 'mosaic pattern'. Bony trabeculae are lined by a layer of osteoid and plump osteoblasts. Osteoclasts resorbing bone is also a feature in the resorptive stage of the disease. Connective tissue stroma is vascular and tend to be fibrous.

Identification Points (Fig. 19.1)

Fibrous Dysplasia
- Cellular loose fibrous connective tissue stroma
- Irregular trabeculae of woven bone having 'Chinese letter pattern'
- Absence of osteoblastic rimming of bony trabeculae

Identification Points (Fig. 19.2)

Paget's Disease
- Irregular trabeculae of mature lamellated bone
- Bony trabeculae having a 'mosaic pattern' and 'jigsaw-puzzle' appearance
- Osteoblastic rimming and areas of osteoclastic bone resorption

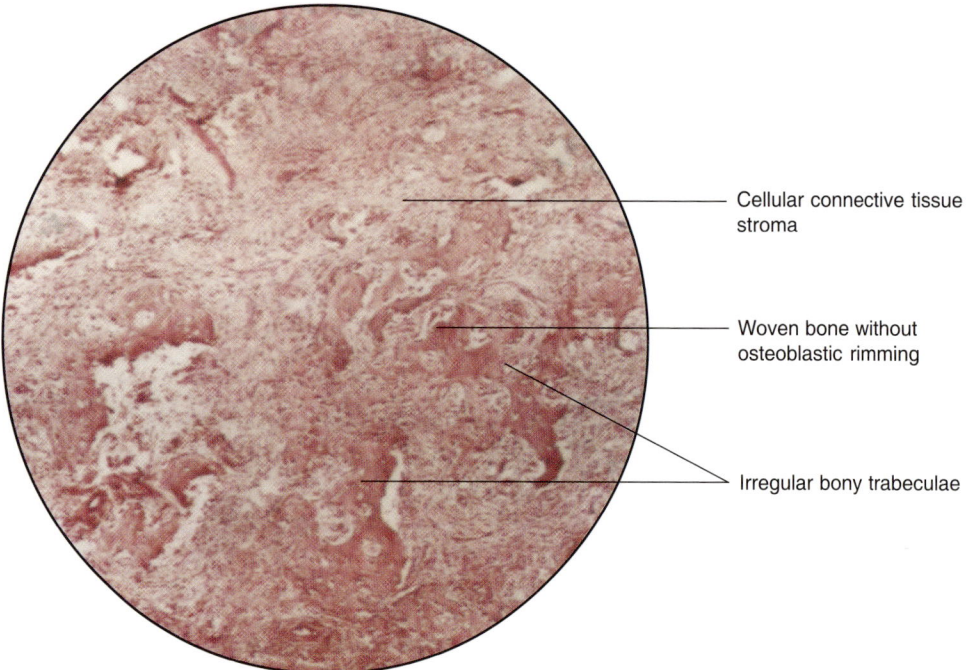

Cellular connective tissue stroma

Woven bone without osteoblastic rimming

Irregular bony trabeculae

Fibrous dysplasia (photomicrograph 10X)

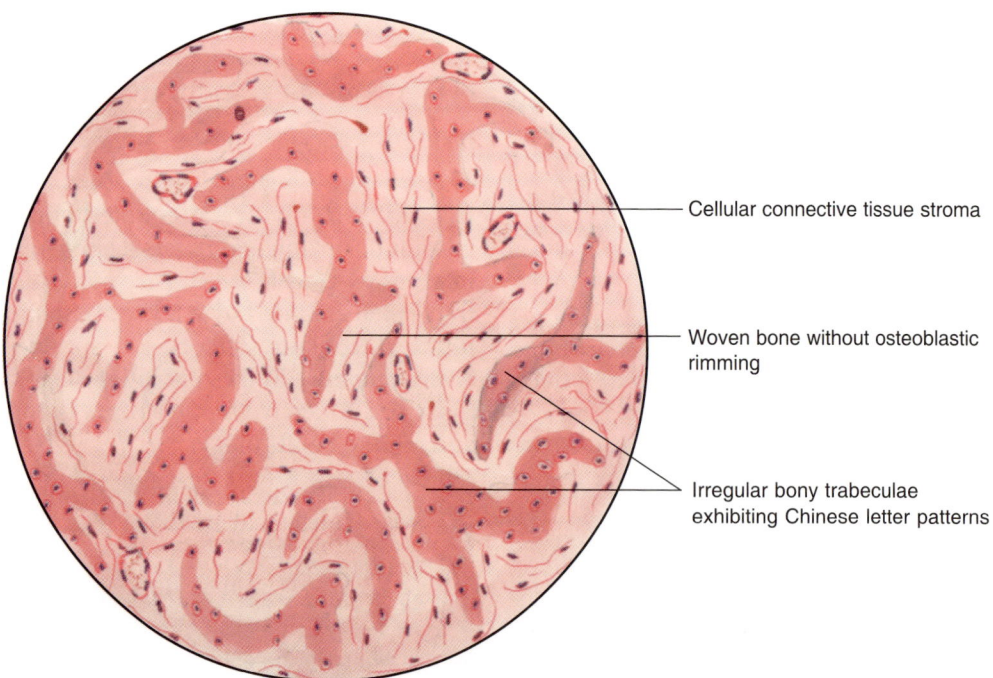

Cellular connective tissue stroma

Woven bone without osteoblastic rimming

Irregular bony trabeculae exhibiting Chinese letter patterns

Fig. 19.1: Fibrous dysplasia

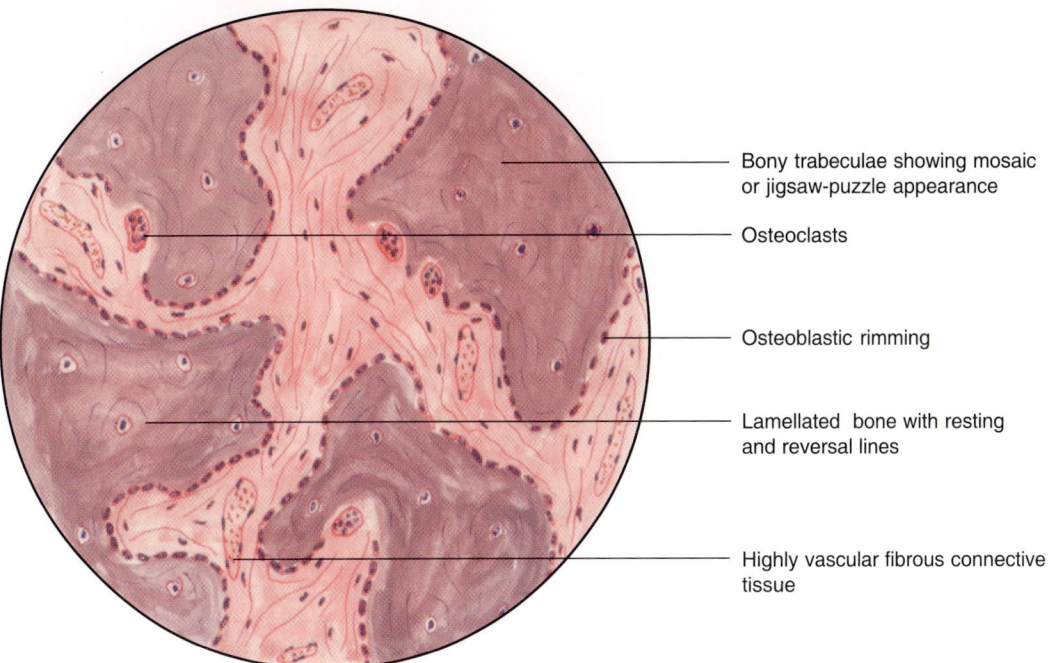

Bony trabeculae showing mosaic or jigsaw-puzzle appearance

Osteoclasts

Osteoblastic rimming

Lamellated bone with resting and reversal lines

Highly vascular fibrous connective tissue

Fig. 19.2: Paget's disease

20

Benign and Malignant Tumors of Oral Cavity

- Benign epithelial tumors
- Potentially malignant disorders of oral mucosa
- Malignant epithelial tumors
- Benign connective tissue neoplasms
- Malignant connective tissue tumors
- Tumor-like lesions

Identification Points (Fig. 20.1)

Papilloma
- Multiple finger-like projections
- Hyperplastic stratified squamous epithelium lining the projections
- Connective tissue forms the core

Tumors of the oral cavity are classified into benign and malignant based on biological behavior. These tumors can originate from both epithelium and connective tissue.

BENIGN EPITHELIAL TUMORS

PAPILLOMA

Papilloma is the commonest benign epithelial tumor of the oral mucosa, that develops due to benign proliferation of stratified squamous epithelium. This lesion clinically presents as a painless exophytic growth with irregular cauliflower or wart-like appearance.

Histopathology (Fig. 20.1)

Papilloma is characterized by finger-like projections lined by hyperplastic stratified squamous keratinized epithelium. Each finger-like projection has a central thin connective tissue core carrying the blood vessels.

MELANOTIC NEVUS

Melanotic nevus is a pigmented lesion which develops due to benign proliferation of nevus cells. Nevus cells are of neural crest origin and functionally similar to melanocytes with the capacity to produce melanin. Unlike melanocytes, nevus cells are not dendritic cells.

Histopathology

Histopathologically melanotic nevus is characterized by proliferation of small ovoid nevus cells arranged to form small round aggregates. These are called thèques. Nevus cells have small uniform nucleus with eosinophilic cytoplasm and indistinct cell boundaries.

Based on location of proliferating nevus cells histopathologically melanotic nevus is divided into:
1. **Junctional nevus (Fig. 20.2):** Nevus cells are arranged in the form of thèques in the basal layers of epithelium especially at the tip of rete ridges. Here the nevi cells are seen in the junction between epithelium

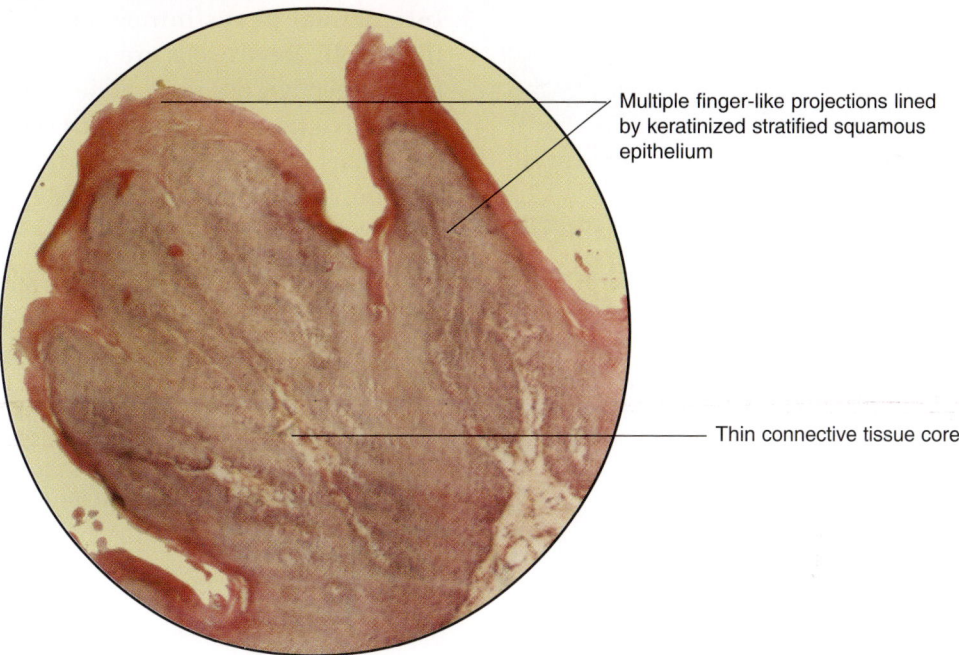

Multiple finger-like projections lined by keratinized stratified squamous epithelium

Thin connective tissue core

Papilloma (photomicrograph 10X)

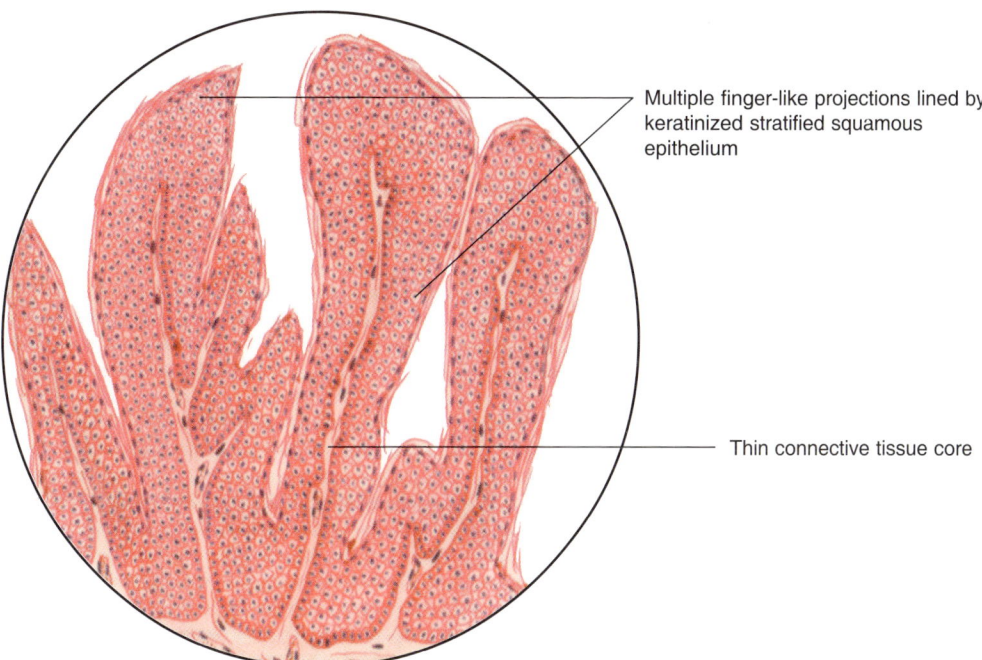

Multiple finger-like projections lined by keratinized stratified squamous epithelium

Thin connective tissue core

Fig. 20.1: Papilloma

Identification Points (Fig. 20.2)

Junctional Nevus
- Nevus cells restricted to epithelium
- Nevus cells arranged to form thèques in the basal layer
- 'Abtropfung' or 'dropping off' effect may be seen

and connective tissue. Junctional activity may be seen with a few cells crossing junction and growing down into connective tissue, which is described as 'abtropfung effect'.

2. **Compound nevus (Fig. 20.3):** In this nevus cell proliferation is seen both in epithelium and connective tissue.

Identification Points (Fig. 20.3)

Compound Nevus
- Proliferating nevus cells in epithelium
- Nests of nevus cells dropping off from the epidermis
- Nests of nevus cells in the connective tissue also

3. **Intradermal nevus/intramucosal nevus (Fig. 20.4):** Nevus cells are found only in the connective tissue. A zone of normal connective tissue is seen which separates the nevus cells from the overlying epithelium. In intramucosal nevus 3 types of cells are seen:

1. Peripheral type A—epithelioid cells
2. Central type B—lymphocyte-like cells
3. Deeper type C—spindle-shaped cells.

Identification Points (Fig. 20.4)

Intradermal Nevus
- Nests of nevus cells in the connective tissue
- Three types of cells are seen—epithelioid, lymphocyte-like and spindle shaped
- Zone of connective tissue separates nevus cells from overlying epithelium

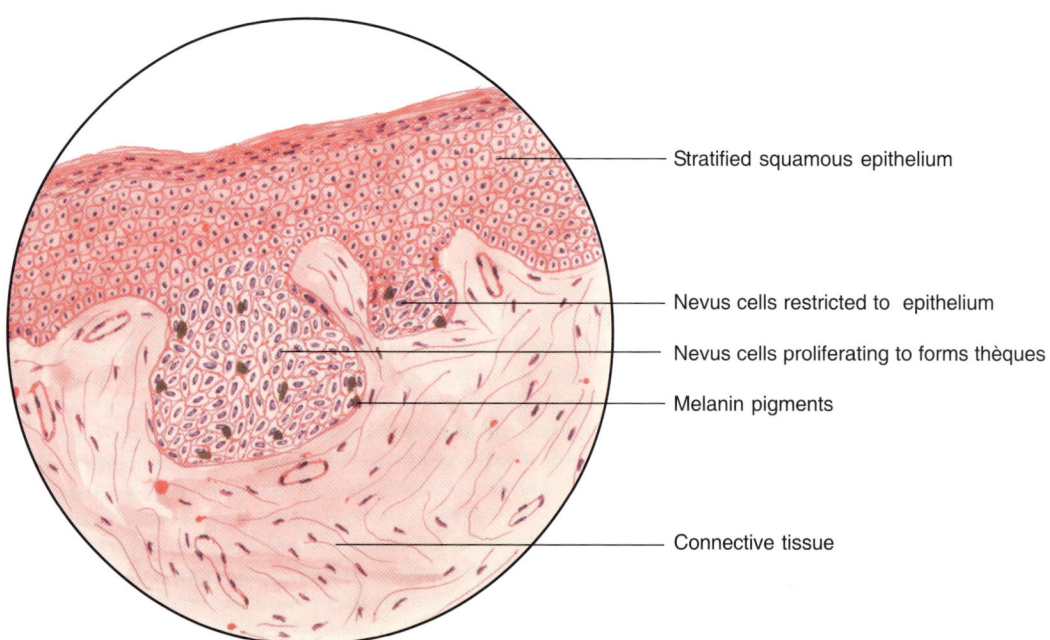

Stratified squamous epithelium

Nevus cells restricted to epithelium

Nevus cells proliferating to forms thèques

Melanin pigments

Connective tissue

Fig. 20.2: Junctional nevus

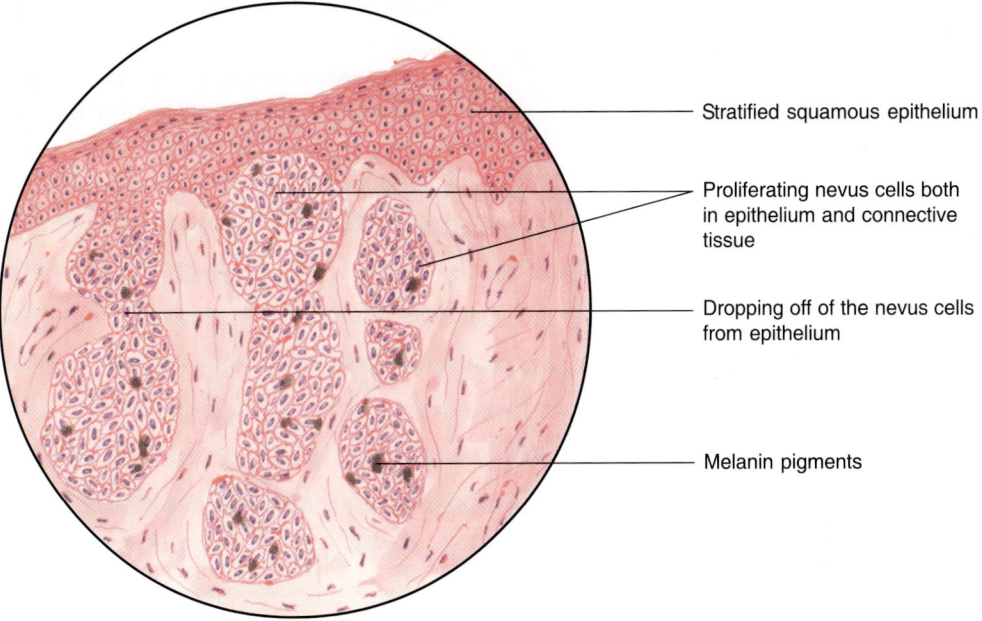

Fig. 20.3: Compound nevus

Stratified squamous epithelium

Proliferating nevus cells both in epithelium and connective tissue

Dropping off of the nevus cells from epithelium

Melanin pigments

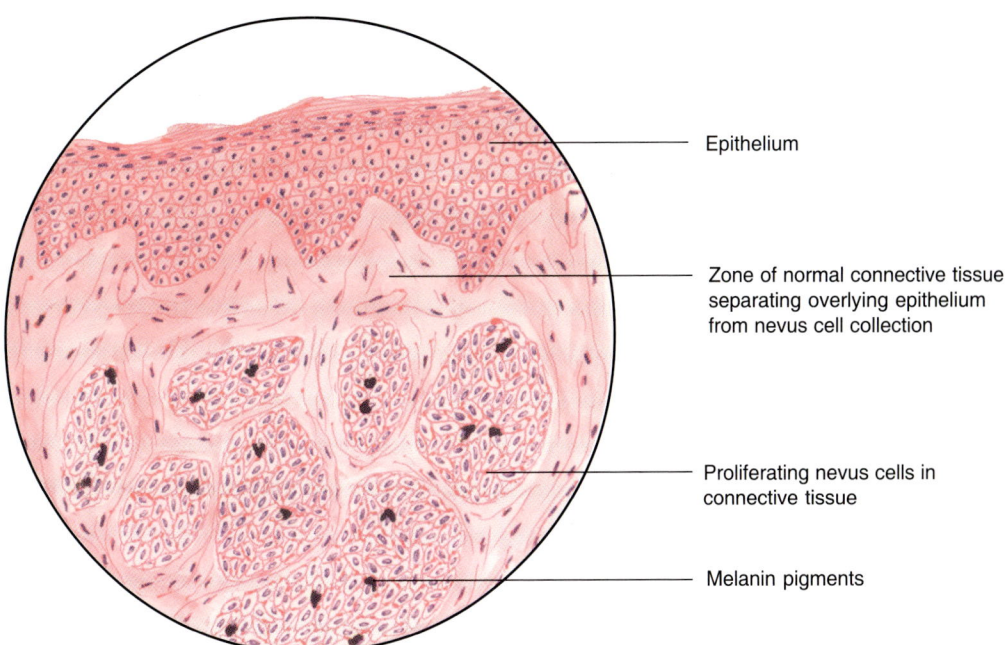

Fig. 20.4: Intradermal nevus

Epithelium

Zone of normal connective tissue separating overlying epithelium from nevus cell collection

Proliferating nevus cells in connective tissue

Melanin pigments

POTENTIALLY MALIGNANT DISORDERS OF ORAL MUCOSA

Potentially malignant disorders of oral mucosa are a group of disorders, some of them may have an increased potential for malignant transformation. These include all the diseases which were earlier considered as premalignant lesions and premalignant conditions.

LEUKOPLAKIA

Leukoplakia is the commonest precancerous lesion that occurs in the oral cavity. It is manifested as a white patch or plaque that cannot be scraped off or rubbed off. Malignant transformation potential is 6–7%.

Histopathology (Figs 20.5 to 20.7)

Microscopically leukoplakia is characterized by:

1. **Hyperkeratosis:** Thickened keratin layer which may be parakeratotic or orthokeratotic. In case of hyper-orthokeratosis a prominent granular layer is seen. Surface of epithelium may be smooth or irregular with papillary projection (verrucous leukoplakia).

2. **Acanthosis:** Most of leukoplakic lesions show thickening of spinous layer which is termed as acanthosis. Some of the leukoplakic lesions may show areas of epithelial atrophy.

3. **Dysplastic features:** The lesions of leukoplakia show dysplastic features of different grades. The features of epithelial dysplasia are:

   - *Bulbous or drop-shaped rete ridges:* Normally the rete ridges taper to the deeper portion or are parallel-sided with blunt ends. In dysplasia, the deepest portion of rete ridges become wider. This occurs to accommodate the increased number of cells.

- *Basal cell hyperplasia:* Normally basal cell layer has one to two layers of cells. In dysplasia, the basal cell layer increases to more than two layers thick.

- *Loss of polarity of basal cells:* Normally the nucleus of basal cells is arranged perpendicular to the basement membrane. When this arrangement is lost, the nuclei are in different angles. This is called loss of polarity.

- *Irregular epithelial stratification:* In normal epithelium distinct layers (strata) are seen. Disturbance in this arrangement is called irregular stratification.

- *Loss of intercellular adhesion:* In normal epithelium the cells are attached to each other by desmosomes. As the dysplasia progresses the cell loses their attachment to each other due to desmosomal changes.

- *Cellular pleomorphism or anisocytosis:* In dysplastic epithelium cells show variation in shape and size.

- *Alteration in nuclear cytoplasmic ratio:* Normal ratio between nucleus and cytoplasm is 1 : 4 or 1 : 6. When the nucleus increases in size, in dysplasia the nuclear cytoplasmic ratio changes to 1 : 1.

- *Nuclear hyperchromatism:* Hyperchromatism is increased or dark staining of nucleus. This occurs, due to increased DNA content of highly active cells in dysplasia.

- *Prominent nucleoli:* In dysplastic epithelial cells nucleoli become prominent and larger.

- *Increased mitosis:* In dysplasia, due to active division of cells more number of mitotic figures are seen when compared to normal epithelium.

- *Level of mitosis:* In normal epithelium only basal and para basal cells have the ability of mitotic division. In dysplastic epithelium mitotic activity is seen even in higher levels of epithelium.

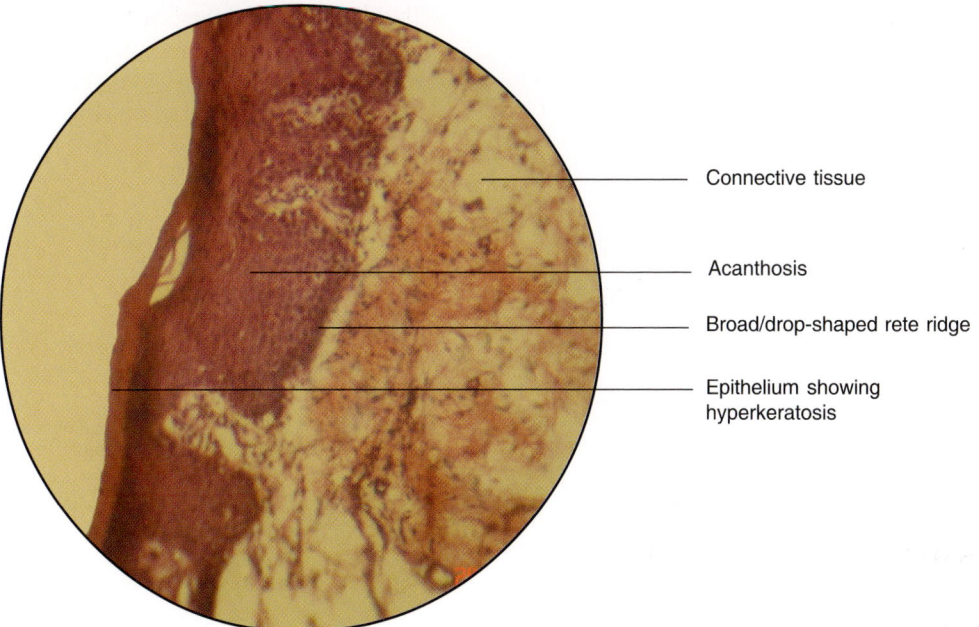

Connective tissue

Acanthosis

Broad/drop-shaped rete ridge

Epithelium showing
hyperkeratosis

Leukoplakia (mild dysplasia) (photomicrograph 10X)

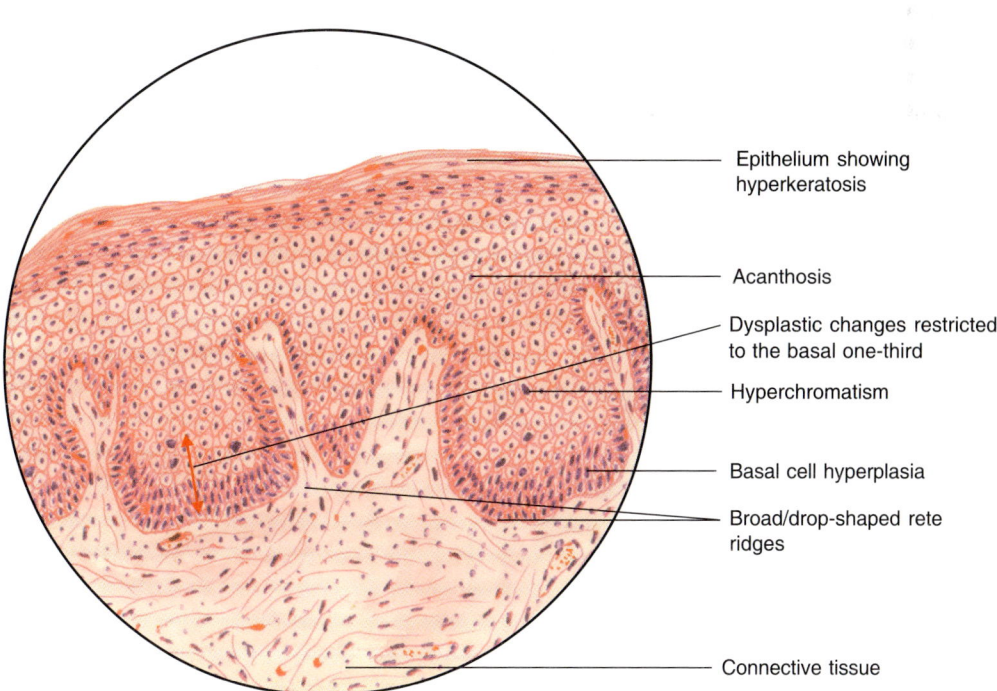

Epithelium showing
hyperkeratosis

Acanthosis

Dysplastic changes restricted
to the basal one-third

Hyperchromatism

Basal cell hyperplasia

Broad/drop-shaped rete
ridges

Connective tissue

Fig. 20.5: Leukoplakia (mild dysplasia)

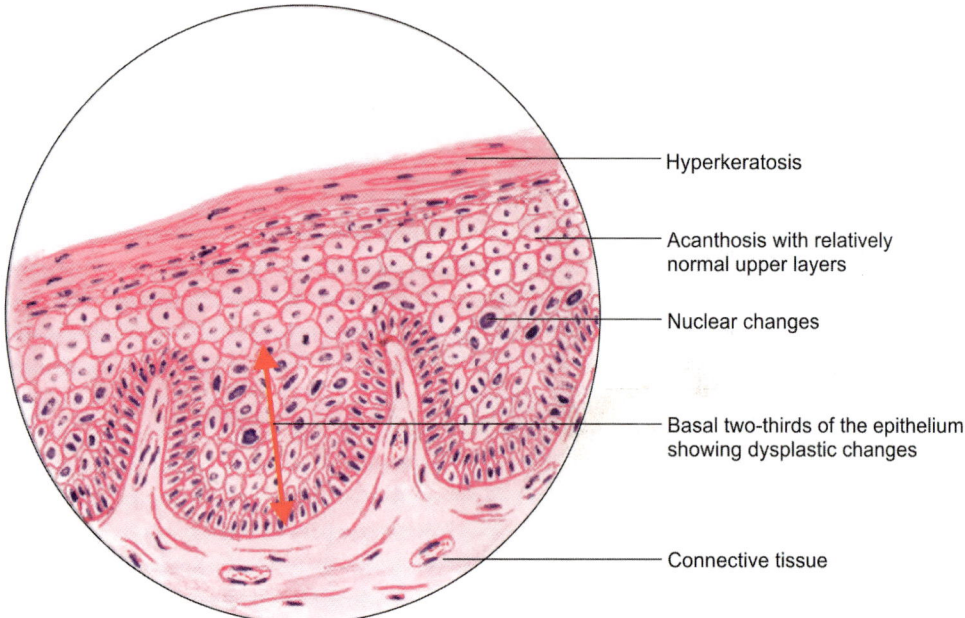

Hyperkeratosis

Acanthosis with relatively normal upper layers

Nuclear changes

Basal two-thirds of the epithelium showing dysplastic changes

Connective tissue

Fig. 20.6: Leukoplakia (moderate dysplasia)

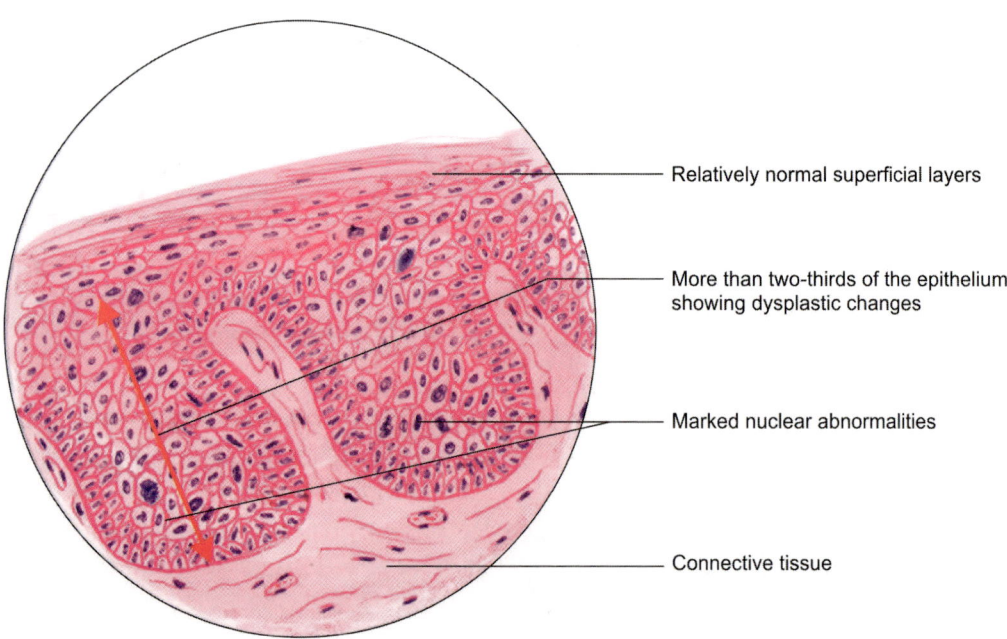

Relatively normal superficial layers

More than two-thirds of the epithelium showing dysplastic changes

Marked nuclear abnormalities

Connective tissue

Fig. 20.7: Leukoplakia (severe dysplasia)

Identification Points (Fig. 20.5)

Leukoplakia with Mild Dysplasia
- Hyperkeratosis
- Acanthosis
- Dysplastic features restricted to basal one-third of epithelium

- *Abnormal mitosis*: Mitotic figures in various forms other than normal is seen in dysplastic epithelium, e.g. tripolar mitotic figures.
- *Dyskeratosis or abnormal keratinization*: Normally keratinization occurs only in the superficial layers of epithelium. In dysplasia keratinization of individual cells or even keratin pearl formation is seen in deeper layers.

Epithelial dysplasia is graded into mild, moderate or severe.

Mild dysplasia: The dysplastic changes are minimal, restricted to basal one-third and rest of the epithelium is normal.

Moderate dysplasia: Basal two-thirds of the epithelium exhibit marked nuclear abnormalities and upper layers showing normal cell maturation and stratification.

Severe dysplasia: More than two-thirds of the epithelium show marked nuclear abnormalities and loss of maturation. Superficial layers exhibit some stratification.

Identification Points (Fig. 20.6)

Leukoplakia with Moderate Dysplasia
- Hyperkeratotic, acanthotic epithelium
- Dysplastic features up to basal two-thirds of epithelium
- Upper layers showing normal cell maturation and stratification

Identification Points (Fig. 20.7)

Leukoplakia with Severe Dysplasia
- Hyperkeratotic, acanthotic epithelium
- More than two-thirds of the epithelium showing dysplastic features
- Superficial layers exhibit some stratification

CARCINOMA IN SITU (INTRAEPITHELIAL CARCINOMA) (Fig. 20.8)

This is a histological term used to describe an epithelium which is exhibiting dysplastic changes throughout its thickness (top to bottom changes). In this, dysplastic features are evident from basal cell layer to the superficial layer, but strictly restricted to the epithelium. The basement membrane is intact.

Identification Points (Fig. 20.8)

Carcinoma in situ
- Top to bottom dysplastic changes from basal layer to superficial layer
- Intact basement membrane

ORAL SUBMUCOUS FIBROSIS

This is a common precancerous condition seen in India, related to betel quid chewing. This disease is characterized by progressive mucosal rigidity caused by fibrosis of connective tissue.

Histopathology (Fig. 20.9)

In oral submucous fibrosis the epithelium is atrophic with short or flat rete ridges. Connective tissue just beneath the epithelium shows hyalinization (juxta-epithelial hyalinization). Connective tissue exhibits fibrosis with dense bundles of collagen fibers. Because of fibrosis of connective tissue the blood vessels become narrow. Focal collections of chronic inflammatory cells are present. In severe cases, muscle undergoes degenerative changes.

Identification Points (Fig. 20.9)

Oral Submucous Fibrosis
- Atrophic epithelium
- Juxta-epithelial hyalinization
- Fibrosed connective tissue

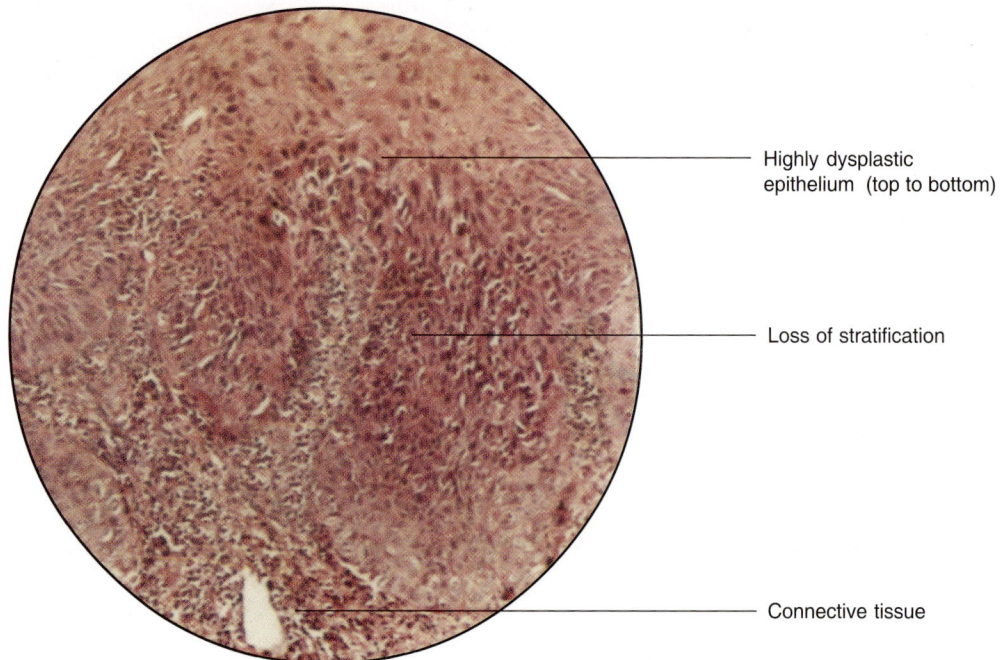

Highly dysplastic epithelium (top to bottom)

Loss of stratification

Connective tissue

Carcinoma in situ (photomicrograph 10X)

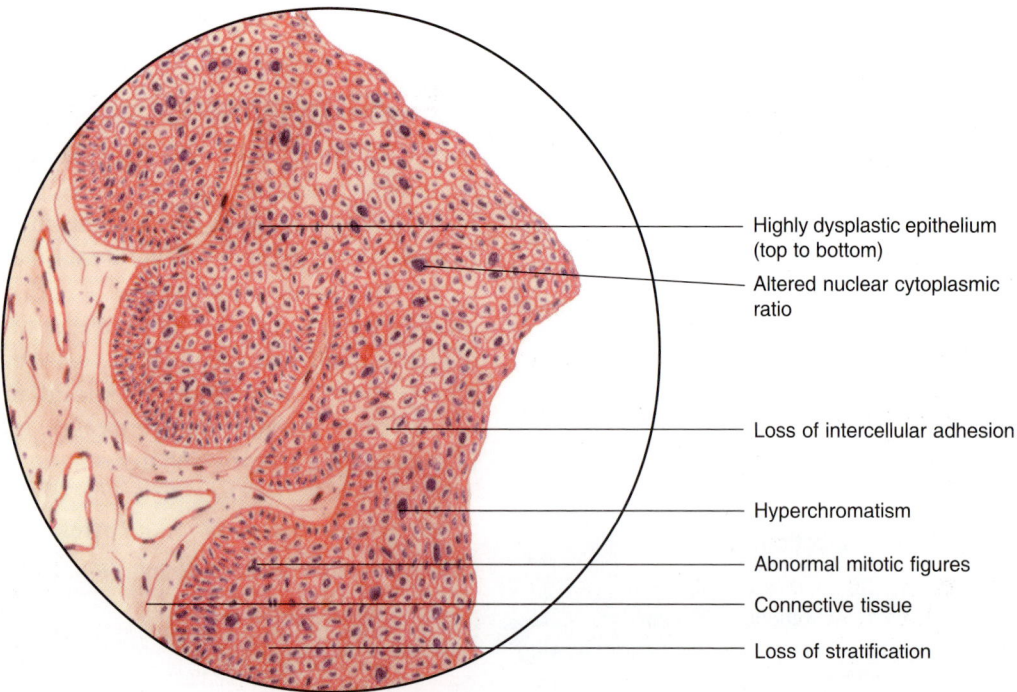

Highly dysplastic epithelium (top to bottom)

Altered nuclear cytoplasmic ratio

Loss of intercellular adhesion

Hyperchromatism

Abnormal mitotic figures

Connective tissue

Loss of stratification

Fig. 20.8: Carcinoma in situ

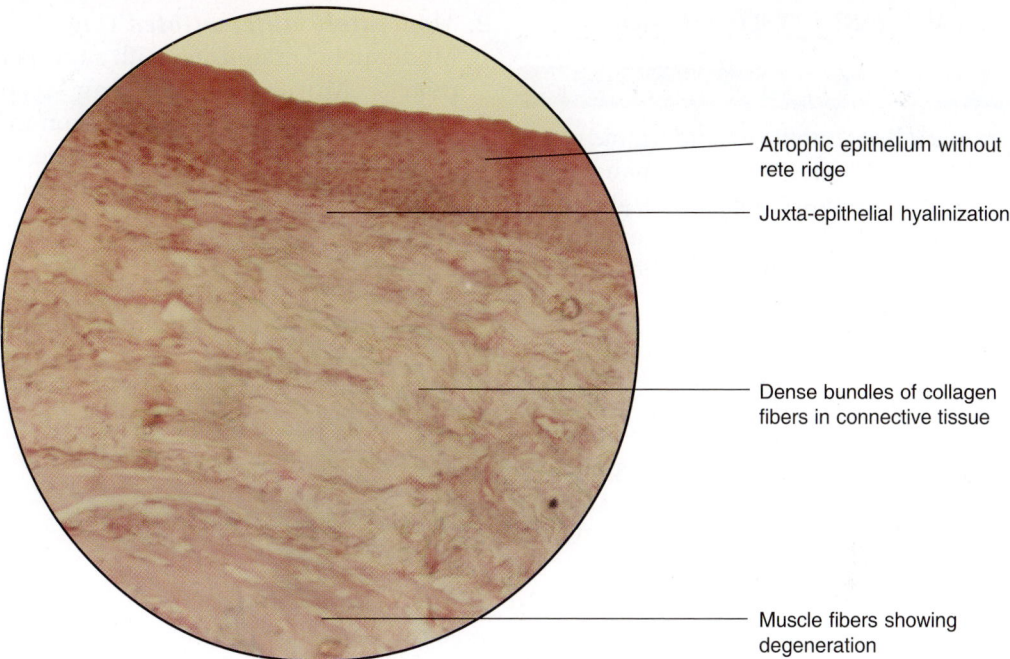

Atrophic epithelium without rete ridge

Juxta-epithelial hyalinization

Dense bundles of collagen fibers in connective tissue

Muscle fibers showing degeneration

Oral submucous fibrosis (photomicrograph 10X)

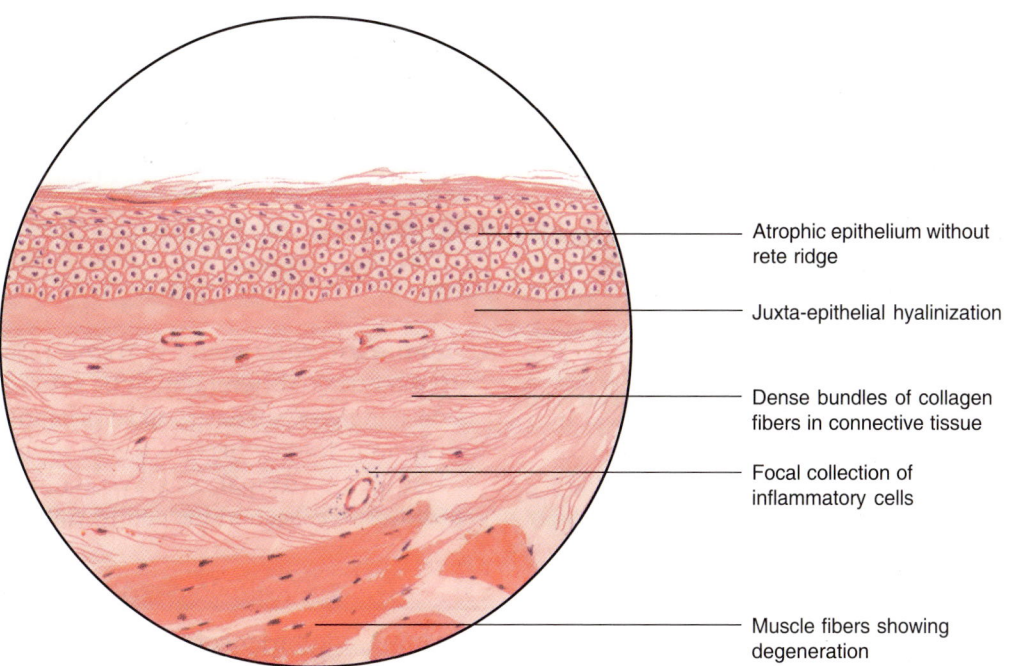

Atrophic epithelium without rete ridge

Juxta-epithelial hyalinization

Dense bundles of collagen fibers in connective tissue

Focal collection of inflammatory cells

Muscle fibers showing degeneration

Fig. 20.9: Oral submucous fibrosis

MALIGNANT EPITHELIAL TUMORS

SQUAMOUS CELL CARCINOMA

Squamous cell carcinoma or epidermoid carcinoma is the commonest epithelial malignancy that occurs in the oral cavity. Clinically these lesions may manifest as ulcers, exophytic growth and red or white patches of oral mucosa.

Histopathology

The most significant microscopic feature of squamous cell carcinoma is dysplastic epithelial cells invading into the connective tissue. These cells may be arranged in the form of cords, sheets or islands. Dysplastic features seen are hyperchromatism of nuclei, alteration of nuclear cytoplasmic ratio, pleomorphism of cells and nuclei, prominent nucleoli, many normal and abnormal mitotic figures, individual cell keratinization and keratin pearl formation. Overlying epithelium will be highly dysplastic and a break in basement membrane can be seen allowing the cells to invade into connective tissue.

Squamous cell carcinoma is graded histologically based on degree of differentiation (keratin formation), dysplastic changes of cells, depth of invasion and host response.

1. *Well differentiated (Fig. 20.10a):* Highly keratinized, with multiple keratin pearl formation and a few cells showing atypical changes. These lesions have well delineated infiltrating boarder and marked lymphocytic infiltration of connective tissue.

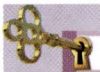

Identification Points (Fig. 20.10a)

Squamous Cell Carcinoma (Well Differentiated)
- Break in basement membrane
- Dysplastic cells invading connective tissue
- Well differentiated cells with multiple keratin pearl formation

2. *Moderately differentiated (Fig. 20.10b):* Moderately keratinized, with a few keratin pearls. More cells showing atypical changes. Dysplastic cell infiltration is seen in the superficial connective tissue in the form of strands and islands with moderate lymphocytic infiltration.

Identification Points (Fig. 20.10b)

Squamous Cell Carcinoma (Moderately Differentiated)
- Break in basement membrane
- Dysplastic cells invading connective tissue
- Moderately differentiated cells with a few keratin pearl formation

3. *Poorly differentiated (Fig. 20.10c):* Minimal keratinization with scanty keratin pearls and abundant atypical changes with more than 50% of the cells showing changes. Small group of cells infiltrating deep into the connective tissue with atypical cells being found adjacent to muscle and salivary gland. Connective tissue shows only very minimal lymphocytic infiltration.

Identification Points (Fig. 20.10c)

Squamous Cell Carcinoma (Poorly Differentiated)
- Break in basement membrane
- Dysplastic cells invading connective tissue
- Poorly differentiated cells with scanty keratinization

4. *Anaplastic carcinoma:* Extreme cellular atypia but no differentiation or keratinization. Single or small group of cells invade deep into the connective tissue replacing most of the stromal cells. No lymhocytic infiltration is seen in the connective tissue.

VERRUCOUS CARCINOMA

It is a low grade variant of squamous cell carcinoma which commonly manifest as painless, thick plaque with a warty or verrucous surface.

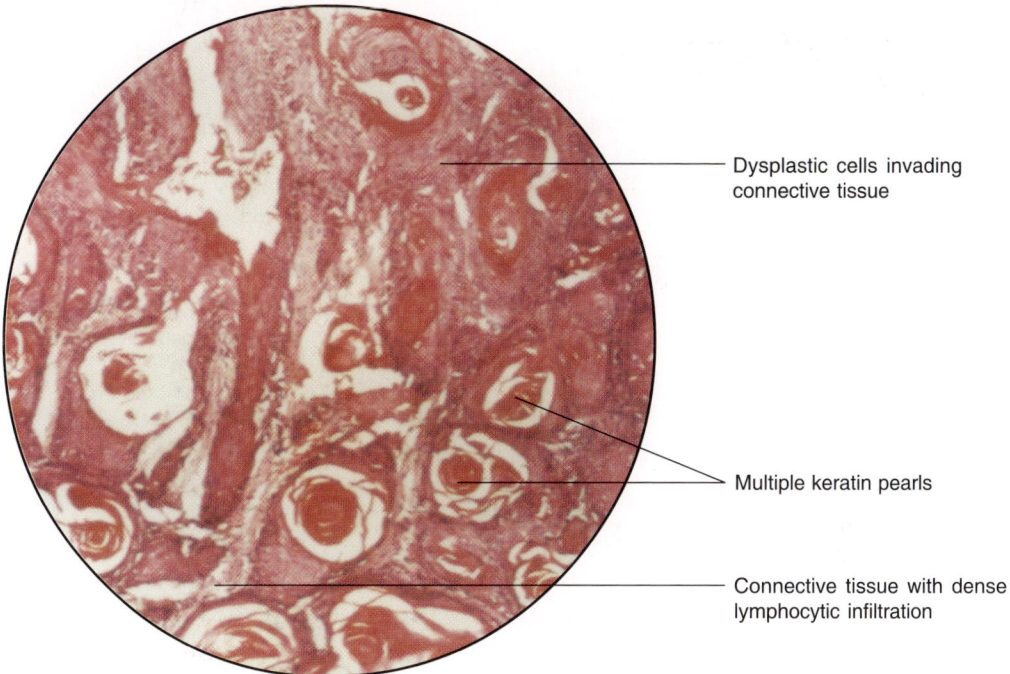

Dysplastic cells invading connective tissue

Multiple keratin pearls

Connective tissue with dense lymphocytic infiltration

Squamous cell carcinoma—well differentiated (photomicrograph 10X)

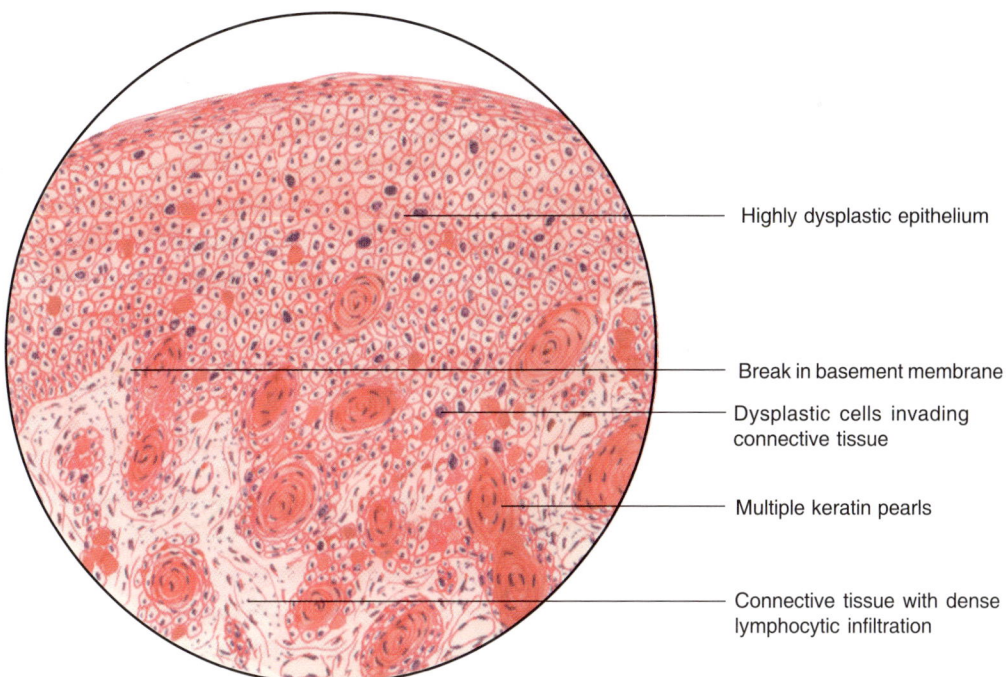

Highly dysplastic epithelium

Break in basement membrane

Dysplastic cells invading connective tissue

Multiple keratin pearls

Connective tissue with dense lymphocytic infiltration

Fig. 20.10a: Squamous cell carcinoma—well differentiated

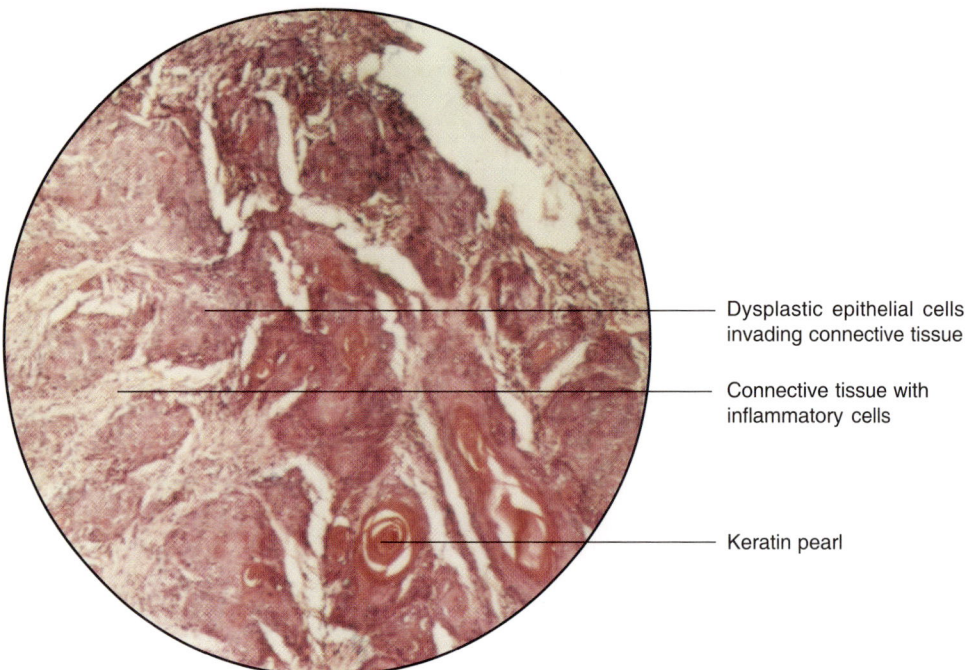

Dysplastic epithelial cells invading connective tissue

Connective tissue with inflammatory cells

Keratin pearl

Squamous cell carcinoma—moderately differentiated (photomicrograph 10X)

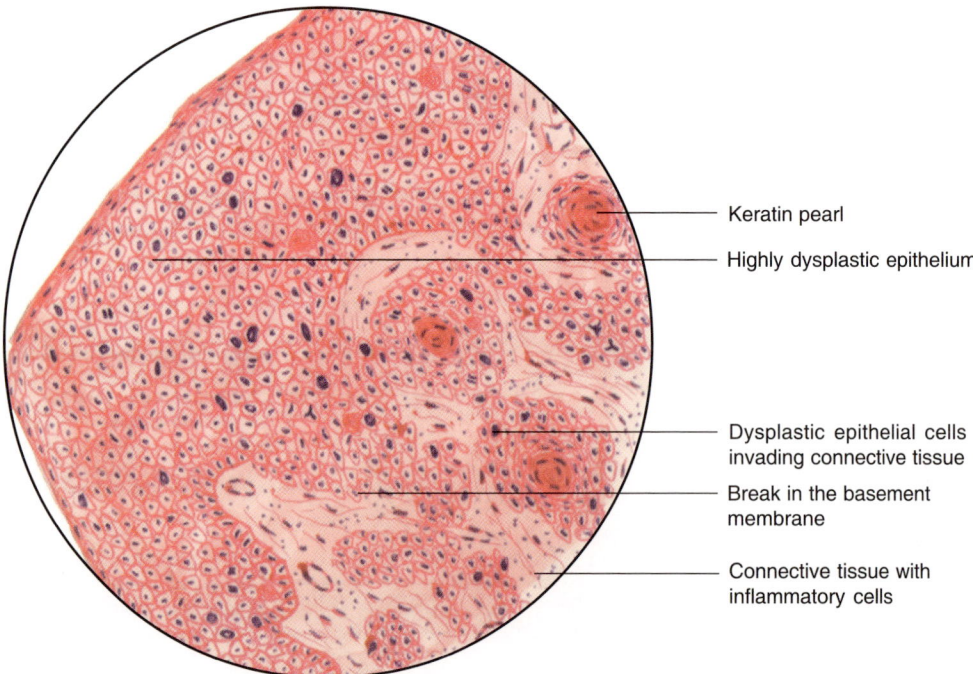

Keratin pearl

Highly dysplastic epithelium

Dysplastic epithelial cells invading connective tissue

Break in the basement membrane

Connective tissue with inflammatory cells

Fig. 20.10b: Squamous cell carcinoma—moderately differentiated

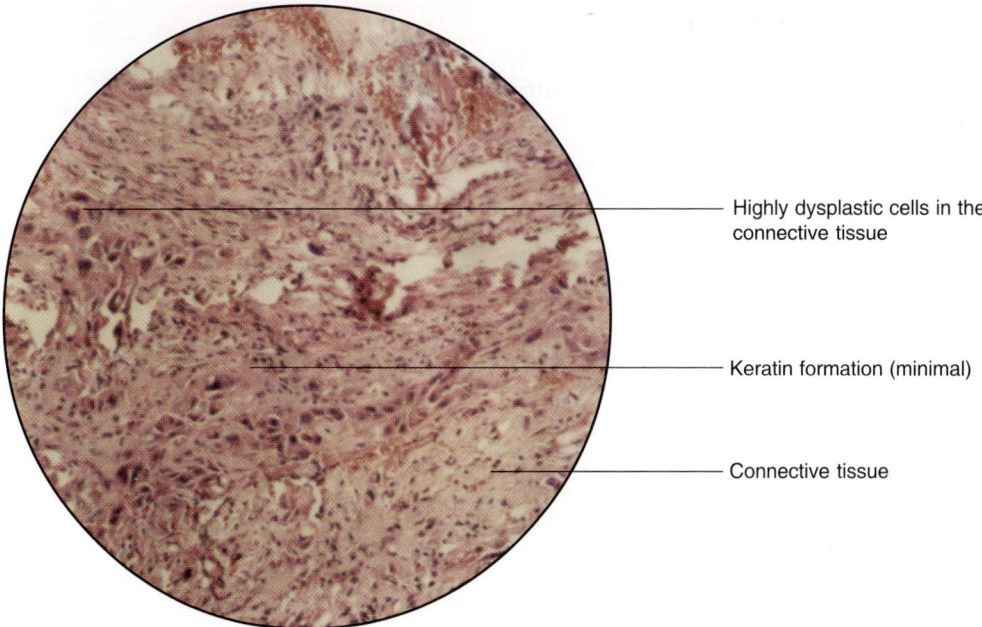

Highly dysplastic cells in the connective tissue

Keratin formation (minimal)

Connective tissue

Squamous cell carcinoma—poorly differentiated (photomicrograph 10X)

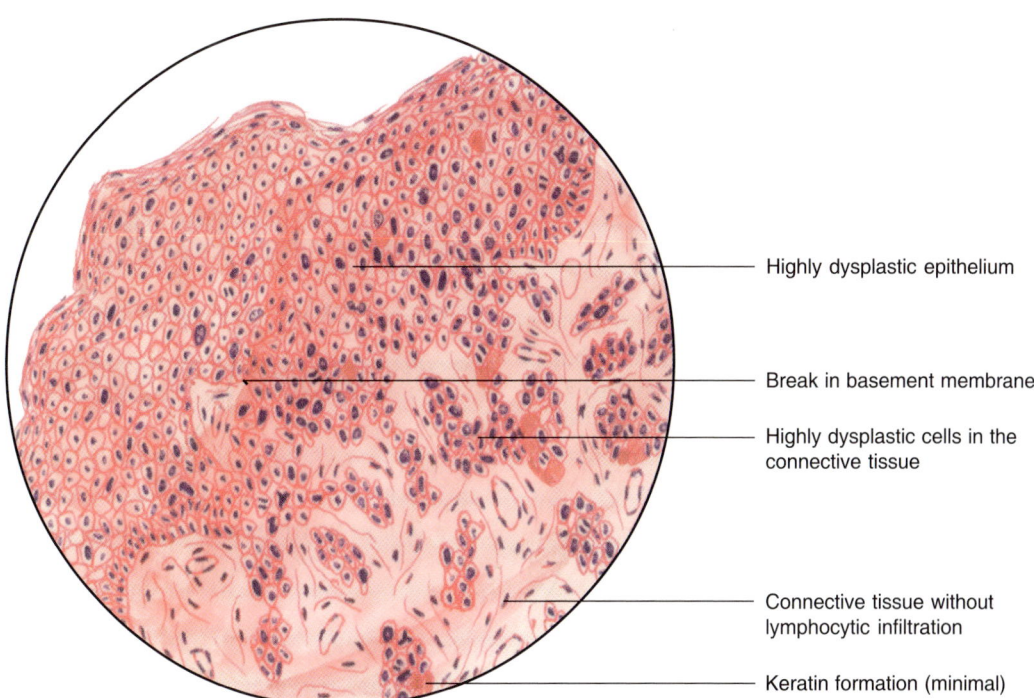

Highly dysplastic epithelium

Break in basement membrane

Highly dysplastic cells in the connective tissue

Connective tissue without lymphocytic infiltration

Keratin formation (minimal)

Fig. 20.10c: Squamous cell carcinoma—poorly differentiated

Histopathology (Fig. 20.11)

Epithelium is hyperplastic with minimal cellular atypia. The rete ridges are broad with pushing border into the deeper connective tissue described as 'elephant foot'-shaped rete ridges. Epithelium is hyperkeratotic with numerous clefts filled with parakeratin (parakeratin plugging) that extends into deep spinous cell layer. Basement membrane is intact. Frequently the connective tissue exhibits dense chronic inflammatory cell infiltration.

Identification Points (Fig. 20.11)

Verrucous Carcinoma
- Hyperplastic epithelium with minimal dysplastic features
- Broad rete ridges with pushing border
- Intact basement membrane
- Chronic inflammatory cells in the connective tissue

BASAL CELL CARCINOMA (RODENT ULCER)

This is an epithelial malignancy arising from the basal layer of skin and its appendages. Clinically this lesion begins as nodules that ulcerate with a rolled out border. The lesion invades into deeper tissue like a rodent. In the oral cavity basal cell carcinoma is not seen unless infiltrated from overlying skin.

Histopathology (Fig. 20.12)

Basal cell carcinoma is characterized by islands, sheets, or epithelial cells in the connective tissue. These epithelial cells resemble basal cells with large deeply staining nuclei and variable number of mitotic figures. The peripheral cells of the islands are distinct with palisading arrangement of nucleus.

Identification Points (Fig. 20.12)

Basal Cell Carcinoma
- Islands of epithelial cells invading connective tissue
- Cells resemble basal cells
- Peripheral cells having palisading arrangement of nuclei

MALIGNANT MELANOMA

Malignant melanoma is a malignant neoplasm arising from melanocytes. This may develop in a benign melanocytic lesion or from melanocytes of otherwise normal mucosa. Clinically this lesion usually present as deeply pigmented area, sometimes ulcerated and hemorrhagic which tend to increase progressively in size.

Histopathology (Fig. 20.13)

Characteristic feature of malignant melanoma is proliferation of atypical melanocytes. In the initial stage, these cells are seen within the basal layer spreading laterally (radial growth). Atypical melanocytes are larger than normal and show varying degrees of pleomorphism and hyperchromatism. As the lesion progresses further to cause vertical growth phase atypical melanocytes invade into the connective tissue. These cells may be epithelioid or spindle-shaped and arranged in the form of loosely aggregated cords or sheets.

Identification Points (Fig. 20.13)

Malignant Melanoma
- Atypical melanocytes invading connective tissue
- Melanocytes may be epithelioid or spindle-shaped with marked pleomorphism
- Melanin pigments may be present

BENIGN CONNECTIVE TISSUE NEOPLASMS

FIBROMA

Fibroma is a benign tumor arising from fibrous connective tissue. Clinically fibroma presents as a painless slow growing, sessile or pedunculated lesion with smooth surface, and firm consistency, pink color, ranging in size from a few millimeters to 1 cm.

Histopathology (Fig. 20.14)

The lesional tissue comprises dense fibrous connective tissue with a few fibroblasts and fibrocytes and scanty blood vessels. Collagen

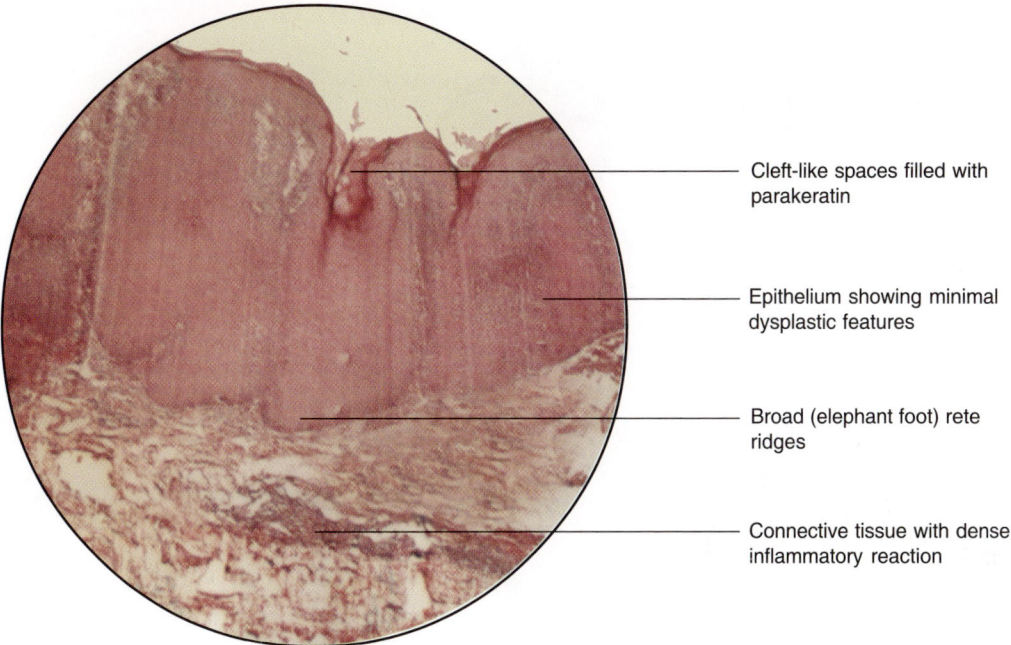

Cleft-like spaces filled with parakeratin

Epithelium showing minimal dysplastic features

Broad (elephant foot) rete ridges

Connective tissue with dense inflammatory reaction

Verrucous carcinoma (photomicrograph 10X)

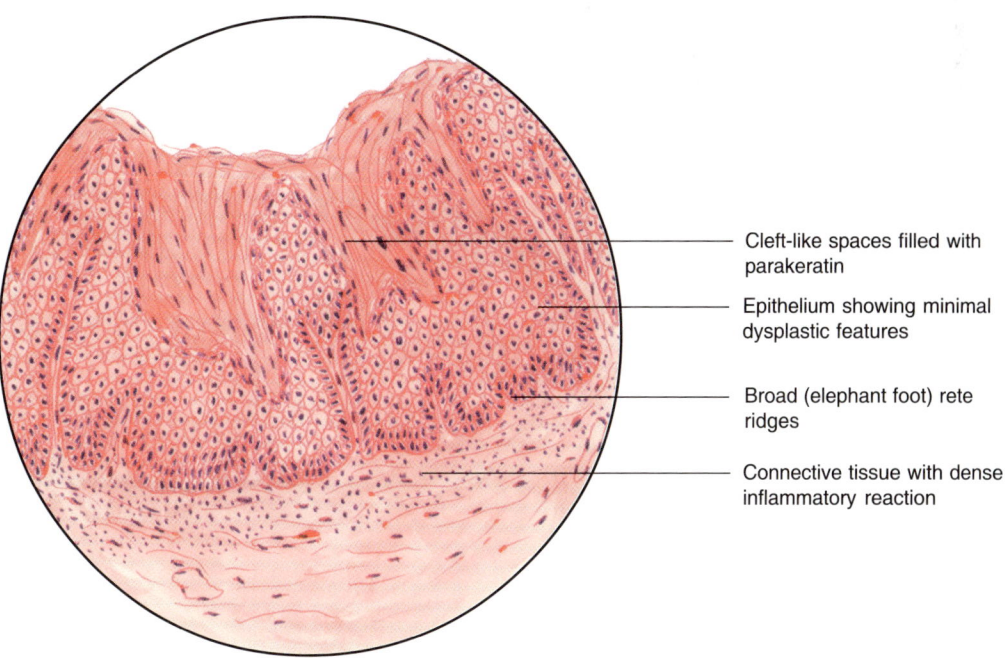

Cleft-like spaces filled with parakeratin

Epithelium showing minimal dysplastic features

Broad (elephant foot) rete ridges

Connective tissue with dense inflammatory reaction

Fig. 20.11: Verrucous carcinoma

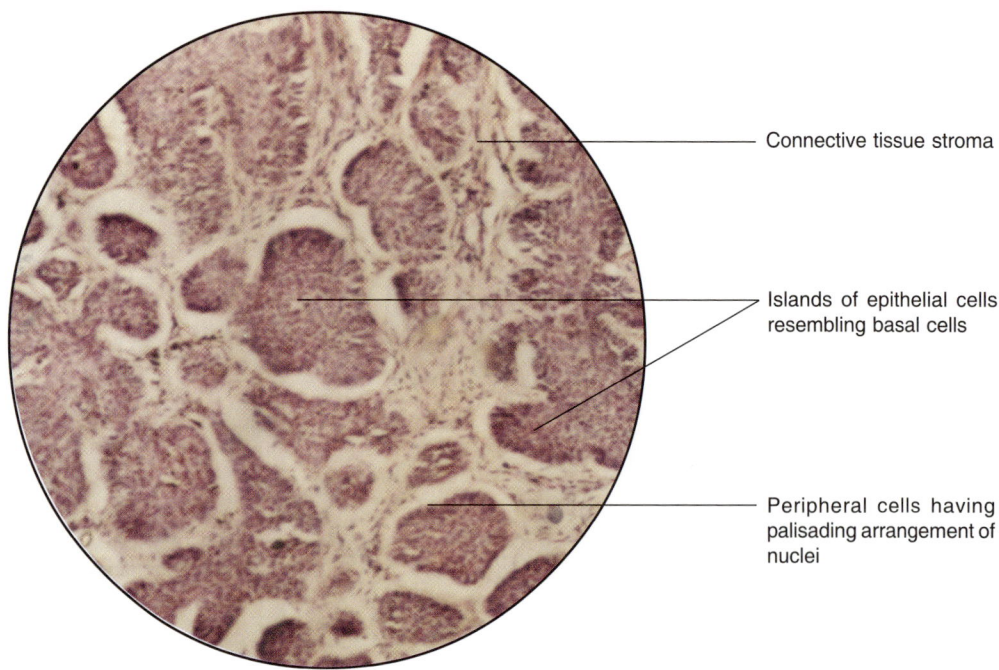

Connective tissue stroma

Islands of epithelial cells resembling basal cells

Peripheral cells having palisading arrangement of nuclei

Basal cell carcinoma (photomicrograph 10X)

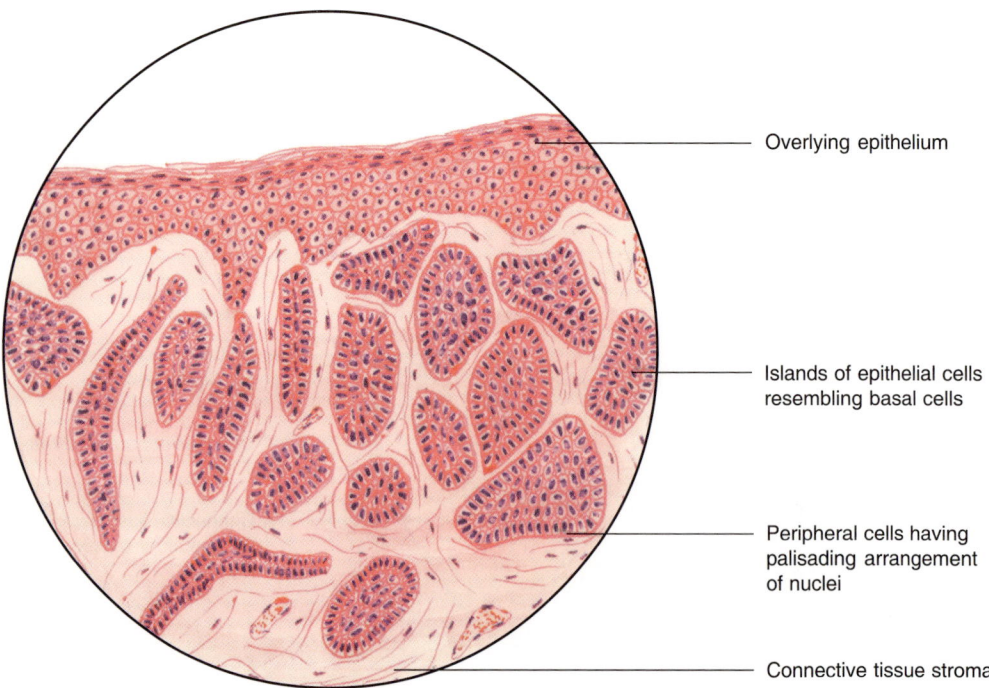

Overlying epithelium

Islands of epithelial cells resembling basal cells

Peripheral cells having palisading arrangement of nuclei

Connective tissue stroma

Fig. 20.12: Basal cell carcinoma

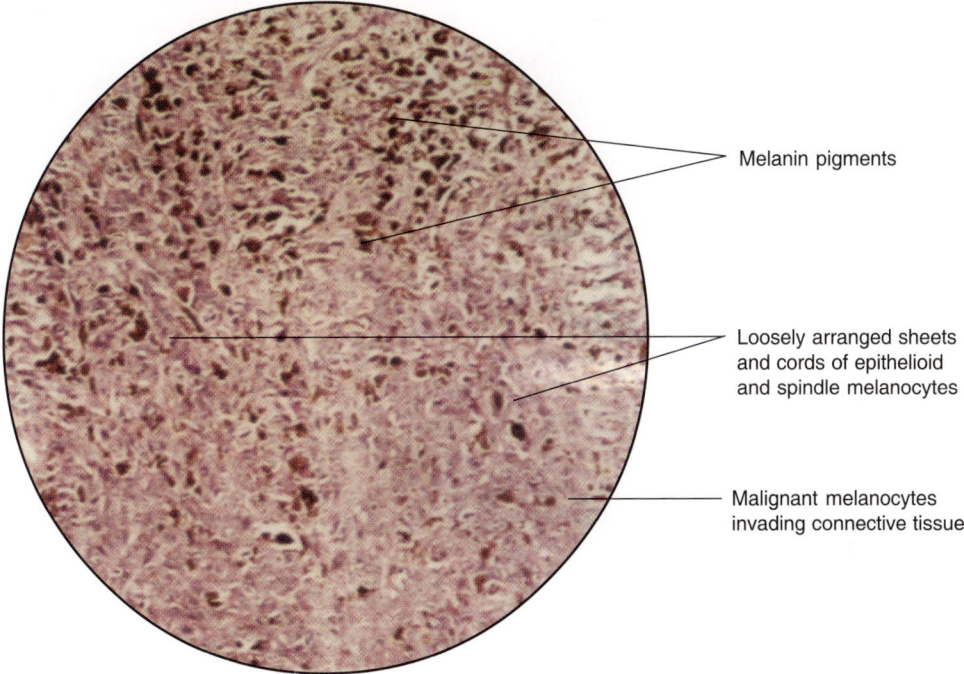

Melanin pigments

Loosely arranged sheets
and cords of epithelioid
and spindle melanocytes

Malignant melanocytes
invading connective tissue

Malignant melanoma (photomicrograph 10X)

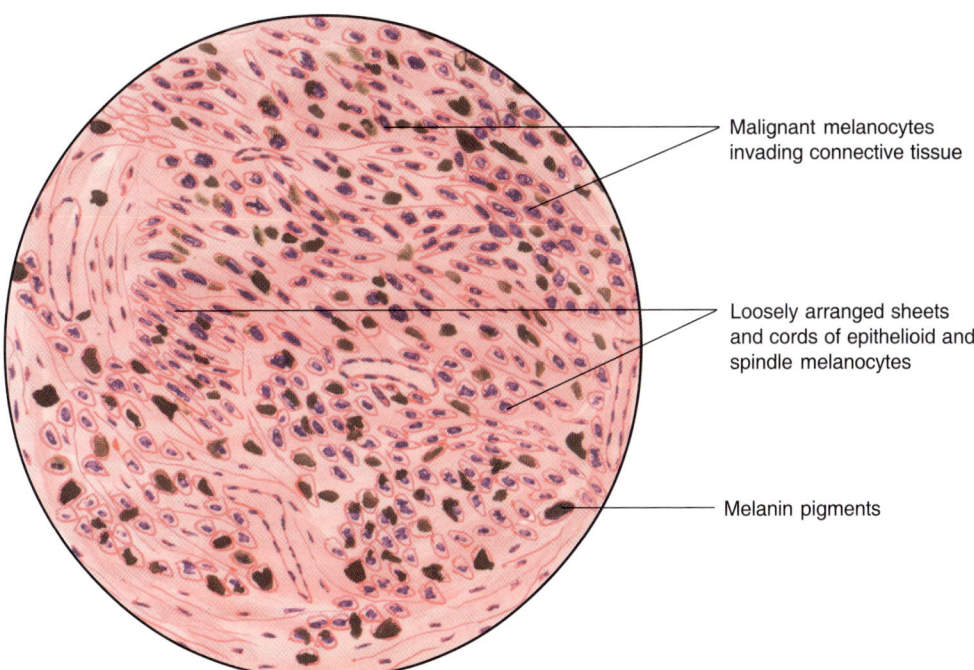

Malignant melanocytes
invading connective tissue

Loosely arranged sheets
and cords of epithelioid and
spindle melanocytes

Melanin pigments

Fig. 20.13: Malignant melanoma

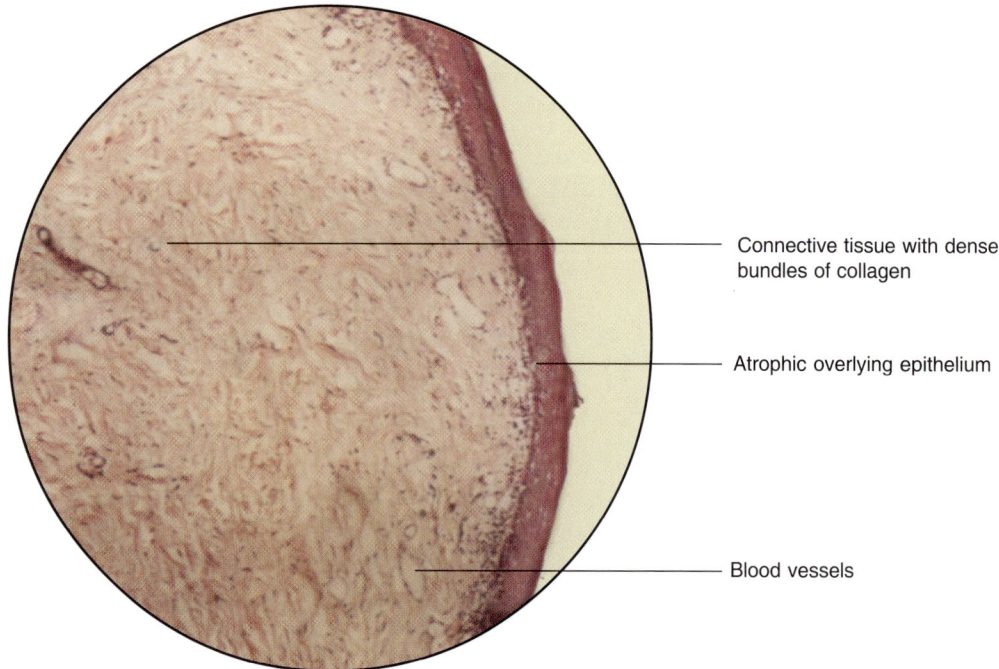

Connective tissue with dense bundles of collagen

Atrophic overlying epithelium

Blood vessels

Fibroma (photomicrograph 4X)

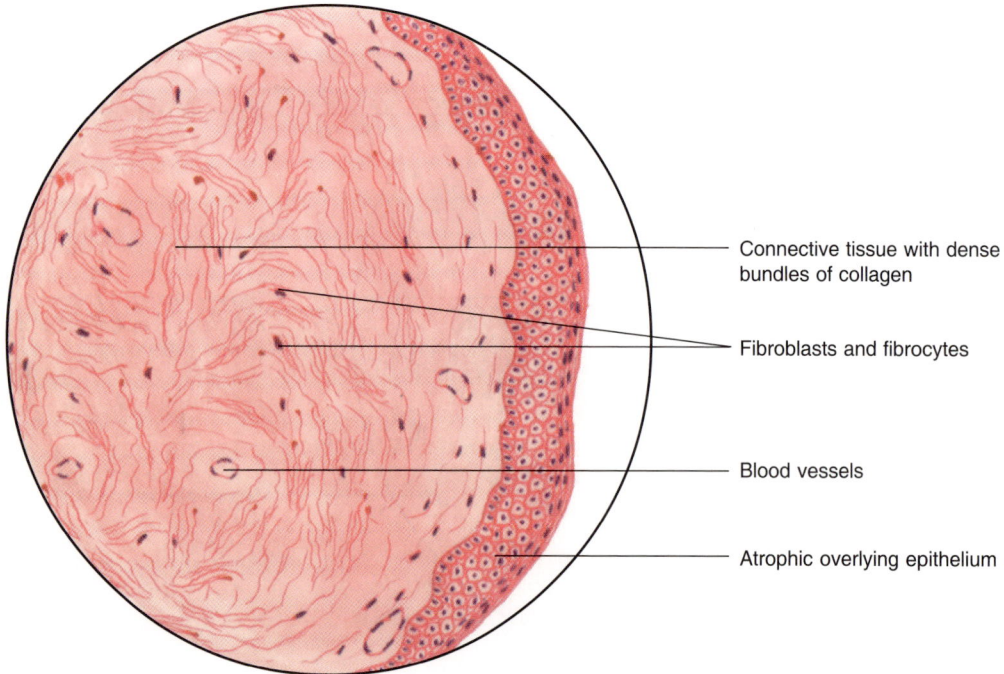

Connective tissue with dense bundles of collagen

Fibroblasts and fibrocytes

Blood vessels

Atrophic overlying epithelium

Fig. 20.14: Fibroma

Identification Points (Fig. 20.14)

Fibroma
- Dense fibrous connective tissue
- Atrophic epithelium

fibers are arranged in bundles in a circular, radiating or haphazard fashion. Overlying stratified squamous epithelium is usually atrophic with flat or short rete ridges.

PERIPHERAL OSSIFYING FIBROMA

This lesion is predominantly a nodular mass of gingiva involving the interdental papilla. Clinically peripheral ossifying fibroma is similar to fibroma; the color may vary from red to pink and frequently with an ulcerated surface.

Histopathology (Fig. 20.15)

Microscopic features are similar to fibroma but associated with formation of mineralized product. Connective tissue is highly cellular specifically in the regions of mineralization. Mineralization may be in the form of osteoid, bony trabeculae or cementum like material. Overlying stratified squamous epithelium may be intact or ulcerated.

Identification Points (Fig. 20.15)

Peripheral Ossifying Fibroma
- Highly cellular connective tissue
- Presence of calcifications

LIPOMA

Lipoma is a benign tumor of fat tissue origin and it is present as an asymptomatic, slow growing nodular mass, soft in consistency, with smooth surface, varying in size usually up to 2 to 3 cm. Color of the lesion may be yellowish.

Histopathology (Fig. 20.16)

Lipoma is composed of mature fat cells. Cells are round or ovoid, with empty looking

Identification Points (Fig. 20.16)

Lipoma
- Composed of mature fat cells
- Fat cells appear empty with nucleus pushed to periphery
- Presence of connective tissue septa

cytoplasm and eccentrically placed nucleus that is pressed against the cell membrane. The lesion is well circumscribed, may have a connective tissue capsule. Connective tissue septa is often seen dividing the lesion into many lobules.

Along with fat cells if fibrous connective tissue is significant it is called fibrolipoma and highly vascular lipoma lesions are called angiolipoma.

HEMANGIOMA

Hemangioma is characterized by benign proliferation of blood vessels and is considered as a hamartoma (tumor-like malformation native to the site). These lesions usually present as red or purplish, flat or slightly raised lesions.

Histopathology (Fig. 20.17)

The most characteristic histopathological feature of hemangioma is presence of numerous endothelium lined vascular channels containing RBCs. Lesions also show numerous proliferating plump endothelial cells. Based on size of the blood vessels, hemangioma can be capillary hemangioma where the vessels are of smaller size or cavernous hemangioma where the vessels are larger.

Identification Points (Fig. 20.17)

Hemangioma
- Multiple blood-filled vascular channels
- Proliferating endothelial cells

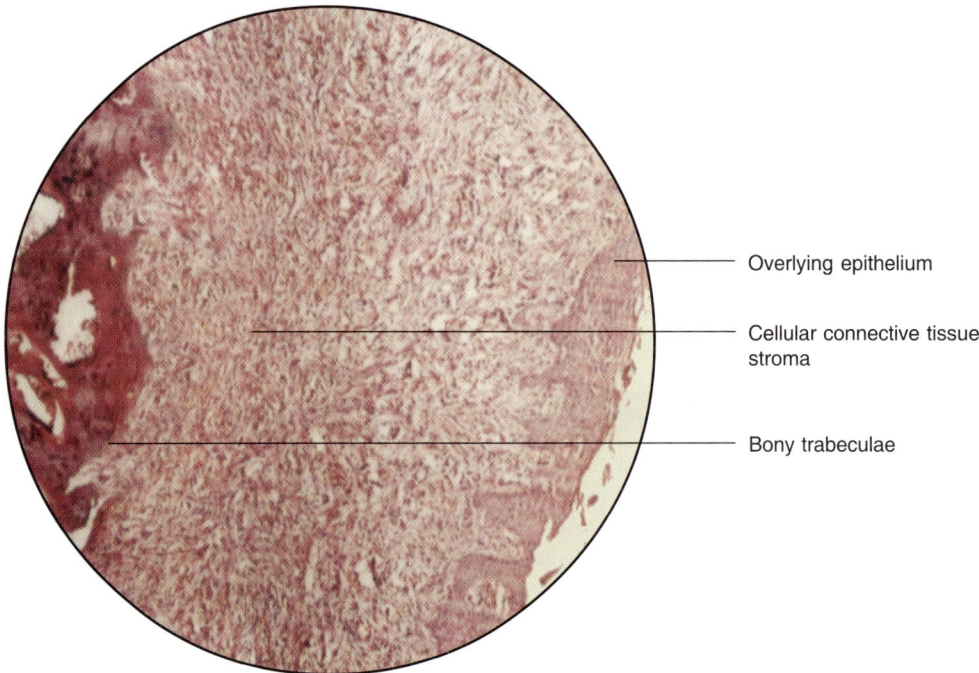

Overlying epithelium

Cellular connective tissue stroma

Bony trabeculae

Peripheral ossifying fibroma (photomicrograph 4X)

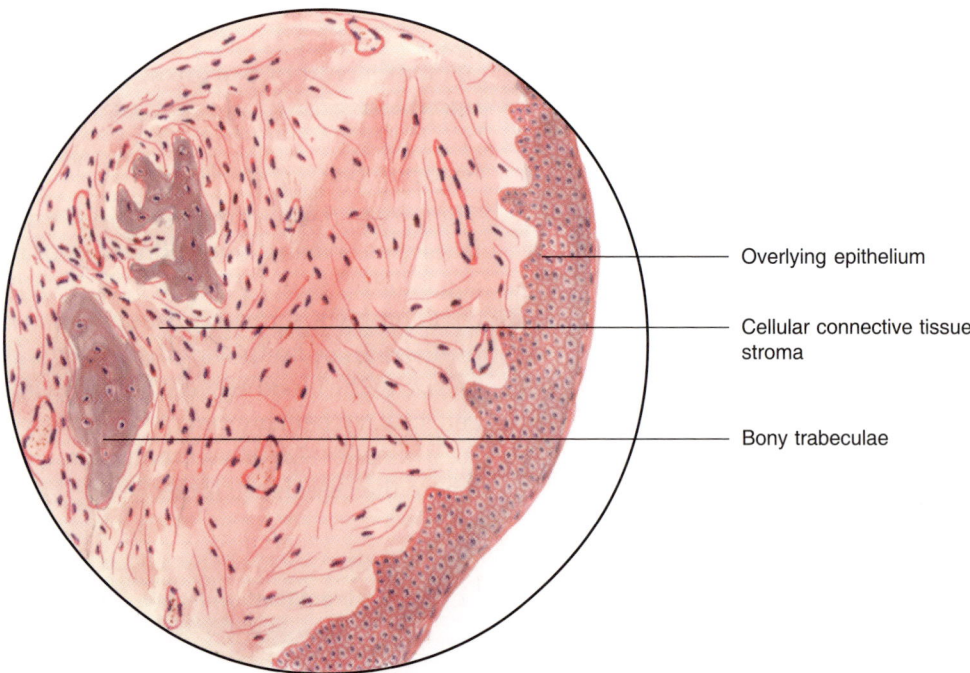

Overlying epithelium

Cellular connective tissue stroma

Bony trabeculae

Fig. 20.15: Peripheral ossifying fibroma

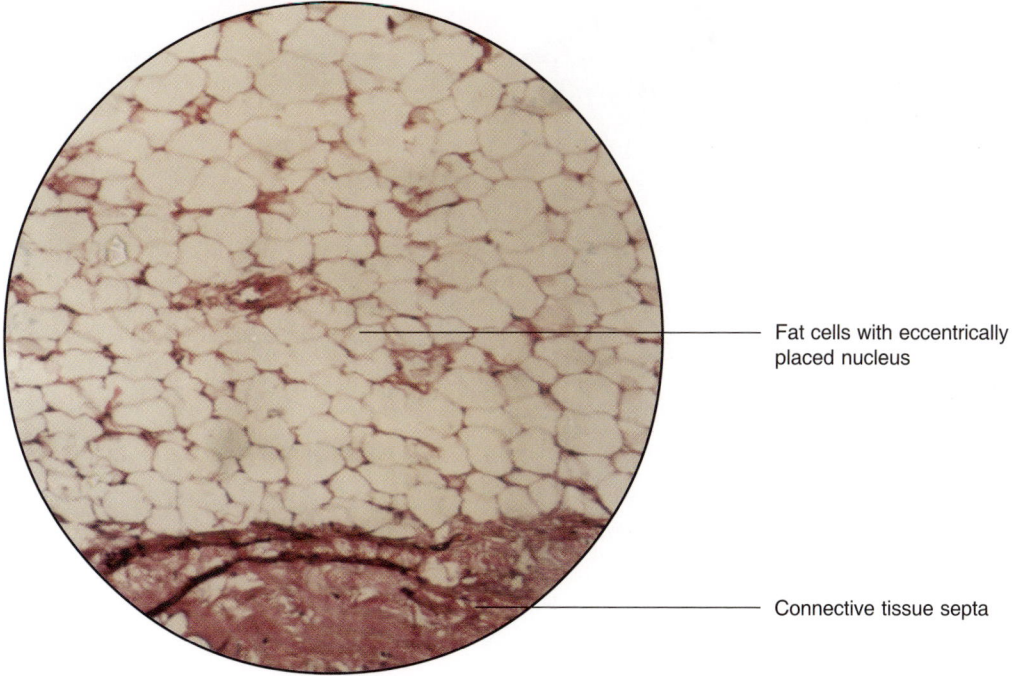

Fat cells with eccentrically placed nucleus

Connective tissue septa

Lipoma (photomicrograph 10X)

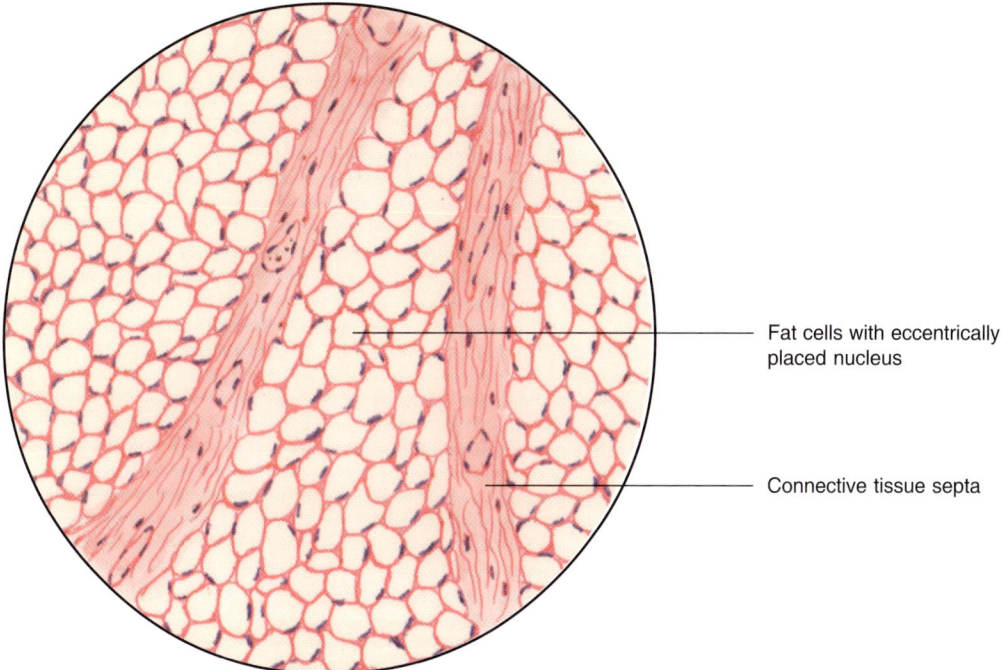

Fat cells with eccentrically placed nucleus

Connective tissue septa

Fig. 20.16: Lipoma

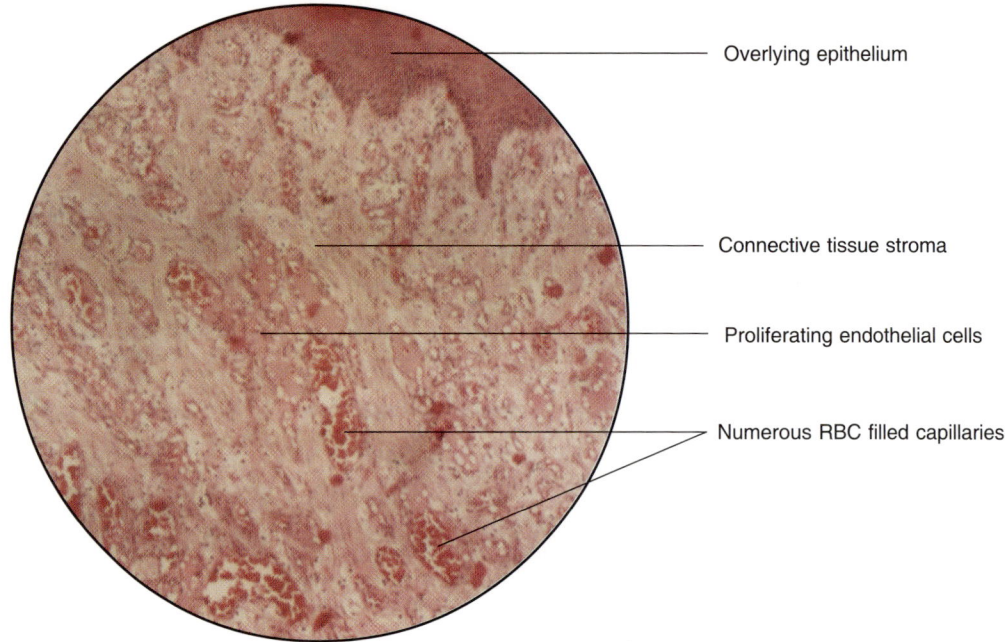

Overlying epithelium

Connective tissue stroma

Proliferating endothelial cells

Numerous RBC filled capillaries

Capillary hemangioma (photomicrograph 10X)

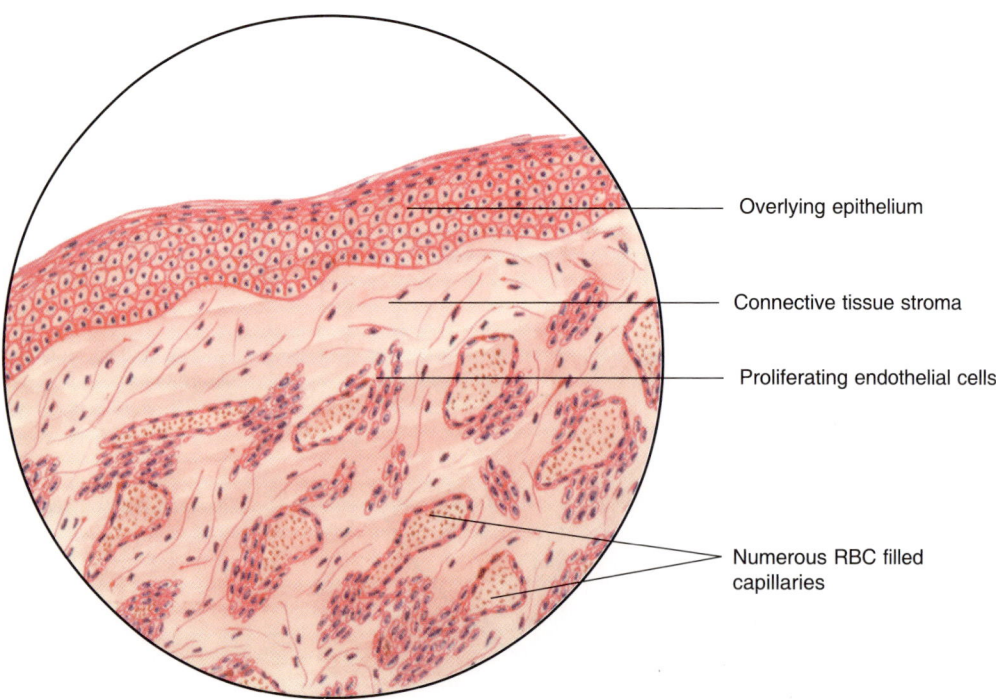

Overlying epithelium

Connective tissue stroma

Proliferating endothelial cells

Numerous RBC filled capillaries

Fig. 20. 17: Capillary hemangioma

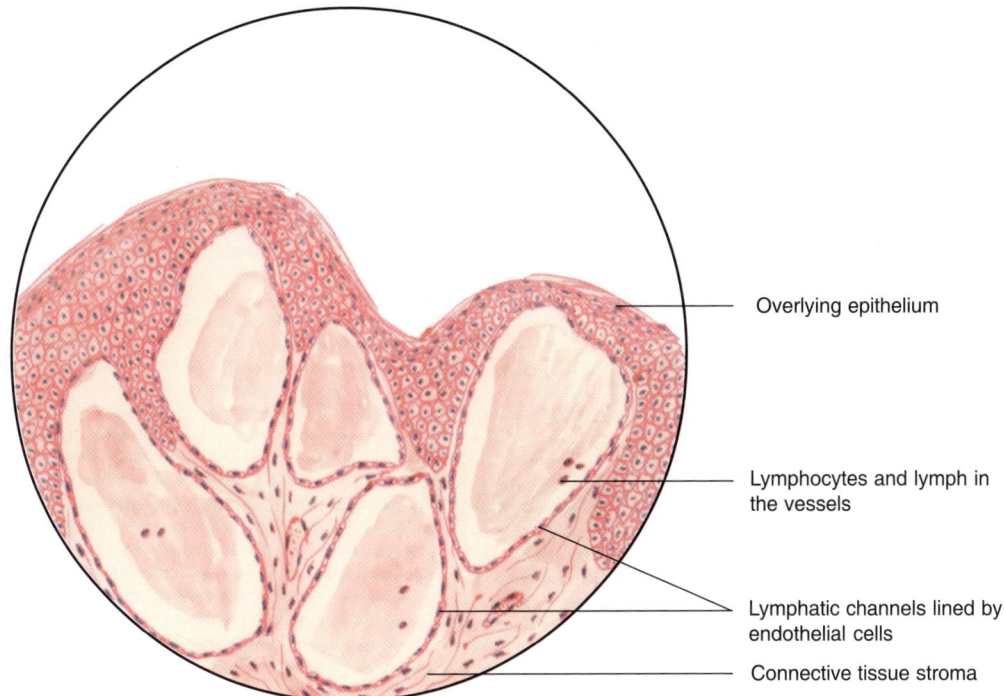

— Overlying epithelium

— Lymphocytes and lymph in
the vessels

— Lymphatic channels lined by
endothelial cells

— Connective tissue stroma

Fig. 20.18: Lymphangioma

LYMPHANGIOMA

Lymphangioma is a benign tumor of lymphatic vessels. This is also considered as hamartoma. Oral lymphangioma usually presents as a lesion of the tongue that manifests as macroglossia. Tongue lesions show pebbly surface.

Histopathology (Fig. 20.18)

Microscopically lymphangioma shows multiple lymphatic channels lined by endothelial cells and containing proteinaceous fluid and occasional lymphocytes. The lesion is typically located just beneath the epithelium and lymphatic channels replaces the connective tissue papillae.

Identification Points (Fig. 20.18)

Lymphangioma
- Multiple lymphatic channels containing lymph
- Lymphatic channels replacing the connective tissue papillae

NEURILEMMOMA (SCHWANNOMA)

Neurilemmoma is a benign tumor of nerve tissue, originating from the Schwann cells. Clinically this lesion presents as an asymptomatic slow growing nodular swelling in association with a nerve trunk, pushing the nerve aside.

Histopathology (Fig. 20.19)

Microscopically neurilemmoma presents as an encapsulated lesion showing two different patterns described as Antoni type A and Antoni type B. In Antoni type A spindle-shaped cells have a regular palisading arrangement. These cells may be arranged

Identification Points (Fig. 20.19)

Neurilemmoma
- Two patterns; Antoni type A and Antoni type B
- Antoni type A with palisading arrangement of cells enclosing 'Verocay bodies'
- Antoni type B with disorderly arrangement of cells

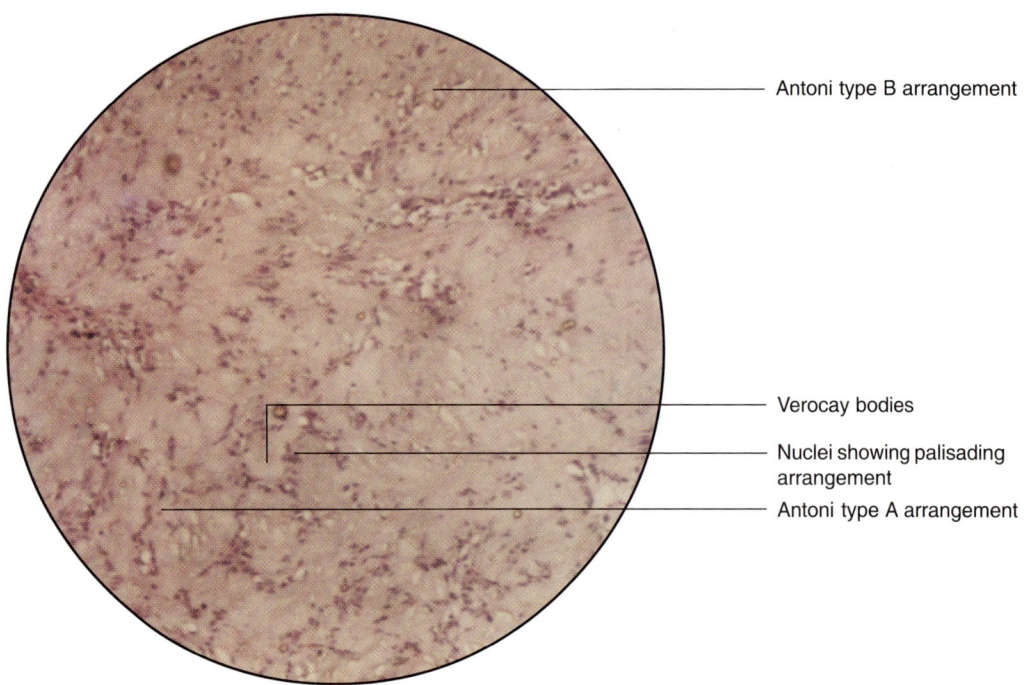

Antoni type B arrangement

Verocay bodies

Nuclei showing palisading arrangement

Antoni type A arrangement

Neurilemmoma (photomicrograph 10X)

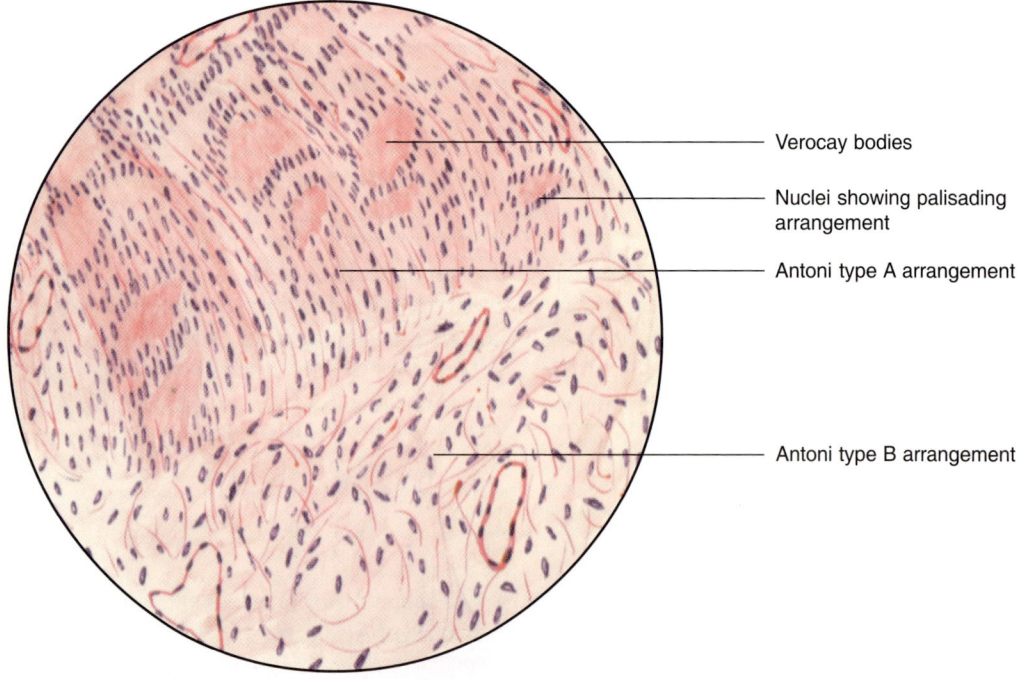

Verocay bodies

Nuclei showing palisading arrangement

Antoni type A arrangement

Antoni type B arrangement

Fig. 20.19: Neurilemmoma

around a central eosinophilic acellular area called as 'Verocay bodies'. In Antoni type B spindle cells are randomly arranged without palisading arrangement. Tissue is less cellular and cells are arranged in a disorderly manner in a loose myxomatous stroma.

NEUROFIBROMA

Neurofibroma is a benign tumor of nerve tissue arising from Schwann cells and perineural fibroblasts. Solitary neurofibroma is seen as a slow growing soft painless nodular mass. Multiple neurofibromas are seen in neurofibromatosis.

Histopathology (Fig. 20.20)

Neurofibroma is characterized by proliferation of elements of peripheral nerves. It comprises interlacing bundles of delicate collagen fibers with spindle-shaped cells including Schwann cells and fibroblasts. Schwann cells have wavy nuclei with pointed ends. Connective tissue stroma may show areas of myxoid degeneration and numerous mast cells.

Identification Points (Fig. 20.20)

Neurofibroma
- Proliferating spindle-shaped cells having wavy nuclei
- Presence of numerous mast cells

MALIGNANT CONNECTIVE TISSUE TUMORS

FIBROSARCOMA

Fibrosarcoma is a malignant neoplasm of fibroblasts. This lesion clinically presents as a slow or sometimes rapidly growing mass invading the local tissue.

Histopathology (Fig. 20.21)

Fibrosarcoma is characterized by proliferation of fibroblasts, showing varying degrees of atypical changes. In well differentiated lesions

Identification Points (Fig. 20.21)

Fibrosarcoma
- Proliferating atypical fibroblasts
- Cells and fibers arranged to form 'herringbone pattern'
- Presence of mitotic figures

fibroblasts are spindle-shaped and arranged to form fascicles that form a 'herringbone pattern'. The cells are less organized and show considerable pleomorphism in poorly differentiated lesions. Variable number of mitotic figures can be identified. The amount of collagen produced is lesser in poorly differentiated tumors than in well differentiated tumors.

OSTEOSARCOMA

Osteosarcoma is a malignant neoplasm of the bone. Early clinical manifestations of this disease are pain and swelling. When jaw bones are involved, loosening of teeth and paresthesia may be noted. Characteristic radiographic presentation is 'sunray' or 'sunburst' appearance.

Histopathology (Fig. 20.22)

The characteristic microscopic feature is proliferation of atypical osteoblasts. These cells are arranged in a disorderly fashion about trabeculae of bone and show considerable pleomorphism and hyperchromatism. Areas of tumor osteoid deposited by these osteoblasts can be seen. Histological variants are osteoblastic, fibroblastic, and chondroblastic osteosarcomas.

Identification Points (Fig. 20.22)

Osteosarcoma
- Proliferating atypical osteoblasts
- Formation of tumor osteoid
- Histological variants are—osteoblastic, chondroblastic and fibroblastic osteosarcomas

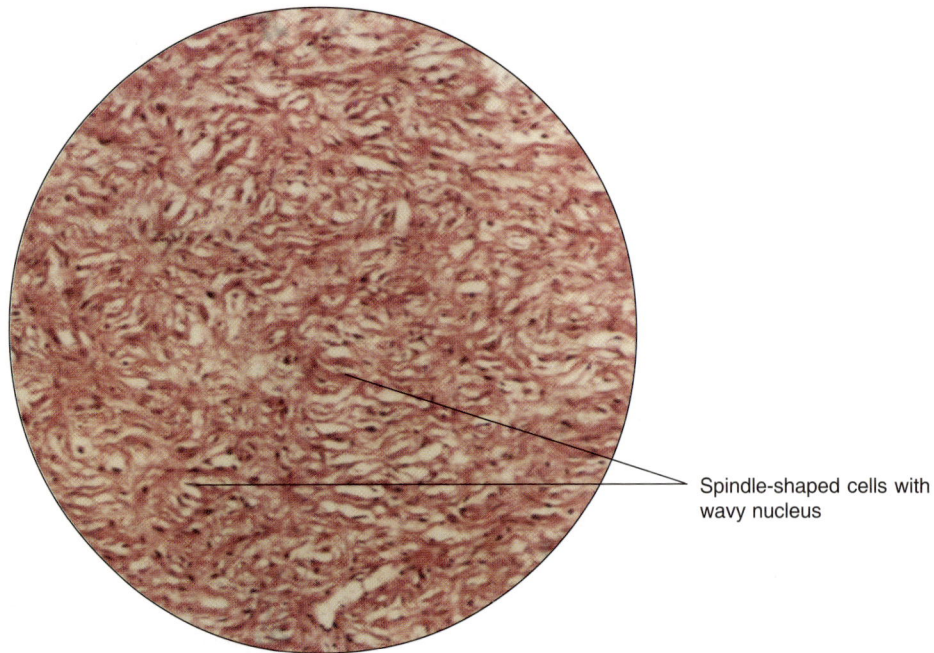

Spindle-shaped cells with wavy nucleus

Neurofibroma (photomicrograph 10X)

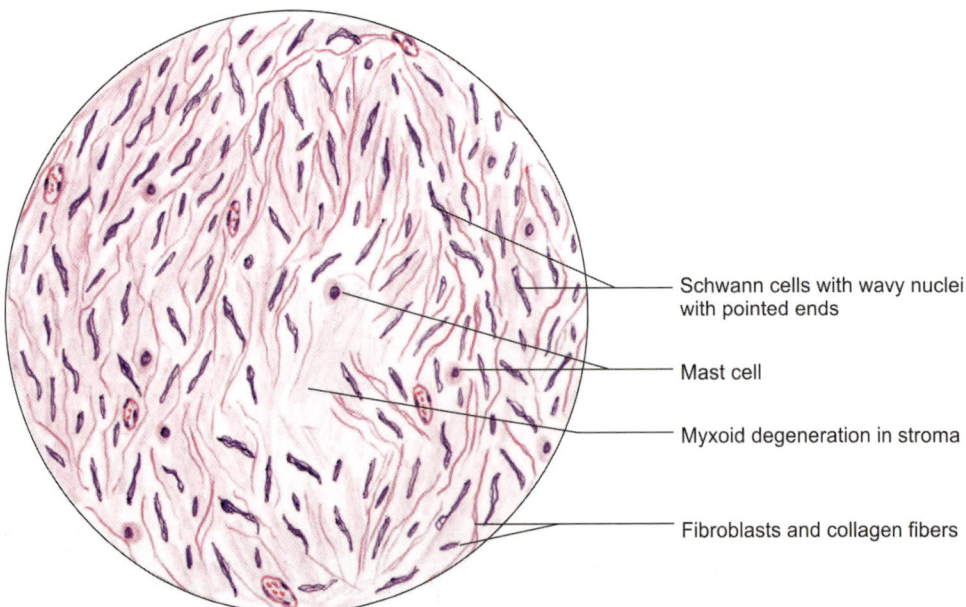

Schwann cells with wavy nuclei with pointed ends

Mast cell

Myxoid degeneration in stroma

Fibroblasts and collagen fibers

Fig. 20.20: Neurofibroma

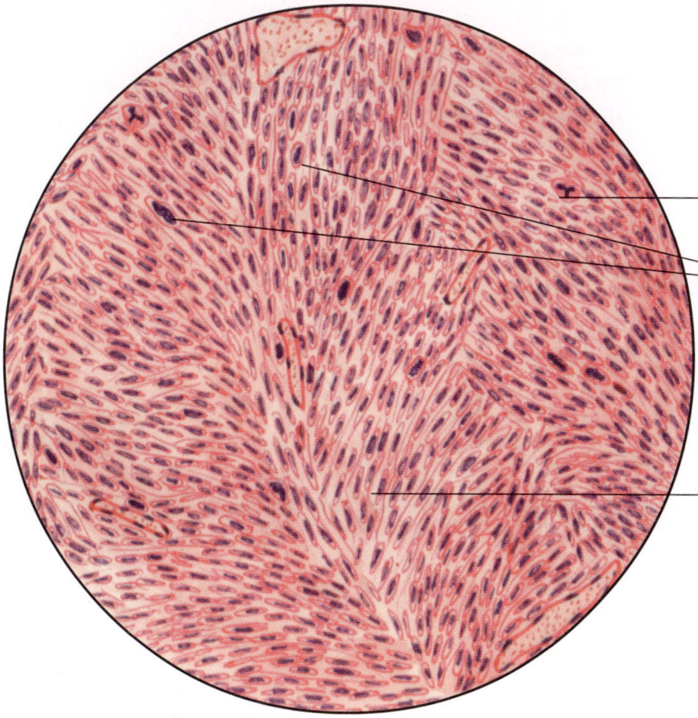

Mitotic figures

Cells exhibiting
hyperchromatism
and pleomorphism

Proliferating fibroblasts
arranged to form herring-
bone pattern

Fig. 20.21: Fibrosarcoma

TUMOR-LIKE LESIONS

CENTRAL GIANT CELL GRANULOMA

This is a destructive lesion of the jaw bones initially asymptomatic, slowly causing bony expansion and facial asymmetry. Radiographic presentation is in the form of unilocular or more frequently as multilocular radiolucency.

Histopathology (Fig. 20.23)

Lesional tissue is composed of highly cellular connective tissue stroma with numerous spindle-shaped cells. Multinucleated giant cells are distributed in this connective tissue. Giant cells are large cells with many nuclei up to 20 or more. Giant cells are usually aggregated close to the blood vessels.

PERIPHERAL GIANT CELL GRANULOMA

This lesion is a tumor-like growth that occurs predominantly in the gingiva presents as a red or reddish blue nodular mass. Clinically these lesions resemble pyogenic granuloma.

Histopathology (Fig. 20.24)

Lesional tissue is composed of many multinucleated giant cells distributed in a highly cellular connective tissue having numerous spindle-shaped cells.

Identification Points (Fig. 20.23)

Central Giant Cell Granuloma
- Highly cellular connective tissue stroma
- Presence of multiple giant cells
- Giant cells arranged close to blood vessels

Identification Points (Fig. 20.24)

Peripheral Giant Cell Granuloma
- Highly cellular connective tissue stroma
- Presence of multiple giant cells
- Zone of connective tissue separating lesional tissue from epithelium

Giant cells are large round or irregular cells with a few or many nuclei. Many blood vessels and extravasated RBCs are seen. One of the characteristic features of this lesion is a zone of dense fibrous connective tissue separating the lesional tissue from overlying stratified squamous epithelium.

PYOGENIC GRANULOMA

Pyogenic granuloma is a common tumor-like lesion usually occurring on gingiva. These lesions present as sessile or pedunculated mass with a smooth or lobulated surface, soft in consistency, red or pinkish in color ranging in size from a few mm to cm.

Histopathology (Fig. 20.25)

Microscopically pyogenic granuloma resembles granulation tissue. The lesion is composed of proliferating fibroblasts, endothelial cells and budding capillaries. Numerous endothelium lined vascular channels filled with RBCs are seen. Lesional tissue is densely infiltrated with chronic inflammatory cells predominantly plasma cells and lymphocytes. Overlying epithelium is usually ulcerated and this ulcerated region is covered with a fibrinous exudates densely infiltrated with acute and chronic inflammatory cells.

Identification Points (Fig. 20.25)

Pyogenic Granuloma
- Granulation tissue containing proliferating fibroblasts, endothelial cells and inflammatory cells
- Ulcerated overlying epithelium

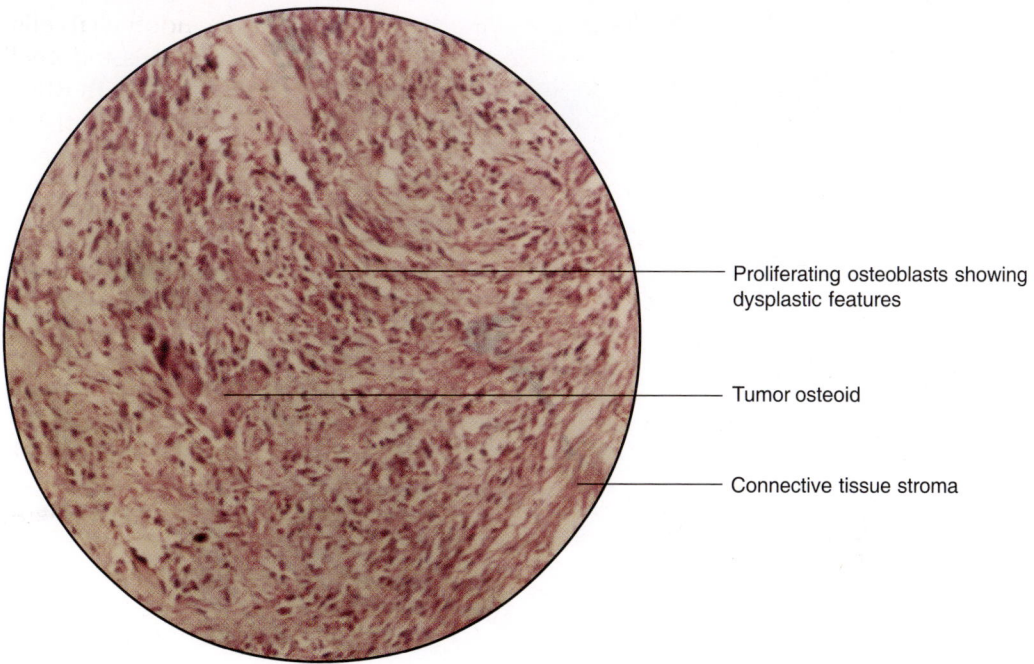

Proliferating osteoblasts showing dysplastic features

Tumor osteoid

Connective tissue stroma

Osteosarcoma (photomicrograph 10X)

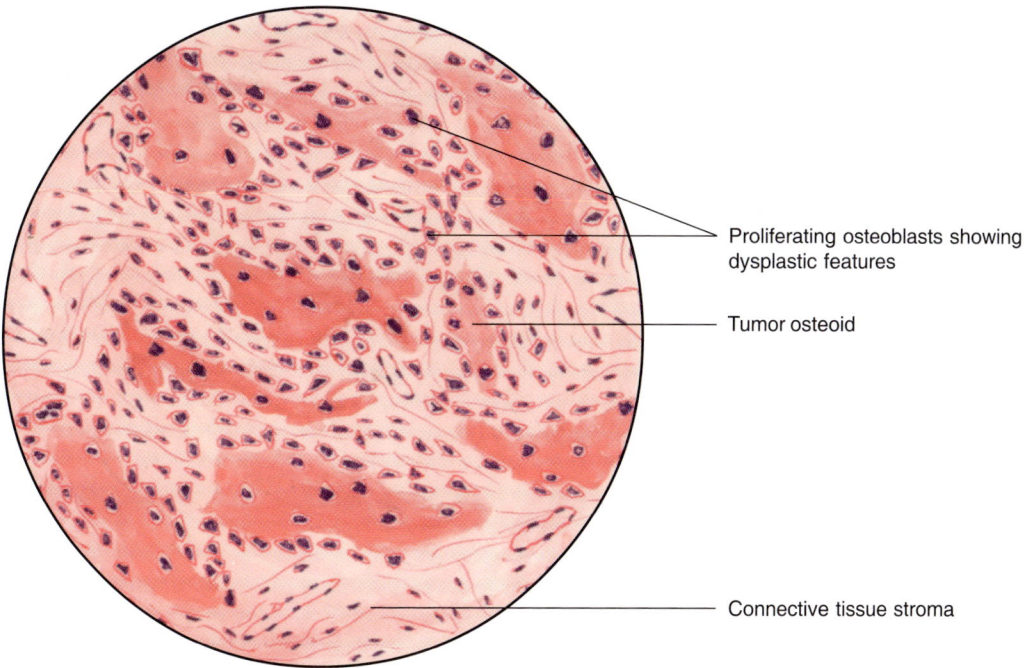

Proliferating osteoblasts showing dysplastic features

Tumor osteoid

Connective tissue stroma

Fig. 20.22: Osteosarcoma

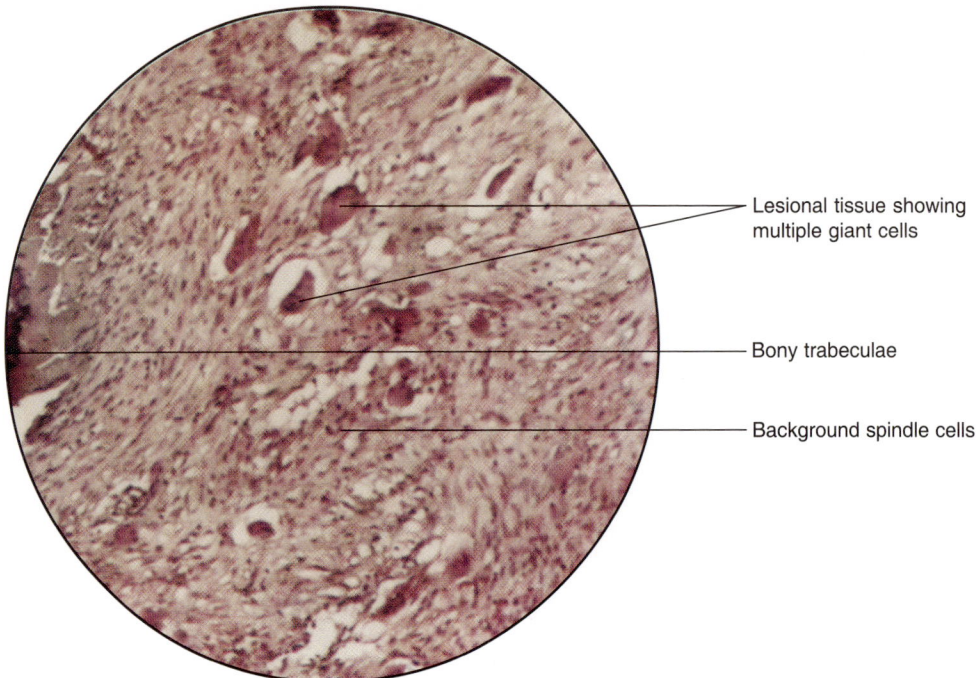

Lesional tissue showing
multiple giant cells

Bony trabeculae

Background spindle cells

Central giant cell granuloma (photomicrograph 10X)

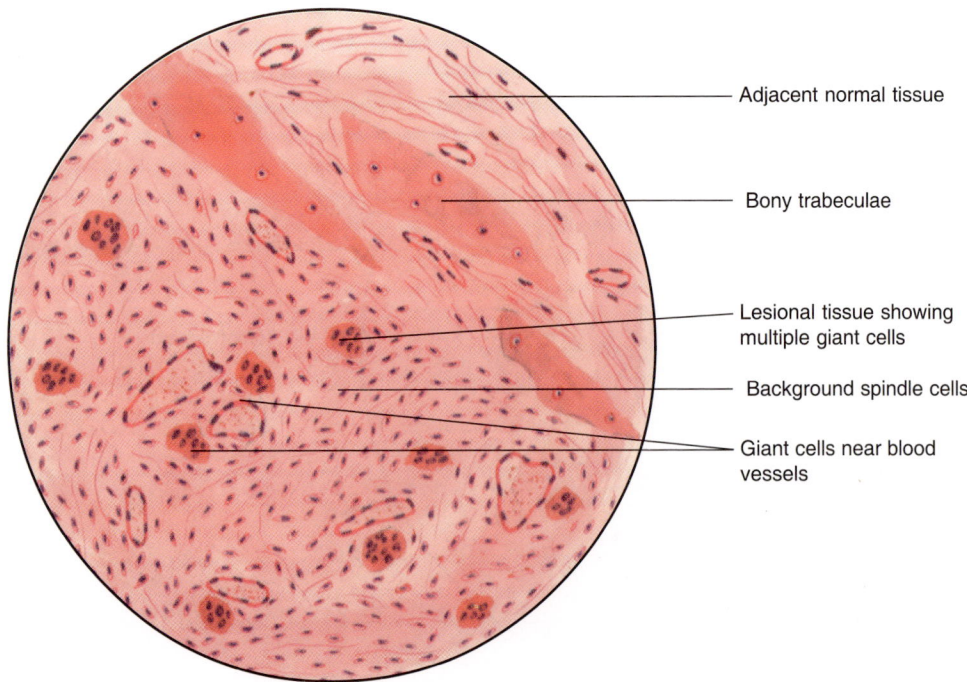

Adjacent normal tissue

Bony trabeculae

Lesional tissue showing
multiple giant cells

Background spindle cells

Giant cells near blood
vessels

Fig. 20.23: Central giant cell granuloma

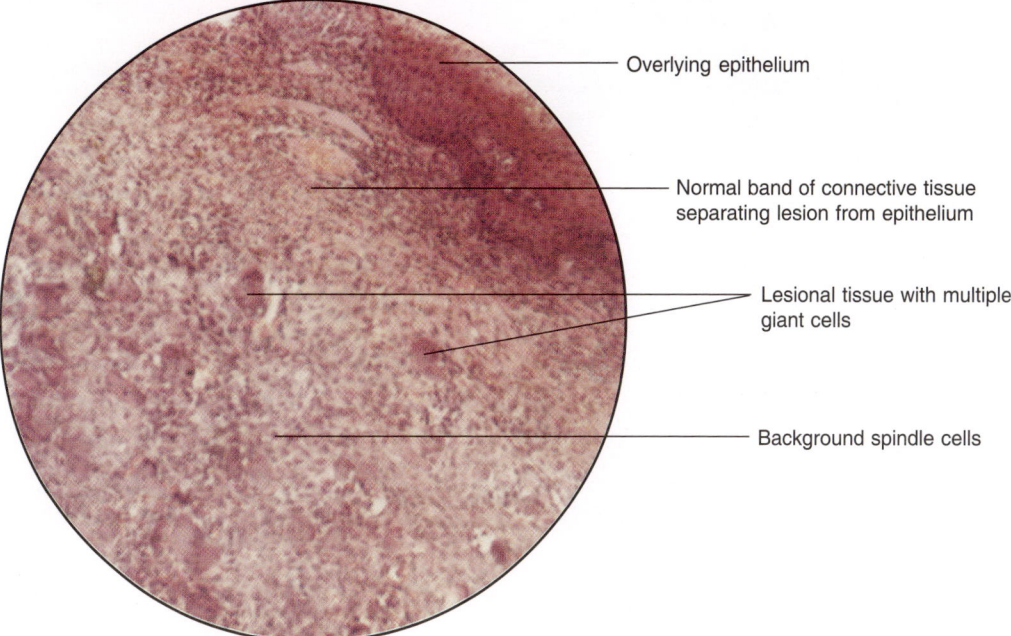

Overlying epithelium

Normal band of connective tissue separating lesion from epithelium

Lesional tissue with multiple giant cells

Background spindle cells

Peripheral giant cell granuloma (photomicrograph 10X)

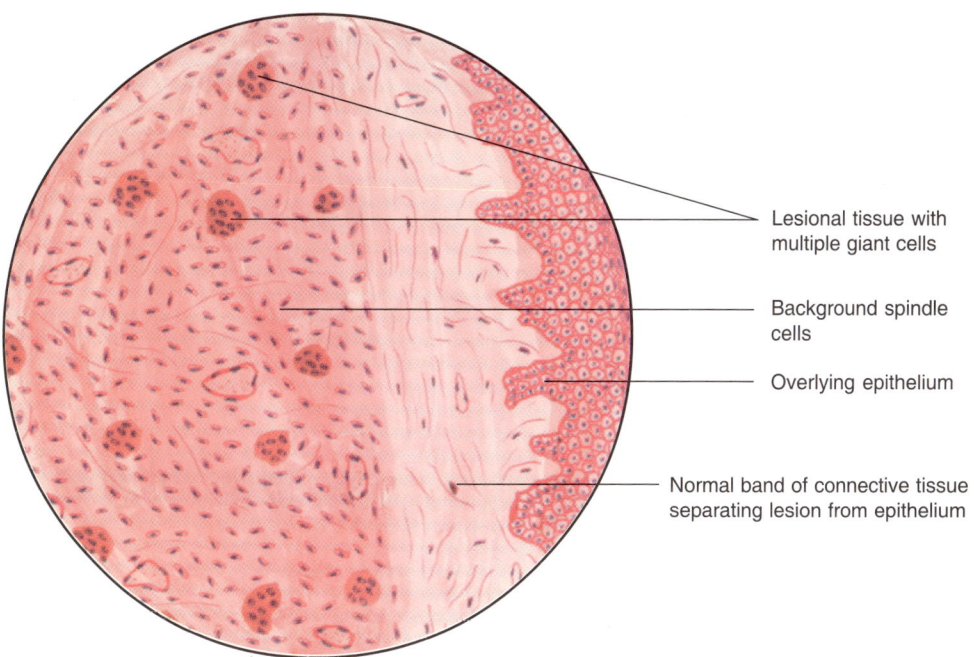

Lesional tissue with multiple giant cells

Background spindle cells

Overlying epithelium

Normal band of connective tissue separating lesion from epithelium

Fig. 20.24: Peripheral giant cell granuloma

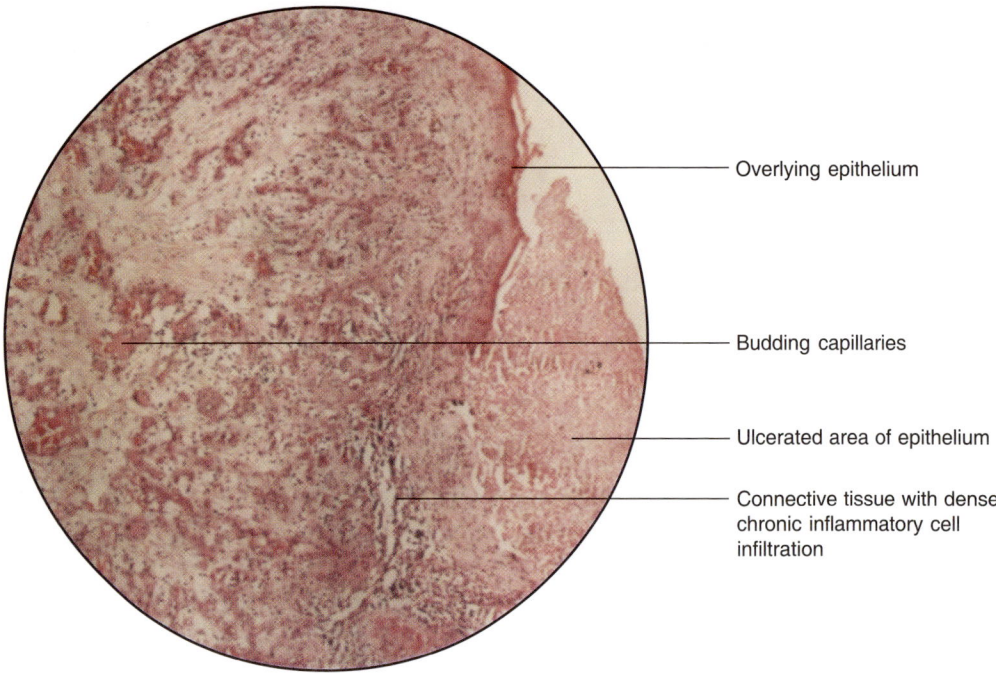

Overlying epithelium

Budding capillaries

Ulcerated area of epithelium

Connective tissue with dense chronic inflammatory cell infiltration

Pyogenic granuloma (photomicrograph 10X)

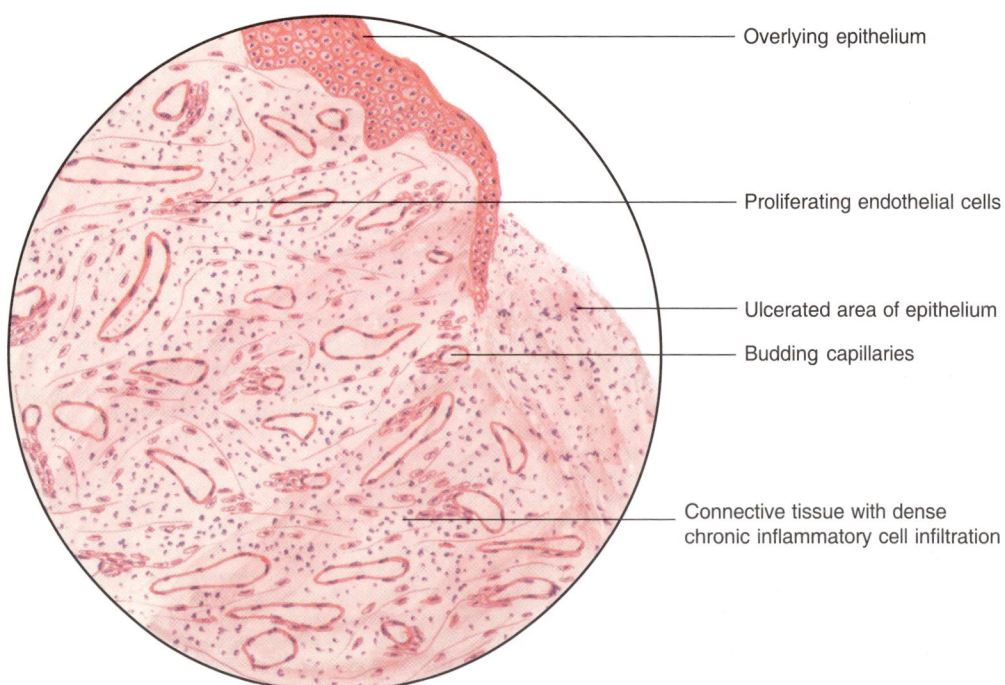

Overlying epithelium

Proliferating endothelial cells

Ulcerated area of epithelium

Budding capillaries

Connective tissue with dense chronic inflammatory cell infiltration

Fig. 20.25: Pyogenic granuloma

21

Developmental Disturbances

- Fordyce's spots or Fordyce's granules
- Developmental disturbances affecting the teeth
  - Gemination
  - Twinning
  - Fusion
  - Concrescence
  - Dilaceration
  - Talon cusp
  - Taurodontism
  - Dens evaginatus
  - Dens invaginatus
  - Supernumerary teeth or hyperdontia
  - Anodontia or hypodontia
  - Supernumerary cusp and roots
  - Enameloma
  - Micro- and macrodontia

FORDYCE'S SPOTS OR FORDYCE'S GRANULES

Fordyce's granules are the developmental anomaly affecting the oral mucosa, which clinically appear as yellowish white papular lesions. They are characterized by heterotopic collection of sebaceous glands in the oral mucosa and considered as normal anatomic variation.

Histopathology (Fig. 21.1)

Fordyce's granules are characterized by the presence of lobules of sebaceous cells beneath the epithelium, often with a central duct communicating to the surface. The sebaceous cells are polygonal with centrally located nucleus and abundant foamy cytoplasm. In contrast to the sebaceous glands of the skin Fordyce's granules lack hair follicle.

DEVELOPMENTAL DISTURBANCES AFFECTING THE TEETH

Gemination

This is a developmental anomaly affecting shape of tooth in which a single tooth germ is attempting to divide, by an invagination, resulting in incomplete formation of two teeth. So the affected tooth has a bifid crown (completely or incompletely separated crown) with a single root. In mild cases only a deep groove is seen extending from incisal edge to the cervical portion. Clinically there is no change in the number of teeth in the oral cavity.

Twinning

If the invagination leads to complete division of tooth into two, that result in formation of two smaller teeth which are identical in appearance. Clinically there is an increase in number of teeth in dental arch.

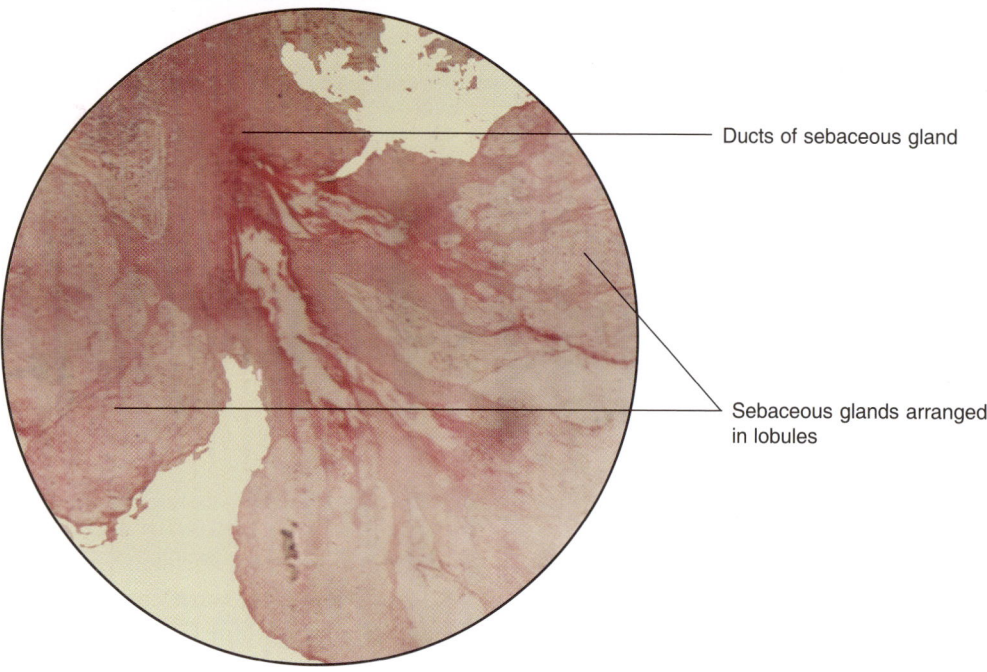

Ducts of sebaceous gland

Sebaceous glands arranged in lobules

Fordyce's granules (photomicrograph 4X)

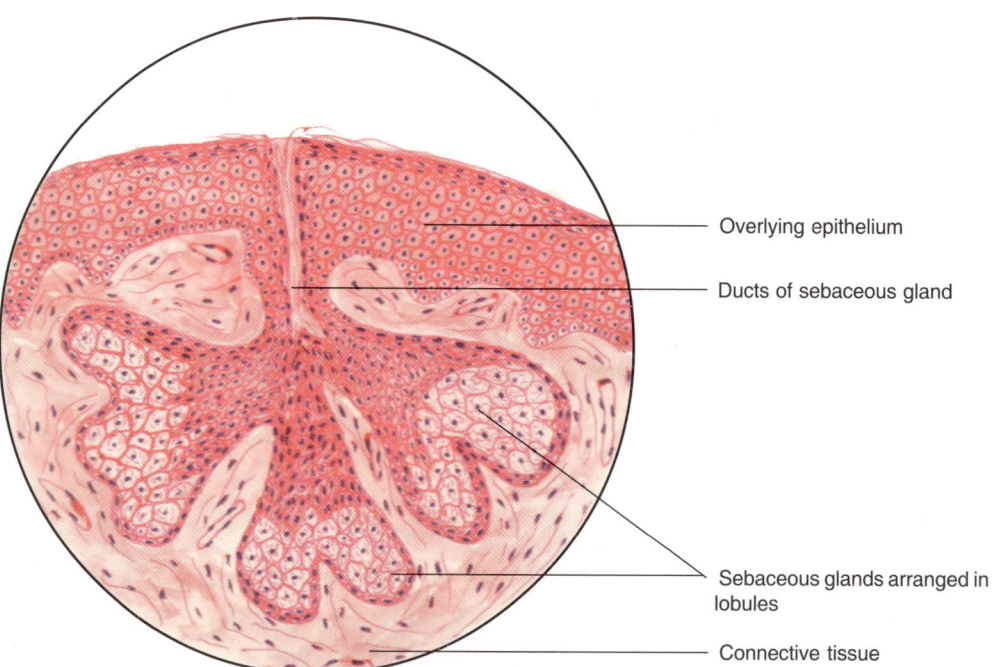

Overlying epithelium

Ducts of sebaceous gland

Sebaceous glands arranged in lobules

Connective tissue

Fig. 21.1: Fordyce's granules

Fusion (Fig. 21.2)

In this anomaly two normally separated tooth germs fuse (join) together to form a single tooth. Depending on time of fusion the resulting tooth may be a completely fused tooth with single crown and root or separated crown with single root. In case of fusion the number of teeth in dental arch is less with a large tooth. This fusion results from a physical force or pressure resulting in contact between two developing tooth germs. One characteristic feature of true fusion is that dentin is always confluent (fusion at dentin level).

Concrescence (Fig. 21.3)

When fusion of two teeth occurs by the deposition of cementum, it is called concrescence. This fusion occurs after the complete formation of root. This can also occur due to traumatic injury, crowding with resorption of interdental bone so that roots of the adjacent teeth are approximated. This particular condition can cause complications at the time of extraction resulting in fracture of bone, etc.

Dilaceration (Fig. 21.4)

Any sharp bend or curve in the root or crown of the tooth is called dilaceration. This occurs due to trauma to the developing tooth resulting in change in the position of already formed portion of the tooth and the remaining part of the tooth form at a different angle. The bend can occur at any region of tooth depending on the amount of tooth formed before injury. Clinical significance of this condition can be difficulty in extraction of affected tooth.

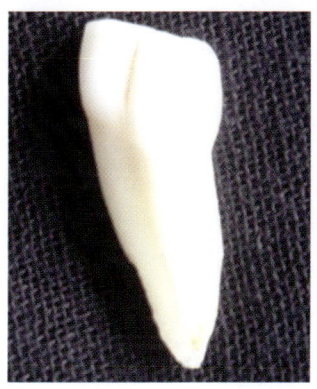

Fig. 21.2: Fusion

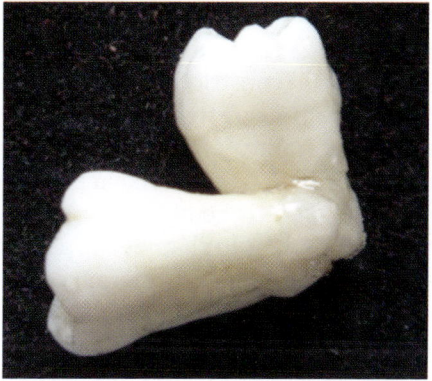

Fig. 21.3: Concrescence

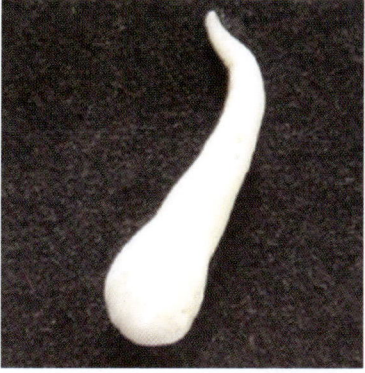

Fig. 21.4: Dilaceration

Talon Cusp

This is an anomalous cusp-like structure projecting from the lingual aspect, in the region of cingulum of maxillary and mandibular incisors. This resembles eagle's talon, hence called talon cusp. This structure has an enamel cover with dentin and a central core of pulp. This is separated from the tooth by a groove. Talon cusp may cause inter-ference in occlusion or make the tooth more prone to caries because of the groove.

Talon cusp is a common feature in Rubinstein-Taybi syndrome.

Taurodontism (Fig. 21.5)

Taurodontism is a developmental anomaly affecting the shape of the tooth in which body of the tooth is enlarged at the expense of root. This condition arises due to failure of Hertwig's epithelial root sheath to invaginate at the proper horizontal level.

The affected tooth appears rectangular without cervical constriction and the bifurca-tion of the root is shifted more apical than normal. The name taurodontism is given because the tooth appears like a bull's tooth (similar to the tooth of cud-chewing animals). In the radiograph pulp chamber appears to be extremely enlarged with increased apico-occlusal height. Based on the level of bifurcation these affected tooth can be:

- *Hypotaurodont*: Bifurcation is slightly apical to normal.

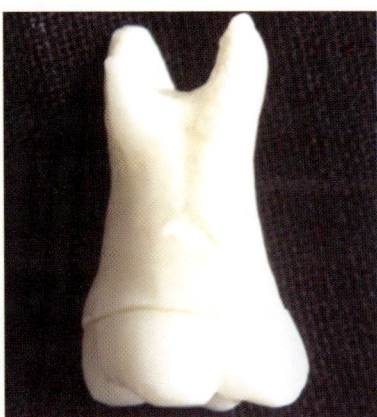

Fig. 21.5: Taurodontism

- *Mesotaurodont*: Bifurcation in the middle of root.
- *Hypertaurodont*: Bifurcation at the apical one-third or no bifurcation at all.

Dens Evaginatus (Leong's Premolar)

Dens evaginatus is a developmental anomaly characterized by the presence of a globule of enamel or an extra cusp on the occlusal aspect between the buccal and lingual cusps of premolars. This condition develop due to evagination of inner enamel epithelium and dental papilla into the enamel organ. This extra cusp may interfere with occlusion and may cause pulp exposure following attrition.

Dens Invaginatus (Dens in Dente)

This is a developmental anomaly affecting the shape of the tooth which occur due to invagination of enamel organ into the dental papilla during odontogenesis. The affected tooth shows an invagination that varies from slightly accentuated lingual pit to a deep folding reaching the root of the tooth. The term 'dens in dente' is given to a severe invagination that gives the appearance of a tooth within a tooth. In a radiograph this condition is seen as a 'pear-shaped' radiolucency in enamel and dentin with a narrow constriction at the opening on the surface.

Supernumerary Teeth or Hyperdontia

This refers to a condition where extra teeth than normal are present. Supernumerary tooth develop from an additional dental lamina near the permanent tooth bud or by splitting of the permanent tooth bud itself. When the supernumerary teeth are located in the dental arch, assisting the normal teeth in function they are called supplementary teeth.

The most common supernumerary tooth is **'mesiodens'** (Fig. 21.6). Mesiodens is an extra tooth located between the two maxillary central incisors. This is a small conical tooth with a small root. Mesiodens may occur singly or paired, erupted or unerupted. This tooth can cause esthetic problems.

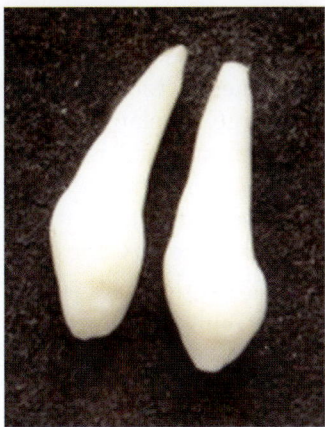

Fig. 21.6: Mesiodens

Distomolar is the second most common supernumerary tooth. They are situated distal to the third molar and may be smaller or of the same size.

Paramolars are the supernumerary teeth present either buccal or palatal to the molars. This may be single or multiple and smaller or of the normal size.

Multiple supernumerary teeth are present in 'Gardner's syndrome' and 'cleidocranial dysplasia'.

Anodontia or Hypodontia

This refers to absence of all or some teeth. True anodontia is congenital absence of teeth which may be total or partial. In total anodontia all the teeth are missing and is usually a feature of hereditary ectodermal dysplasia. The term partial anodontia is used when one or more teeth are missing. Most commonly missing tooth is third molars followed by maxillary laterals and second premolars. The condition in which multiple teeth are impacted is referred to as pseudoanodontia. False or induced anodontia occurs as a result of extraction of all the teeth.

Supernumerary Cusps or Roots

Supernumerary root (Fig. 21.7) refers to a condition where a tooth has extra root than normally expected. This condition is seen mainly in mandibular canines and premolars. These extra roots can cause difficulties in extraction and an unrecognized broken root that is not removed may cause infection

Any extra cusp on a tooth is called supernumerary cusp. Rarely this may interfere with occlusion.

Enameloma (Enamel Pearl) (Fig. 21.8)

Enamel pearl is a globule of enamel seen on the root near cementoenamel junction or close to furcation area. These structure may have a central core of pulp covered by dentin and enamel. Enamel pearl is formed by a group of displaced ameloblasts or cells of Hertwig's epithelial root sheath that have attained a capacity to form enamel.

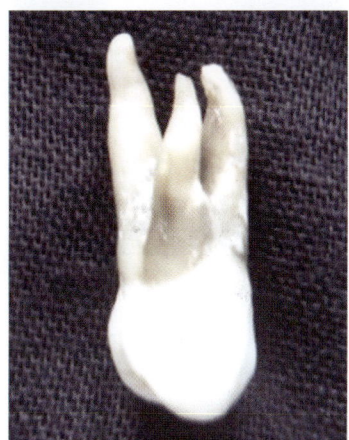

Fig. 21.7: Supernumerary root

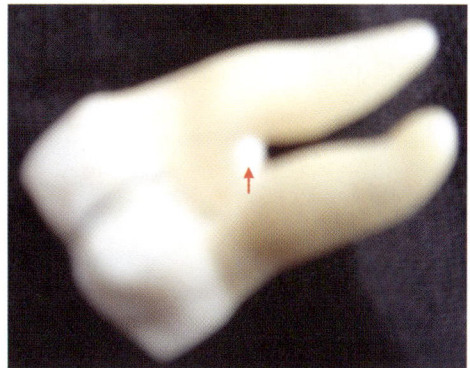

Fig. 21.8: Enameloma

Microdontia and Macrodontia

Microdontia is a condition wherein the teeth are smaller than normal. This condition may be true or relative. In true microdontia the actual size of the tooth is small. In relative microdontia the actual size is within normal range but appears smaller because of larger jaws. Generalized microdontia is seen in pituitary dwarfism. Peg-shaped lateral incisor is the most common single tooth that appear as microdont.

Macrodontia is a condition in which teeth are larger than normal. This also may be true or relative. In true macrodontia the actual size of the tooth is large. In relative microdontia the actual size is within normal range but appears larger because of smaller jaws. Generalized microdontia is seen in pituitary gigantism. In hemifacial hypertrophy the teeth on the affected side may be larger than normal.

The term Rhizomicry (Fig. 21.9) is used when the roots are smaller than normal. Rhizomegaly (Fig. 21.10) refers to abnormally larger roots.

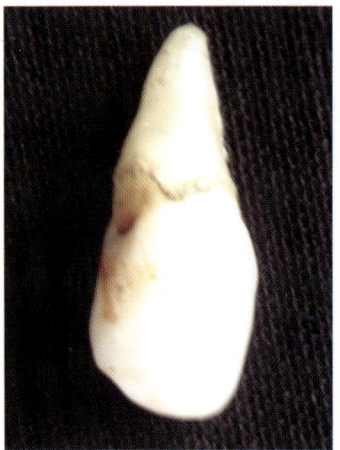

Fig. 21.9: Rhizomicry

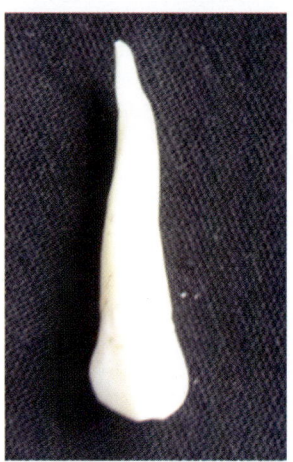

Fig. 21.10: Rhizomegaly

Index